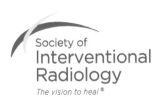

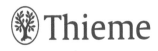

Pocketbook of Clinical IR

A Concise Guide to Interventional Radiology

Shantanu Warhadpande, MD
Resident Physician
Department of Radiology
University of Pittsburgh Medical Center
Pittsburgh, PA, USA

Alex Lionberg, MD
Resident Physician
Department of Radiology
University of Chicago Medicine
Chicago, IL, USA

Kyle J. Cooper, MD, RPVI
Assistant Professor
Department of Radiology
Division of Interventional Radiology
Loma Linda University
Loma Linda, CA, USA

165 illustrations

Thieme
New York • Stuttgart • Delhi • Rio de Janeiro

Acquisitions Editor: William Lamsback
Managing Editor: Madhumita Dey
Director, Editorial Services: Mary Jo Casey
Production Editor: Rohit Bhardwaj
International Production Director: Andreas Schabert
Editorial Director: Sue Hodgson
International Marketing Director: Fiona Henderson
International Sales Director: Louisa Turrell
Senior Vice President and Chief Operating
    Officer: Sarah Vanderbilt
President: Brian D. Scanlan

Library of Congress Cataloging-in-Publication Data

Names: Warhadpande, Shantanu, editor. | Lionberg, Alex,
    editor. | Cooper, Kyle (Kyle James), editor.
Title: Pocketbook of clinical IR: a concise guide to
    interventional radiology / [edited by] Shantanu
    Warhadpande, Alex Lionberg, Kyle Cooper.
Description: New York: Thieme, [2019] | Includes
    bibliographical references and index.
Identifiers: LCCN 2018058258 (print) | LCCN
    2018058961 (ebook) | ISBN 9781626239241 (ebook) |
    ISBN 9781626239234 (pbk.)
Subjects: | MESH: Radiology, Interventional—methods |
    Handbook
Classification: LCC RD33.55 (ebook) | LCC RD33.55
    (print) | NLM WN 39 | DDC 617.05—dc23
LC record available at https://lccn.loc.gov/2018058258

Important note: Medicine is an ever-changing science undergoing continual development. Research and clinical experience are continually expanding our knowledge, in particular our knowledge of proper treatment and drug therapy. Insofar as this book mentions any dosage or application, readers may rest assured that the authors, editors, and publishers have made every effort to ensure that such references are in accordance with **the state of knowledge at the time of production of the book.**

Nevertheless, this does not involve, imply, or express any guarantee or responsibility on the part of the publishers in respect to any dosage instructions and forms of applications stated in the book. **Every user is requested to examine carefully** the manufacturers' leaflets accompanying each drug and to check, if necessary in consultation with a physician or specialist, whether the dosage schedules mentioned therein or the contraindications stated by the manufacturers differ from the statements made in the present book. Such examination is particularly important with drugs that are either rarely used or have been newly released on the market. Every dosage schedule or every form of application used is entirely at the user's own risk and responsibility. The authors and publishers request every user to report to the publishers any discrepancies or inaccuracies noticed. If errors in this work are found after publication, errata will be posted at www.thieme.com on the product description page.

Some of the product names, patents, and registered designs referred to in this book are in fact registered trademarks or proprietary names even though specific reference to this fact is not always made in the text. Therefore, the appearance of a name without designation as proprietary is not to be construed as a representation by the publisher that it is in the public domain.

© 2019 Thieme Medical Publishers, Inc.
Thieme Publishers New York
333 Seventh Avenue, New York, NY 10001 USA
+1 800 782 3488, customerservice@thieme.com

Thieme Publishers Stuttgart
Rüdigerstrasse 14, 70469 Stuttgart, Germany
+49 [0]711 8931 421, customerservice@thieme.de

Thieme Publishers Delhi
A-12, Second Floor, Sector-2, Noida-201301
Uttar Pradesh, India
+91 120 45 566 00, customerservice@thieme.in

Thieme Publishers Rio de Janeiro,
Thieme Publicações Ltda.
Edifício Rodolpho de Paoli, 25º andar
Av. Nilo Peçanha, 50 – Sala 2508
Rio de Janeiro 20020-906 Brasil
+55 21 3172 2297

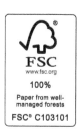

FSC
www.fsc.org
100%
Paper from well-managed forests
FSC® C103101

Cover design: Thieme Publishing Group
Typesetting by DiTech Process Solutions, India

Printed in USA by King Printing Company, Inc.

ISBN 978-1-62623-923-4

Also available as an e-book:
eISBN 978-1-62623-924-1

543

Contents

Contents

Foreword

"...for the secret of the care of the patient is in caring for the patient."

Francis Peabody, MD

The field of Interventional Radiology (IR) continues to grow and change. There has been unprecedented growth in this field as compared to any other in medicine. The expansion of minimally-invasive image-guided interventions continues, but more importantly, the clinical care of the patients undergoing these therapies is now receiving an equal importance in our training. There is no better practitioner who understands the appropriateness of our procedures and knows how to care for the patients receiving these therapies than the providers who perform these interventions. IR has distinguished itself as a primary specialty due to these three unique factors: Interventional radiologists are experts in medical imaging, authorities in image-guided procedures, and provide the clinical care to patients receiving these image-guided procedures. It is perhaps this last distinguishing factor that requires the maximum attention in training the future interventional radiologists. Much work is being focused on transformational changes to the training of interventional radiologists. These efforts will focus on expansion from a one-year fellowship to a five-year training program, where the clinical care of the patient is fundamental to the procedures that the radiologists are trained to perform.

With the recognition of IR as its own primary specialty, the recruitment of trainees into our specialty has shifted. For example, during the recruitment of medical students early in their training, many of them may have otherwise chosen clinical procedural specialties other than interventional radiology. As some would say, we are no longer fishing from the same pond. There is tremendous interest in our specialty among medical students. These young aspiring clinicians seek not only to diagnose but also to treat their patient's ailments in a manner that is less invasive, less painful, with faster recovery, and often less expensive. This should be the future of medicine. To better understand and consider IR as a future career, many of these trainees have elected to "shadow in IR" or take an M3 IR elective or an M4 sub-internship in IR. The path to IR is not limited to medical students as many junior residents in diagnostic radiology will pursue IR through the new independent pathway. Therefore, a need for a resource like a pocketbook targeted for these groups is paramount. Appropriately so, this pocketbook focuses on clinical care as the foundational base of our specialty. The authors are themselves young, aspiring interventional radiologists who saw the need for such a resource.

I congratulate Shantanu, Alex, and Kyle for their outstanding and much needed contribution in imparting training to young interventional radiologists. This pocketbook is well-organized and reader-friendly. It is targeted for senior medical students and junior residents who are interested to know about IR. It provides a natural progression from start to finish, with foundational chapters preceding the more clinically oriented chapters. My message for all aspiring interventional radiologists: 'The secret to good IR training is the clinical care of the patient.'

Parag J. Patel, MD, MS, FSIR
Associate Professor
Department of Radiology and Surgery
Medical College of Wisconsin
Milwaukee, WI, USA

Preface

Our decision to write this book began when we were medical students and were shadowing and completing IR electives. IR confronts the trainee with a steep learning curve, and our experience during those early days made that clear. While there were some IR resources available to help medical students get oriented to the specialty, they all tended to be procedure-oriented. The books we were reading fell short of providing the much-needed context to make sense of the busy workings of the IR department. Though we could learn and follow the steps during a chemoembolization procedure, we had an obvious lack of understanding of the matter related to diagnosis of patients and management decisions that usually took place behind the scenes.

In contrast, when we spent time rotating in a surgical oncology clinic, our preceptor (and soon-to-be mentor) Dr. Carl Schmidt at Ohio State University changed our view. He was an outstanding surgeon, compassionate with his patients, and dedicated to teaching. Knowing our goals of pursuing IR in residency, he encouraged us to think about the management of oncology patients through the eyes of a clinician, and taught us to recognize the interplay of medical, surgical, and IR treatment for these patients.

Later, while discussing our shared experience of that rotation, we experienced our 'Aha!' moment. We recognized that despite the technical nature of interventional radiology, it was incredibly important for trainees to understand the clinical context prior to investigating into the fundamentals of procedures.

We decided to put this philosophy into action and write a book that reflected this thought process. As trainees ourselves, we also knew how important it was for us to keep it concise enough to be read before or during a rotation in IR.

This book focuses on the clinical care of patients who undergo IR treatment. As far as the technical description of procedures are concerned, we have provided a concise summary in the form of 'procedure boxes' throughout the book. We believe that these to-the-point descriptions will help young interventional radiologists watch and participate in cases early in their training. Readers will get better at procedures as they progress by simply watching and handling more cases. Even the best books that describe *how* to do a procedure are no substitute for seeing and learning for yourself under the supervision of an attending or senior resident. For now, the goal of aspiring interventional radiologists should be to focus on familiarizing themselves with the tools, the lingo, and the general conceptual steps of IR procedures.

To help them attain this, the first three chapters describe the workflow in the IR department, as well as the tools and equipment used.

The primary purpose of this pocketbook is to give the interventional radiologists a clinical foundation and working understanding of most of the disease processes that IR encounters. We have prioritized concision and readability rather than attempting to provide an exhaustive resource. This book should be used during days of IR training to build a strong foundation. Readers may then turn to other texts and resources to increase their knowledge in the field.

The book is meant to be read start-to-finish. Each chapter builds on the previous chapter. We have intentionally kept the style relatively informal to make it easier to read and to get through the material quickly. Additionally, we have tried our best to organically cite evidence based studies in-text rather than with footnotes to make this book as practical as possible.

We hope the readers will find this book a helpful resource.

Shantanu Warhadpande, MD
Alex Lionberg, MD
Kyle J. Cooper, MD, RPVI

Acknowledgments

This book is the product of countless hours of work over several years. Despite the hectic schedule of internship years, Shantanu's wedding planning, and we being based out in three different cities and having to communicate via conference calls, we managed to take this book from idea to completion in a relatively short time. Bringing out this book would not have been possible without the early mentorship of Dr. Carl Schmidt. His passion for teaching and support for our idea inspired us to write this book. Dr. Sarah White gave us invaluable guidance on how to fine-tune our ideas. She was also one of the first persons to provide us feedback on our first chapter.

Joy Gornal believed in us from the very beginning. She constantly fought for us to make this book a reality. She probably has heard this a thousand times, but IR is truly lucky to have her. When it came to finding a publisher, Celia Bucci, our friend and a published author herself, gave us a crash course on the logistics of book writing, for which we are immensely grateful.

Dr. Paul Rochon helped us in recruiting attendings and also helped with the chapters. Dr. Geogy Vatakencherry has been our mentor for years (not to mention many others as well!). We cannot say enough about his infectious passion for practicing clinical IR. His vote of confidence and positive energy motivated us when we needed it the most. Dr. Rakesh Navuluri is another attending who went beyond what was asked from him, helping us at many crucial points throughout the process of writing this book.

We would like to thank all our authors who have dedicated their time and effort in contributing chapters for this book. We truly appreciate the hard work.

Finally, we are grateful to our families and friends for the patience they showed towards us over the past three years and for allowing us to work on the book when seemingly everyone was out living life. Without our wives, parents, siblings, and friends we would not have made it this far. Thank you for the support and thank you for believing in us.

Shantanu Warhadpande, MD
Alex Lionberg, MD
Kyle J. Cooper, MD, RPVI

Contributors

Ashley Altman, MD
Resident
Department of Radiology
University of Chicago
Chicago, IL, USA

Victor Nicholas Becerra, MD
Resident Physician
Department of Radiology
Abany Medical Center
Albany, NY, USA

Rajat Chand, MD
Resident
Department of Radiology
John H. Stroger Jr. Hospital of Cook County
Chicago, IL, USA

Orrie Close, MD
Fellow
Department of Interventional Radiology
Northwestern Memorial Hospital
Chicago, IL, USA

Kyle J. Cooper, MD, RPVI
Assistant Professor
Department of Radiology
Division of Interventional Radiology
Loma Linda University
Loma Linda, CA, USA

John Do, MD
Interventional Radiology Resident
Department of Radiology
UC San Diego Medical Center
La Jolla, CA, USA

Alexander Maad El-Ali, MD
Chief Resident
Department of Radiology
University of Pittsburgh Medical Center
Pittsburgh, PA, USA

Aaron M. Fischman, MD, FSIR, FCIRSE
Associate Professor
Department of Radiology and Surgery
Icahn School of Medicine at Mount Sinai
New York, NY, USA

Joseph J. Gemmete, MD, FACR, FSIR, FAHA
Professor
Departments of Radiology, Neurosurgery,
    Neurology, and Otolaryngology
University of Michigan Hospitals
Ann Arbor, MI, USA

Patrick Grierson, MD, PhD
Clinical Fellow
Department of Internal Medicine
Washington University School of Medicine
Saint Louis, MO, USA

Gregory E. Guy, MD
Interventional Radiology Specialist
Department of Radiology
Ohio State University Wexner Medical Center
Columbus, OH, USA

Trilochan Hiremath, MD
Resident (PGY-5)
Department of Radiology
University of Pittsburgh Medical Center
Pittsburgh, PA, USA

Junjian Huang, MD
Resident Physician
Department of Radiology
Pennsylvania Hospital of the University of
    Pennsylvania Health System
Pittsburgh, PA, USA

Alexandria S. Jo, MD
Resident Physician
Department of Radiology
University of Michigan
Ann Arbor, MI, USA

Andrew Klobuka, MD
Chief Resident
Department of Radiology
University of Pittsburgh Medical Center
Pittsburgh, PA, USA

Matthew Evan Krosin, MD
Resident
Department of Radiology
University of Pittsburgh Medical Center
Pittsburgh, PA, USA

Alex Lionberg, MD
Resident Physician
Department of Radiology
University of Chicago Medicine
Chicago, IL, USA

Lisa Liu, MD
Medical Student
Rush University
Calabasas, CA, USA

Juan Domingo Ly Liu, MD
Resident
Department of Radiology
University of Pittsburgh Medical Center
Pittsburgh, PA, USA

Bill Saliba Majdalany, MD
Assistant Professor
Department of Radiology
University of Michigan
Ann Arbor, MI, USA

David J. Maldow, MD
Resident Physician (PGY-4)
IR/DR Integrated Residency Program
University of Rochester Medical Center
Rochester, NY, USA

Jonathan G. Martin, MD
Assistant Professor
Department of Radiology
Duke University
Durham, NC, USA

Jason W. Mitchell, MD, MPH, MBA
Assistant Professor
Department of Radiology and Imaging Sciences
Emory University School of Medicine
Atlanta, GA, USA

Rakesh Navuluri, MD
Associate Professor
Department of Radiology
University of Chicago
Chicago, IL, USA

Andrew Niekamp, MD
Radiology Resident (PGY-5)
Department of Diagnostic and Interventional
  Imaging
McGovern School of Medicine
University of Texas
Houston, TX, USA

Zachary Nuffer, MD
Resident
Department of Imaging Sciences
University of Rochester
Rochester, NY, USA

James K. Park, MD, PhD
Assistant Professor
Division of Interventional Radiology
University of Pittsburgh Medical Center
Pittsburgh, PA, USA

Mangaladevi Patil, MD
Integrated Interventional Radiology
  Resident
Department of Radiology
Emory University School of Medicine
Atlanta, GA, USA

Joshua Pinter, MD
Radiologist
Department of Interventional Radiology
University of Pittsburgh
Pittsburgh, PA, USA

Suraj Prakash, MD, MBA
Resident
Department of Interventional Radiology
Medical College of Wisconsin
Milwaukee, WI, USA

Carl Schmidt, MD
Professor of Surgery
Chief
Division of Surgical Oncology
Department of Surgery
West Virginia University School of Medicine
Morgantown, WV, USA

L. C. Alexander Skidmore, MD
Resident
Department of Radiology
University of Pittsburgh Medical Center
Pittsburgh, PA, USA

Kurt Stahlfeld, MD
Surgeon
Department of Surgery
UPMC Mercy
Pittsburgh, PA, USA

Deepak Sudheendra, MD, FSIR, RPVI
Assistant Professor of Clinical Radiology and
  Surgery
Department of Radiology
University of Pennsylvania Perelman School of
  Medicine
Philadelphia, PA, USA

Devdutta Warhadpande, MD, MS
Clinical Assistant IV
Department of Medical Imaging
University of Arizona
Tucson, AZ, USA

Shantanu Warhadpande, MD
Resident Physician
Department of Radiology
University of Pittsburgh Medical Center
Pittsburgh, PA, USA

Gregory J. Woodhead, MD, PhD
IR Physician
Assistant Professor
Section of Vascular and Interventional Radiology
Department of Medical Imaging
University of Arizona College of Medicine
Banner University Medical Center
Tucson, AZ, USA

Geogy Vatakencherry, MD, FSIR
Chief
Department of Vascular and Interventional
  Radiology
Kaiser Permanente Los Angeles Medical Center
Los Angeles, CA, USA

Nicholas Zerona, MS, MD
Resident
Department of Radiology
Cleveland Clinic
Cleveland, OH, USA

Board of Review

1 The Basics of IR

Alex Lionberg, Shantanu Warhadpande, and Joshua Pinter

Being a trainee in IR can be intimidating. The specialty sees a wide variety of pathology, and performs over a hundred different procedures. The equipment and imaging techniques used require some time to get acclimated to. All of this can be overwhelming. However, with some fundamental knowledge and the tips outlined in this book, you can hit the ground running on your first IR rotation.

When it comes to learning IR procedures, there's no substitute for getting your feet wet and participating in cases. While it is important to get as much procedural experience as you can, you'll also need to be attentive to the clinical responsibilities expected of you as a trainee on the service. This includes answering the phone, fielding consults, and interfacing with other clinical teams. You should take full ownership of patients scheduled for procedures during the day, postprocedure patients, and the new consults as they come in.

Your day starts with reviewing the scheduled cases. This includes reviewing the indication for the procedure, any relevant imaging available, and any pertinent progress notes. You'll learn quickly that IR is a fast-paced specialty. Preparing ahead of time will make the day run much smoother.

Consults for IR can come at any time; some are urgent or emergent, while others may be routine. A good habit to get into is to follow the same set of steps for each new consult so that you don't overlook any important details (▶ Table 1.1).

1.1 The IR Consult

What Is the Reason for the Consult?

Determine the nature of the clinical problem and the expectations of the referring service. There should be a conversation where you gather from the referring team the underlying clinical problem, the interventions that have been performed thus far, and the urgency. You'll need to make sure you understand what they are hoping to gain from the IR procedure. If the consult is for a diagnostic procedure, what information is being sought? Good communication will ensure that both the IR team and the referring service have an understanding of what will be done.

Does the Patient Need to Be Seen Immediately?

If an urgent consult is requested, gather the bare bones information (clinical history, hemodynamic status, laboratory values, imaging), but don't delay in notifying your attending. He or she may decide to bring the patient straight to IR. If the consult is nonurgent, you have time to perform a more thorough work-up before staffing the

Table 1.1 Consult checklist

What is the reason for the consult?
Does the patient need to be seen immediately?
Are there alternatives to IR treatment that are more appropriate, and have they already been attempted?
Is the procedure technically feasible?
Are there any safety concerns that need to be addressed?

case. An ideal presentation will include the clinical history, imaging findings, your final assessment, and a proposed plan of action.

Are There Alternatives to IR Treatment That Are More Appropriate, and Have They Already Been Attempted?

It is important to have some foundational knowledge of the diseases commonly treated by IR, and how the IR procedure fits into the bigger picture. Unfortunately, this is not always cut and dry. Many IR procedures do not fall neatly into an algorithm. A good understanding of the clinical context is required to determine if and when IR should get involved.

Is the Procedure Technically Feasible?

If an IR intervention is potentially indicated, review the relevant imaging available to you. As radiologists, our expertise in imaging interpretation allows us to learn a great deal about the patient before we even meet them. We can plan out a procedural approach, identify anatomic variants, and look for potential pitfalls. As a trainee, you may not have a strong foundation in imaging, so it's okay to ask your senior residents or an attending for help.

Are There Any Safety Concerns That Need to Be Addressed?

If the conditions above are met, the next step is completing a basic preprocedure work-up. This can be time consuming, but it is important to review before officially approving a procedure. This is part of what separates clinicians from technicians.

Bleeding Risk

Bleeding risk should be assessed for any patient undergoing an interventional procedure. Society of Interventional Radiology (SIR) guidelines stratify procedures into low, moderate, and high risk of bleeding. **Low-risk procedures** are those which are either minimally traumatic with small access devices, or those in which access is obtained into a space in which bleeding would be easily detected and controlled. Examples include paracentesis, drainage catheter exchange, superficial biopsies, peripherally inserted central catheter (PICC) placement, and IVC filter placement. **Moderate-risk procedures** include the majority of interventional procedures, including most arterial and venous interventions, and tunneled line placement. **High-risk procedures** are those in which a solid organ is traversed, including transjugular intrahepatic portosystemic shunt (TIPS), biliary interventions, and nephrostomy access.

The two laboratory tests that are most important in determining the bleeding risk are platelets and international normalized ratio (INR). For all procedures, platelets need to be greater than 50,000. For low-risk procedures, the INR needs to be below 2. For moderate- and high-risk procedures, the INR needs to be below 1.5 (▶ Table 1.2).

The number of patients on long-term anticoagulation has increased in recent years, and there are now a wide variety of medications used for this purpose (see Chapter 9). The preprocedural assessment should look into any history of bleeding or clotting disorders, as well as review use of warfarin, heparin, antiplatelet agents, or the newer factor Xa or direct thrombin inhibitors. Screening laboratory tests should include INR, partial thromboplastin time (PTT), and platelets (+/– anti-Xa levels). Note that PTT/INR takes into account only a portion of the overall clotting cascade.

Thromboelastography (TEG) is a relatively quick blood test that measures the functionality of the *entire* blood clotting cascade (platelet function, clot formation, fibrin cross-linking, etc.). TEG is presented as a graph of clot formation and fibrinolysis (called a TEG tracing), with several parameters measured, each corresponding to different parts of the coagulation cascade. In IR, the two patient populations that you'll see getting a TEG include bleeding patients, (especially in the setting of traumatic or obstetric bleeds), and cirrhotics. In the setting of trauma, coagulopathy is one of the components of the "deadly triad" (along with hypothermia and metabolic acidosis). In cirrhotics, poor synthetic function of the liver leads to low levels of coagulation factors. Abnormal PTT/INR in these patients only tells one part of the story. By identifying the specific dysfunctional components of the coagulation cascade, a TEG study can determine which types of blood products should be transfused. The details of interpreting TEGs is beyond what you need to know. For now, simply know when and how it can be used.

For those patients on anticoagulation, reversal agents may be necessary in order to expedite an IR procedure. These include protamine sulfate for heparin, idarucizumab for dabigatran, and vitamin K for warfarin. In some cases, reversal is accomplished with the use of blood products. Options include fresh frozen plasma (FFP), prothrombin complex concentrate (PCC), platelets, and cryoprecipitate (▶ **Table 1.3**).

Table 1.2 IR procedure risk stratification based on the bleeding risk

Risk category	Procedures	Laboratory thresholds
Low risk	PICC insertions, dialysis interventions, IVC filters, thora-/paracentesis, superficial biopsies	INR < 2 Platelets > 50,000
Moderate risk	Any procedure requiring an arterial stick and intervention up to 7 Fr, venous interventions, embolizations, tunneled central catheter, port placements, perc chole, liver biopsy, abscess drainage, lung biopsy, spine procedures	INR < 1.5 Platelets > 50,000
High risk	TIPS, PTC/PTBD, percutaneous renal procedures (nephrostomy tube, biopsy)	INR < 1.5 Platelets > 50,000

Abbreviations: perc chole, percutaneous cholecystostomy; PICC, peripherally inserted central catheter; PTBD, percutaneous transhepatic biliary drainage; PTC, percutaneous transhepatic cholangiography; TIPS, transjugular intrahepatic portosystemic shunt.

Table 1.3 Reversal agents for common anticoagulants

Anticoagulant	Reversal agent
Warfarin	Immediate reversal: FFP or PCC + vitamin K Semiurgent reversal: vitamin K
Heparin (including enoxaparin/LMWH)	Protamine sulfate
Dabigatran	Idarucizumab
All other novel oral anticoagulants	PPC; new reversal agents being studied

Abbreviations: FFP, fresh frozen plasma; LMWH, low-molecular-weight heparin; PPC, prothrombin complex concentrate.
Source: Adapted from Patel IJ, Davidson JC, Nikolic B, et al. Consensus guidelines for periprocedural management of coagulation status and hemostasis risk in percutaneous image-guided interventions. J Vasc Interv Radiol 2012;23(6):727–736.

For routine procedures, anticoagulants can simply be stopped beforehand to reduce the risk of bleeding. Here are some general rules about when to stop anticoagulants:

- Aspirin does not need to be stopped for low- and moderate-risk procedures. Aspirin should be held for 5 days prior to a high-risk procedure.
- Clopidogrel should be held for 5 days prior to *all* procedures.
- Most direct oral anticoagulants (DOACs) should be stopped 2 to 3 days before a procedure.
- Unfractionated heparin can be stopped approximately 6 hours prior to a procedure.
- Enoxaparin (low-molecular-weight heparin) should be held for 24 hours prior to *all* procedures.
- Warfarin should be held for 3 to 5 days before a procedure. INR should be monitored and brought below 2 (for low-risk procedures) or below 1.5 (for moderate- and high-risk procedures). For patients at high risk for thrombotic complications, this may require bridging with a shorter-acting agent such as enoxaparin or heparin.

When stopping anticoagulation, discuss with the referring service the risks of holding the medication versus the risk of bleeding associated with the procedure. In some cases, holding a medication can be dangerous. For example, holding an antiplatelet agent in the setting of a recently placed coronary stent can lead to stent thrombosis. In some cases, rules on holding medications or the acceptable thresholds for coagulation labs can be bent, but this is at the discretion of the attending who will be doing the case. When exceptions are made, it should be documented in the electronic medical record (EMR) and discussed with the patient and referring service.

Aspiration Risk

Aspiration risk is another important consideration prior to any interventional procedure, as most are performed using moderate sedation. Narcotic pain medication given during the procedure slows gastric motility and can be associated with nausea and vomiting. This introduces a risk of aspiration, especially with the patient lying flat on the table.

The best way to reduce the risk of aspiration is to keep the patient's stomach empty. The American Society of Anesthesiologists recommends a minimum of 2 hours fasting for clear liquids and 8 hours of fasting for meals, though institutional guidelines for moderate sedation may vary.

Contraindications to Contrast

Severe allergic reactions to low osmolar, nonionic contrast agents are uncommon, occurring in less than 1 in 2,000 administrations. Risk factors for contrast reaction include prior reaction, unrelated allergies, asthma, anxiety, and usage of β-blockers. Of these, only a prior reaction to the same class of contrast medium is significant enough to prompt premedication or simply avoidance of intravenous contrast. Shellfish allergy or allergy to other iodine-containing compounds should *not* be considered a contraindication to intravenous contrast. Reactions to iodinated contrast are not considered true allergies, since they are thought to be mediated by direct histamine release rather than circulating antibodies. The mechanism of histamine release provides the theoretical basis for contrast premedication. For elective cases, a 13-hour oral premedication is recommended, consisting of 50-mg prednisone at 13, 7, and 1 hour before the procedure, plus 50 mg of diphenhydramine within an hour of the procedure. For urgent cases, intravenous premedication can be performed with 40 mg of methylprednisolone (or equivalent) given every 4 hours until contrast administration, and 50 mg diphenhydramine within one hour of the procedure. Even in urgent cases, premedication should be attempted for a minimum of 4 to 5 hours if at all possible. In emergent situations, involvement of anesthesia in anticipation of an anaphylactic event may be required if there are no alternatives to the use of iodinated contrast.

Iodinated contrast can also adversely affect renal function. Risk factors for contrast-induced nephropathy (CIN) include pre-existing chronic kidney disease, diabetes, heart failure, older age, and large contrast volume administered. Patients at risk should be screened with a serum creatinine level prior to contrast administration. Those with acute kidney injury, or an estimated glomerular filtration rate (GFR) of less than 60 should have the procedure delayed or performed with alternatives to iodinated contrast if possible. Hydration with intravenous fluids prior to and following the procedure can also decrease the risk, with specific protocols varying according to institutional guidelines.

Unstable Patients and the Risk of Decompensation

If the patient is unstable or if there is a significant chance the patient might decompensate in the IR suite, anesthesiology should be involved. Other situations in which general anesthesia may be appropriate include those patients with a significant tolerance to opioids, when the procedure is expected to cause a great amount of pain, or if the patient has severe cardiopulmonary disease.

Should the Patient Be Seen Before Being Brought to IR?

One of the major advantages of being an image-guided procedural specialty is that deciding whether to do a case or not can often be done with the clinical information and imaging available to us in the EMR. While we absolutely encourage it, going to see every consult prior to the patient being brought to the preprocedural area is not always necessary. On the other hand, doing so allows you to ask the patient questions, confirm information in the chart, do a focused examination, and make sure the patient is an active participant in the plan prior to obtaining consent.

Once you've progressed through the consult checklist and all of the necessary information is gathered, you will present the case to an attending. He or she will determine if the case is approved. If approved, let the referring service know and inform the staff in charge of scheduling. If the case is turned down, politely notify the referring team of the reason for the decision, if there is a plan for IR to follow the patient, and then document it in the patient's chart. Generally speaking, consult notes and H&Ps in IR should be focused and to the point. The note communicates the information that was gathered and the plan that was formulated.

In the eyes of referring services, IR has gained a reputation of being able to think outside of the box and find creative ways to solve problems. For this reason, it is not uncommon to encounter some resistance when turning down a procedure. Always be courteous, stick to the facts, and involve your attending in the conversation early to ensure all parties are satisfied with the plan. Remember that the referring physicians just want the best care for their patient and may see IR as the patient's last hope.

1.2 Preprocedure Tasks

Consent

After a case is approved and scheduled, the patient is usually brought to a holding area where nurses check the patient in, take vitals, draw blood if necessary, etc. This is also the time to consent the patient for the procedure if not done already. Depending on the policy at your institution, consents may be done by a resident, a nurse practitioner or physician assistant, a fellow, or the attending. Components of a good consent include a description of the procedure, the risks involved, the benefits, and the alternatives. Consent should also be obtained for any related procedures that *might* be necessary. For example, when consenting a patient for a lung biopsy, also consent for a chest tube in case the procedure is complicated by a pneumothorax.

Antibiotics

Some IR procedures require the patient to receive a dose of antibiotics before getting started. For the most part, vascular procedures are considered clean and do not require antibiotic prophylaxis. The rationale behind prophylaxis in certain circumstances has to do with contamination by the passage of needles and catheters through contaminated parts of the body and into the bloodstream.

Procedures involving the hepatobiliary, genitourinary, or gastrointestinal systems are considered contaminated, and require prophylactic antibiotics with gram-negative coverage. In some cases, antibiotics may be appropriate even in the absence of contamination, such as with placement of a stent-graft or for an embolization procedure. A stent-graft introduces an intravascular foreign body, and an embolization creates an infarcted area of tissue, both of which could be a nidus for bacterial growth. Procedures involving the spine rarely lead to infection, but it can be quite serious when it happens, often requiring surgical debridement. For this reason, vertebroplasty/kyphoplasty and discography patients receive prophylaxis to cover skin flora. Prophylaxis is not routinely recommended for permanent vascular access, including tunneled lines and chest ports, but some IR departments include it as part of their policy, since many of these patients are on immunosuppressive agents or are otherwise above average risk for infection.

As there is a lack of strong, prospectively validated data on the subject, the use of prophylactic antibiotics is based on the SIR standards of practice consensus guidelines. In some cases, the data are not strong enough to offer a consensus, and the practice is instead based on departmental policies. ▶ Table 1.4 breaks down the general guidelines for antibiotic prophylaxis, but note that the antibiotics used and the procedures for which they are indicated may differ from those at your institution.

Table 1.4 Antibiotic prophylaxis for common interventional procedures

Antibiotic	Procedures
No antibiotic prophylaxis necessary	Diagnostic angiography, angioplasty, stenting, IVC filter placement
Cefazolin	Vertebroplasty, lumbar discography, endograft placement, gastrostomy tubes, possibly permanent vascular access lines, and dialysis access interventions
Ceftriaxone or other cephalosporin with gram-negative coverage	Biliary drainage, abscess drainage, nephrostomy tubes, chemoembolization

In general, cefazolin is used for clean procedures to cover against skin flora. For abdominal/genitourinary (GU) procedures, ceftriaxone or another cephalosporin with gram-negative coverage is given. Clindamycin is an option for those with a significant penicillin allergy, and vancomycin may be necessary for those with a high risk of methicillin-resistant *Staphylococcus aureus* (MRSA). If the patient is already on antibiotics, it is important to make sure that it has adequate coverage for the planned procedure. Otherwise, a separate dose may be indicated.

Sedation

Before nursing staff brings the patient into the IR suite, the plan for sedation should be established. Conscious sedation is typically accomplished using **midazolam** and **fentanyl** for the majority of cases. A typical starting dose of midazolam is 0.5 to 1 mg, while the starting dose of fentanyl is 50 mcg. Additional doses of each can be given as necessary during the procedure but should be used conservatively. In general, midazolam is a safe medication, with very high doses required before problems arise. In the rare case when a patient's respiratory or mental status deteriorates from oversedation, reversal agents are available for use. Flumazenil is given for midazolam overdose (benzodiazepine antagonist), and naloxone for opiate overdose.

Oral conscious sedation is safe for most patients. Occasionally, a patient will describe a reaction to sedation medications and there will be a question of whether the procedure can be done without it. For simple procedures, such as line placement, local anesthetic may be sufficient. Trying to perform more complicated procedures without sedation can be risky, as it is important to have the patient remain still while you are working. If there are situations in which sedation needs to be withheld, make sure an attending knows about this ahead of time. Cases that require general anesthesia will also need to be planned ahead of time.

1.3 The IR Suite

After all tasks are completed in holding and consent is obtained, the patient can be brought back to the IR suite. This is a strange environment for newcomers, and the tools used come with a learning curve. Developing an understanding of frequently used terminology, how to use the equipment, and the safety issues involved will facilitate more active participation in IR procedures.

Fluoroscopy is the most commonly used imaging tool in IR. Ultrasound is predominantly used for vascular access and also for some percutaneous procedures. CT is used mainly for biopsies, drains, and ablations.

During fluoroscopically guided procedures, the patient lies on a table underneath an **imaging detector**, often called a "C-arm" (▶ Fig. 1.1). The X-ray beam originates from the X-ray tube, which is located below the patient. The beam exits the tube, enters the patient, and passes through to the detector above the patient.

IR procedures are performed with **pulsed fluoroscopy**—essentially real-time X-rays. Pulsed fluoroscopy takes multiple individual X-rays per second, which appear to be "real-time" motion. Most procedures can be accomplished with surprisingly low frame rates of 4 to 7 frames per second; the lowest frame rate that allows the procedure to be accomplished in the quickest and safest manner should be selected. Contrast materials can be injected into vessels, ducts, organs, and spaces so that they can be visualized by fluoroscopy. The contrast will opacify the lumen or space by absorbing some of the X-rays on their way to the detector, allowing these structures to be visualized.

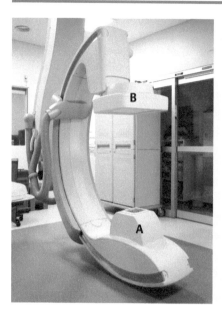

Fig. 1.1 Example of a procedural fluoroscopy unit. The X-ray beam originates at the (A) X-ray tube and is directed toward the (B) image detector.

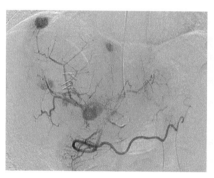

Fig. 1.2 Example of celiac artery digital subtraction angiography where all the surrounding soft tissue and bones have been subtracted out, leaving us only the opacified arterial anatomy.

Digital subtraction angiography (DSA) is a technique commonly used to optimally visualize blood vessels. During DSA, bones and other soft tissue are "subtracted" from the fluoroscopic image, leaving only an image of contrast-filled blood vessels (▶ **Fig. 1.2**). DSA images require the patient to be completely still in order for the surrounding structures to be subtracted. You'll often hear the patient instructed "don't breathe, don't move" when acquiring DSA images. Some respiratory motion is inevitable in most cases, which will lead to motion artifact on DSA images.

For angiography, iodinated contrast and CO_2 gas are the most common classes of contrast agents. **Iodinated contrast** is a positive contrast agent (radiopaque) and can be either ionic or nonionic. *Ionic* contrast is water soluble with a low viscosity. It is nephrotoxic and should be used with caution in patients with a low GFR. It also has the potential to cause adverse reactions that can range from simple itching to anaphylactic shock, though that latter is quite rare. *Nonionic* contrast does not dissolve in blood and is more viscous than ionic contrast. However, it tends to cause fewer adverse effects than ionic contrast. For this reason, nonionic agents are used almost exclusively.

Iodinated contrast can be delivered into the body via hand injection or by power injector. Hand injection is preferred for delivery of controlled contrast boluses or if injecting into smaller vessels. On the other hand, a **power injector** is ideal when a high volume of contrast needs to be delivered quickly (▶**Fig. 1.3**). Power injectors are usually used to opacify large-caliber vessels (like the vena cava or the aorta), or when attempting to opacify a large vascular bed (such as the superior mesenteric artery and its branches). Because contrast is injected at such a high-flow rate, the tubing must be free of air bubbles, otherwise there is a risk of air embolism.

When using a power injector, you may hear "20 for 30," "5 for 15," or some variant of these two numbers. The first number refers to the flow rate (20 mL/s), while the second number refers to the total volume of contrast to be injected. So "20 for 30" means contrast injection at a rate of 20 mL/s for 1.5 s, for a total injected volume of 30 mL. The flow rates and total volume varies depending on the vessel you're trying to opacify and the interventionalist's preference.

CO_2 **gas** can also be used for angiography. Unlike iodinated contrast, CO_2 gas is a *negative* contrast agent, meaning it is *radiolucent* (▶**Fig. 1.4**). Special CO_2 digital subtraction techniques are necessary to visualize CO_2 contrast within the bloodstream. CO_2 gas is water soluble with a low viscosity. It is also buoyant and rises to the least dependent portion of a vessel; in a supine patient, anterior-most structures are preferentially "opacified." CO_2 is not nephrotoxic and rarely causes an adverse reaction. One disadvantage is that it can only be delivered via a hand injection.

CO_2 as a contrast agent is neurotoxic and should never be allowed to enter the cerebral vasculature. Additionally, CO_2 gas can cause ventricular dysfunction. Any procedures that increase the risk of CO_2 entering the cerebral vasculature are contraindicated. This includes procedures in proximity to the thoracic aorta and coronary circulation.

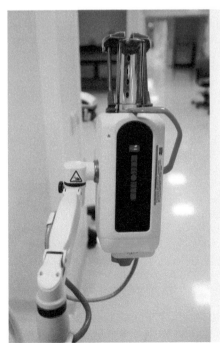

Fig. 1.3 Power injectors are used to deliver a high volume of contrast relatively quickly for large-caliber vessels or large vascular beds.

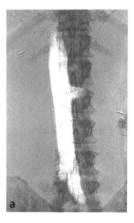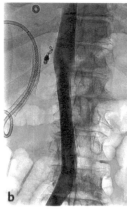

Fig. 1.4 Example of CO_2 angiography. CO_2 angiography uses negative contrast. Compare how (a) a negative contrast image looks compared to a (b) positive contrast image.

Radiation Safety

Radiation safety involves protection for yourself, the staff in the room, and the patient on the table. While you won't do yourself harm after just one procedure, your cumulative risk *will* increase if you don't follow good radiation safety habits procedure after procedure, month after month, year after year. Protect yourself!

Personal protection includes a lead apron, a thyroid shield, and lead glasses. The lead apron should fit well, not too tight or too loose. Lead also needs to be taken care of properly when you are not wearing it. Do not sit on it, drape it over a chair or fold it, since this can cause cracks to form and limit its protective ability. Before and after use, always hang up the lead apron on a hanger or a hook. This is a good habit to form early.

Fluoroscopic technique can make a big difference in the level of exposure to both the patient and staff in the room. The most important factors that you can control when in the angiography suite are time, shielding, and distance. Keep in mind that although exposure to the patient is from the primary X-ray beam, exposure to everyone else in the room is mostly from X-ray scatter. Care should be taken to minimize the amount of radiation used and the amount of scatter generated whenever possible.

Trainees have a tendency of keeping their foot on the fluoro pedal without realizing it. Be aware that this happens and avoid it. Only fluoro when you are looking at the screen.

When using fluoro, always be aware of how you are positioned in relation to the X-ray tube and patient. Radiation exposure decreases inversely with the square of the distance from the source. This means small increases in your distance from the patient make big differences in your level of exposure to scatter from the patient. You can increase your distance by using extension tubing while injecting contrast, avoiding leaning directly on the patient or table, and stepping back when possible. When using fluoro and turning your whole body toward the monitor, you are exposing your unleaded armhole to the table, which provides the scatter radiation a direct route into your chest.

You can minimize scatter radiation by keeping the detector close to the patient. The lead curtain below the table should be in place to minimize side scatter to the operators. Above the table, a transparent lead shield can be maneuvered between you and the X-ray tube (▶ **Fig. 1.5**).

Always be mindful of the other staff in the room. Since they have no control over when the radiation is being used, it is up to you to ensure their safety. First and foremost, look around the room to make sure everyone is wearing lead before starting to

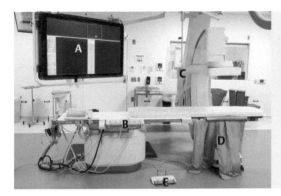

Fig. 1.5 In the IR suite, a patient will lie on table with the region of interest within the C-arm. Other equipment includes **(A)** monitor, **(B)** table/fluoro controls, **(C)** lead shield, **(D)** lead curtains, and **(E)** fluoro pedal.

use fluoro. There are also points during the procedure where staff can leave the room while images are being taken, which further reduces unnecessary exposure.

In addition to protecting yourself and the other staff, it is also your responsibility to minimize radiation exposure to the patient. An important concept in radiology is **ALARA**, which stands for "as low as reasonably achievable." This refers to the fact that we should use as little radiation as possible to obtain adequate images or perform the procedure successfully.

A common way we record radiation exposure to the patient is by recording the fluoroscopy time (FT). However, FT does not measure the radiation dose the patient was exposed to. The radiation dose to the patient is measured by the **air kerma**. Nearly all fluoroscopic equipment will measure reference point air kerma, which is a measure of the energy delivered by the X-ray tube to a volume of air. This is reported in units of **gray** (Gy) and often labeled "cumulative dose." Too high of a radiation dose in a single setting can have an adverse effect on the skin. As a general rule, the dose to the skin will be one-third of the cumulative dose, although this varies.

During complex procedures, the radiation exposure may reach a threshold dose beyond which the patient may suffer skin injury. Skin injuries can appear as early as 2 weeks or as late as 12 weeks after the procedure, and range from transient erythema and hair loss at doses of 2 to 5 Gy, to skin atrophy and ulceration at higher doses of more than 10 Gy.

Patients who have received a dose in which skin injury is possible should be told about the location exposed to the highest dose. Normally the tube is positioned under the table with the image detector over the table, so a patient supine during a procedure will receive the highest skin dose on the back. Patients who receive a very high dose should be scheduled for a skin check soon after the procedure.

There are some general strategies to minimize radiation exposure. **Collimation** involves narrowing the fluoroscopic field of view such that the radiation beam strikes a smaller area of the body. This decreases scatter radiation and keeps the surrounding tissue (including your own hand sometimes) from being directly exposed to the beam. You typically collimate such that only the area of interest is shown on the monitor.

While performing a fluoroscopy-guided procedure, you'll instinctively want to magnify the image to get a better look at the working area. Unfortunately, magnification comes at a cost, as the dose increases significantly with each level of magnification. Magnify when it is necessary, but otherwise avoid doing so. Move the monitor closer to your eyes to improve visualization before magnifying. Digital magnification can be employed on some systems, which does not increase radiation dose.

1.4 The Procedure

With some foundational knowledge about radiation safety and equipment in the IR suite, you're ready to take part in the procedure.

The technicians and nursing staff are in charge of bringing the patients into the room, moving them to the procedure table, prepping the site to be worked on, placing sterile drapes, and setting up the equipment. Depending on the procedure being performed, the patients might be prone or supine, with their arms extended or tucked in.

Before entering the room, you will need to put on a cap, mask, and glasses. Find yourself a set of appropriately sized lead, including a thyroid shield. Inside the room, have a pair of gloves and a sterile gown ready for yourself (if you let the technicians or nurses know ahead of time, they are often kind enough to do this for you). Only once you're leaded up, with gloves and gown ready in the room can you scrub. At least once in your IR training, you'll scrub in and walk into the IR suite without wearing your lead. It's alright, we've all done it.

The policy in most IR departments is that you don't need to do a full-on scrub. Instead, you can use a chlorhexidine/ethyl alcohol hand sanitizer from a dispenser near the room. The specific technique and timing required depends on the solution and institutional policies. Once in the room, gown and glove up. Many IRs advocate wearing two pairs of gloves. If you find a hole in a glove during the procedure, this can help you determine if a puncture went all the way through to your skin or not. You can also remove the top pair and put on a new pair without breaking scrub.

Every IR procedure starts with a time-out. A time-out will identify the patient's name and date of birth, the procedure being performed, and the laterality of the intervention (if necessary). The nurse will go through the patient's allergies, pertinent labs, as well as any sedation medications and antibiotics that have been given.

When first starting out, you can be most helpful by assisting a fellow, senior resident, or attending during the procedure. In order to do this, you should have basic knowledge of the various catheters and wires, and sequences in which they are used (described in Chapter 2).

If you have some time before the procedure starts, you can familiarize yourself with the equipment on the table. An important concept is learning which tools are designed to fit inside of each other. The nice thing is that you can simulate the procedure outside the body, figuring out how each of the pieces are meant to work together. Along with reading up on the procedure, assisting with a case will help you recognize and anticipate the steps, and prepare you to begin performing basic procedures yourself.

Interpreting Fluoroscopic Images

As you spend some time working with attending interventional radiologists, you'll take note of how they are able to interpret fluoroscopic images rapidly and seemingly without effort. Meanwhile, you may not even be certain what part of the body you are looking at. It's not something to be discouraged by. Over time, interpretation of these images will become almost automatic, but only after you have seen plenty of cases and trained your brain to do so.

Until you have mastered this skill, you should have a systematic way of interpreting fluoroscopic images. This is similar to what you have learned about approaching chest X-rays, however, fluoroscopy is even more challenging since you only see a portion of the anatomy (which is often abnormal on top of it). Sometimes you won't even have the benefit of seeing the preceding events that led up to the image in question. Part of IR training is practicing image interpretation by taking unknown cases. Your attending will give you one or more static fluoroscopic images and ask you to explain what is happening. This simple framework can help you work through the case:

1. Identify the type of study: Most fluoroscopic images will have *some* structure opacified in relation to the catheter. Identifying the opacified structure will tell you what kind of study you're looking at.

   First, find the catheter tip and the course it is taking. The location and directionality of the catheter will provide a clue as to what structure has been accessed. Once you've found the catheter, look at what the contrast is opacifying. For example, a catheter circuitously traveling from the midline to the right upper quadrant of the abdomen might be in place for a hepatic angiogram. Similarly, a catheter entering the right upper quadrant from the skin could be a hepatobiliary intervention. If a blood vessel is being shown, decide if the opacified vessel is an artery or a vein, and in which part of the body it is in. The relationship of the opacified vessel to adjacent bones is often helpful. Use the spine as a landmark when in the abdomen (aorta should be to its left, vena cava to its right). Use the extremity bones and pelvic girdle to orient yourself in the arms and legs.

2. Identify the pathology: Once you know what type of study you're looking at and where in the body you are, you can use the pattern of opacification to find the abnormality. Most pathology can be identified when there is contrast opacification where it shouldn't be, or lack of contrast filling when it should normally be seen. Differentiating normal from abnormal takes some time to learn, but it all comes down to pattern recognition. The more you see, the better you'll get.

   If you've identified the arterial system, look for contrast blush/extravasation, narrow segments, aneurysms, etc. In the venous system, look for flow through collateral vessels or filling defects that could indicate thrombosis or occlusion of the vein. In the biliary system, look for dilated or narrow areas in the biliary ducts. Sometimes you can deduce what's happening based on the tools you see in the image. If there's an angioplasty balloon in the image, the problem is likely some sort of narrowing.

3. Put it all together: Seeing what's happening in an image is the biggest hurdle. Once you've collected that information, you can then *think* about what's going on. The cases that will be presented to you are usually picked out because there's some teaching point to be made. Your challenge is to take the imaging findings and make a conclusion about what disease process is present. Why did the person have this IR procedure done in the first place?

   Is the biliary duct narrowing due to a benign stricture or is there a compressive mass? Is the venous occlusion due to a hypercoagulable state or is there an underlying venous compression? Is the renal artery narrowing due to atherosclerosis or are we dealing with fibromuscular dysplasia? These are the types of questions you can consider once you have an idea what you're looking at.

   Taking cases can be a humbling experience when you have to struggle through it. The more you see and the more you know about IR procedures, the easier it will become. Bear in mind that it is rare to find yourself in a real-life scenario where you have to interpret a single image. When doing a case, you have the benefit of knowing the steps you took to get there, not to mention pre-existing imaging for the patient that can be reviewed when necessary. With that said, the real benefit of taking unknown cases is training your brain to look at fluoroscopic images and take in a great deal of information at once. This will help you considerably as you transition to performing procedures yourself.

1.5 Postprocedure Care

Once the procedure is complete, this is now *your* patient. You will care for him or her not only in the postprocedure holding area, but potentially for days after the procedure as well. Since we are predominantly a consult service, there is a tendency in IR to send the patient back to the referring service for all their future care. While it is true we are not equipped to attend to our patients' every need on the floor, it does not absolve us from the responsibility we have to follow through and ensure that we are providing the best care possible. After the procedure is over, your goals should include: (1) ensuring a safe transition of care, (2) maintaining good communication with the other teams caring for the patient, and (3) being vigilant so that any problems that arise can be dealt with in a timely fashion, and with as little harm to the patient as possible.

In the immediate postprocedure period, you will need to put in relevant orders, complete the postprocedure documentation, and manage any procedure-related problems. It can be tempting to immediately jump to the next case, but all of these postprocedure tasks need to be taken care of.

Relevant orders may include laboratory studies, bed rest or activity level orders, diet and fluid orders, follow-up imaging, etc. As a rule, any labs or imaging you order need to be followed up on by IR (either you or the on-call resident). Do not assume the referring team knows why the order was placed or what to do with the result.

Documenting what was done in the procedure is an important part of our communication. Depending on your institution's policy, this may involve writing a postprocedure note in the chart, including a description of the procedure and any complications encountered. These are usually short and sweet. You may also have to dictate a separate procedure report. For routine procedures, a standard template is typically available for you to use, but you will need to make sure that the steps described reflect what was actually done. In addition, the report should describe any imaging findings during the case, and any challenges or complications that occurred. The impression states whether the procedure was a success and if there is a plan for the patient going forward. For more involved procedures, it is also a good practice to verbally communicate the results to the referring team. In these cases, the dictation alone does not make for good communication. Call the service to tell them what was done and anything to look out for. Speaking over the phone also allows the team to ask you questions.

After the procedure, patients are moved to the postprocedure area. While they are there, you are the one primarily taking care of them. That means you will be called to triage any issue that comes up. Most often these are simple problems, but you should be ready for anything, as delayed complications do occur and can occasionally be quite serious. If the nurse calls you about an issue, go see the patient.

The majority of calls are not serious, but will require you to lay eyes on the patient and make sure everything is okay. Some problems are potentially serious but still within your capability to manage. You'll also need to recognize situations that are serious enough where the primary team needs to be called to assist, or even the rapid response team. Trying to handle these situations that are beyond what you've been trained to do will just delay proper management and cause more harm to the patient. If called about something potentially serious, make an overall assessment of how the patient looks. If he or she looks sick, trust your gut and proceed cautiously. Recognize abnormal vitals, as that is probably the biggest indicator as to whether the situation is something you can handle, or if you need to call for backup.

Shortness of breath is a common postprocedure complaint. For this type of call, go see the patient and assess the severity. A patient speaking in full sentences is reassuring. If appropriate, start the patient on oxygen and check his or her oxygen saturation. In some cases, shortness of breath may be simply due to splinting, especially following hepatobiliary procedures. Better pain control will allow these patients to breathe normally and be more comfortable. For those patients who appear to have a serious problem, you'll need to consider the possibility of complications like pneumothorax or air embolism. If you were in the procedure, ask yourself if there was anything that happened during the case that would introduce this risk. Ordering a chest X-ray is simple enough to do, and can rule out many emergent cardiopulmonary complications. If something is severe enough that you are considering a CT scan for the patient, you'll want to call the primary service and alert them to the situation.

Pain is not uncommon after IR procedures. The difficulty in these situations is determining if it is expected postprocedure pain or a clue that something more serious is going on. A good illustration of this is a patient with abdominal pain after a percutaneous liver biopsy procedure. Some patients do experience a significant amount of pain from the procedure, but you would not want to miss a rapidly-forming hematoma causing pain due to stretching of the liver capsule. *Severe* pain can be a warning that something needs to be done, such as evaluate for occult bleeding, rather than just give more pain medications.

If a patient complains of chest pain and you think the patient is having a myocardial infarction (MI), the first steps are getting an ECG and sending cardiac markers. If it is a ST-elevation myocardial infarction (STEMI), call a rapid response, give the patient sublingual nitroglycerin, oxygen, morphine, and aspirin("NOMA"). Any significant cardiac chest pain should be communicated to the primary team.

Occasionally you'll be called for a patient complaining of chills, which may be accompanied by visible shaking. This is the presentation of postprocedural rigors. It occurs in the setting of transient bacteremia, which is not uncommon following IR procedures, especially when the patient hasn't received prophylactic antibiotics. During GU/hepatobiliary procedures, overdistension of the urinary collecting system, biliary tree, or gallbladder with contrast can also lead to transient bacteremia by forcing bacteria across the lumen wall. The immune response triggered leads to chills and shivering. It can be alarming for the patient, but when recognized, symptomatic treatment with meperidine is often effective while the immune system clears up the bacteremia. A minority of patients may become increasingly septic with dropping blood pressure. In these cases you will need to be more aggressive, which means gaining central access, bolusing with fluids, and starting empiric antibiotics.

Postprocedure bleeding from the access site happens from time to time. The most important determination is whether bleeding is coming from the incision itself or if it could be injury to a superficial vessel. For example, after a G-tube placement, is the bleeding from the skin or could it be injury to the epigastric artery or a gastric vessel during puncture? Keep a close eye on the patient's hemodynamics. If it is serious, the patient may need to be taken back for a diagnostic angiogram. Never send a potentially unstable patient back to anything less than an ICU level of care, and always keep the referring team in the loop.

Hypotension in the postprocedure setting could be the result of a number of different problems. It may be simply due to dehydration and the effect of medications given during the case. If you think the patient may be volume depleted you can try fluid boluses, but do so judiciously unless you know for certain the patient has no risk factors for volume overload. If the pressure is only borderline low and the patient is mentating fine, close monitoring alone is not a bad choice.

The most important thing to think about when evaluating hypotension is determining if it could be the heralding feature of a severe complication. If the blood pressure is rapidly downtrending and the patient is tachycardic, you could be dealing with something like vessel rupture or cardiac tamponade. Two things you will do right away is call a rapid response and have someone grab your attending. For serious complications, sometimes the best action is to roll the patient back to the IR suite and do an angiogram. Your attending can help make that call if there is high enough suspicion for an iatrogenic injury. In the meantime, start fluids, ask for labs to be drawn, and get a STAT chest X-ray. When the rapid response team arrives, you'll need to give a brief patient history, say what procedure was performed, and what steps have been taken thus far. These situations are rare, but be prepared just in case.

Rounding in IR

Rounding is handled differently depending on the institution. Some residents are routinely involved, while in other places there is no expectation for residents to take part. Wherever you train, if you have the opportunity to round, you should. You might even have to go out your way to make this happen if it isn't already set up for you.

There are a few reasons why rounding is important, some practical and others more idealistic. Rounding allows us to follow up on the results of our procedure, as well as catch any delayed complications. We are in a unique position to correlate the findings gained first-hand during the procedure with the patient's clinical response to treatment. If the procedure failed to achieve its goal, we can provide management recommendations to the referring team, including any further IR interventions.

Rounding provides a means of communication with the patient and the referring team. At a minimum you should write a daily progress note. It doesn't need to be long but it should state the procedure that was performed, any relevant objective data, and IR's assessment and plan. Talking directly with the referring team (sometimes even seeking them out in person) is a good habit to form. This allows any questions to be answered and demonstrates to the referring team that IR is invested in our patients.

Finally, rounding and being visible on the floors is good for PR purposes. It allows us to build rapport with the referring teams, which can in turn lead to better referrals and a more collaborative role for the department. Simple things like this can improve IR's standing in the hospital and ensure we continue to have a fruitful practice.

There's an old adage in private practice: a successful and valuable consultant is available, affable, and able. As the face of a clinical IR service, it is the trainee's job to be all three. Our hope is that you use this pocketbook to build a solid clinical foundation and become more *able* . By the end of your training, strive to not just be the best proceduralist, but also the best clinical interventional radiologist you can be.

Suggested Readings

[1]   American College of Radiology. Manual on Contrast Media. Reston, VA: American College of Radiology; 2015

[2]   Balter S, Hopewell JW, Miller DL, Wagner LK, Zelefsky MJ. Fluoroscopically guided interventional procedures: a review of radiation effects on patients' skin and hair. Radiology. 2010; 254(2):326–341

[3]   Patel IJ, Davidson JC, Nikolic B, et al.; Standards of Practice Committee, with Cardiovascular and Interventional Radiological Society of Europe (CIRSE) Endorsement. Standards of Practice Committee of the Society of Interventional Radiology. Addendum of newer anticoagulants to the SIR consensus guideline. J Vasc Interv Radiol. 2013; 24(5):641–645

2 Tools of the Trade

Suraj Prakash, Matthew Evan Krosin, L. C. Alexander Skidmore, and Gregory E. Guy

2.1 Vascular Procedures

Pioneered by Dr. Sven-Ivar Seldinger, the **Seldinger technique** is the most common method used for obtaining vascular access. The technique allows the introduction of instruments into the vessel, starting with a needle and sequentially upsizing to catheters and other tools large enough to perform procedures. It can be used to gain access nearly anywhere in the body with the same basic steps. Comfort with the Seldinger technique and the tools utilized is a must for every IR trainee.

Accessing the Vessel

A variety of different needles are used in IR. The size of a needle is denoted by gauge, which is a measure of its outer diameter. The larger the gauge, the *smaller* the outer diameter. The inner diameter of a needle is dependent on both the gauge and the thickness of the needle.

Hypodermic needles are narrow in diameter and used to administer local anesthesia. They are generally 25-gauge or 27-gauge. Drawing up medication is slow when using these higher gauge needles. For convenience, an 18-gauge needle can be used first when drawing local anesthesia into a syringe, and then exchanged for one of the smaller-diameter (larger gauge) needles prior to injecting.

The Seldinger technique begins with the introduction of an **access needle** into the target vessel. Access needles come in two types. One is a single hollow piece with a beveled tip, and the other is two-pieced, with a sharp central stylet inside of a hollow blunted tip (▶ Fig. 2.1). The most common sizes of vascular access needles are 18-gauge and 21-gauge.

After an access needle has been placed into the vessel lumen, a **guidewire** is inserted through the hollow portion, into the vessel (▶ Fig. 2.2). Guidewires commonly range in diameter from 0.010 to 0.038 inch (you may hear them referred to as "oh-one-eight wire, oh-three-eight," etc.). Guidewires come in different lengths, thickness, and stiffness. They are used to access target vessels and provide a scaffold over which other interventional tools can be inserted. The guidewire *outer* diameter should match the inner diameter of the needle or catheter through which it will pass.

Once the guidewire is in the vessel, the soft tissues and hole in the vessel through which the guidewire passes need to be dilated to allow room for various catheters and

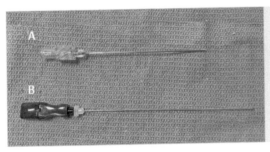

Fig. 2.1 Example of two access needles. The **(A)** 21 gauge micropuncture access needle is a one-piece needle and is most commonly used to access blood vessels. The **(B)** longer Chiba needle is a two-piece needle with an inner stylet; Chiba needles are used for many nonvascular procedures.

other tools. **Dilators** are stiff, hollow tubes with tapered tips. Their purpose is to spread overlying subcutaneous tissue and the vessel wall itself. Dilators of increasing diameter can be sequentially inserted to facilitate gradual tissue spread. They allow even the smallest vessel access to be increased to the appropriate size. By convention, outer dilator diameter is measured in units of **French (Fr)**. Fr size is equivalent to three times the outside diameter in millimeters. For example, a 6 Fr dilator has an outside diameter of 2 mm. Said another way, 1 Fr = 1/3 mm.

Sheaths are tubes inserted into the access site to facilitate insertion and exchange of instruments into the vessel of interest without repeatedly traumatizing the wall (▶ **Fig. 2.3**). **Catheters** are hollow tubes that vary greatly in size, tip shape, and length. Catheters, along with guidewires, are used to navigate and select target vessels. As with dilators, catheters are sized by Fr, which reflects the outer diameter of the catheter, and also by the size of guidewire that passes through. In contrast, the Fr size of sheaths is a reference to their *inner* diameter. This makes it easier to pair appropriately sized catheters and sheaths. For example, a 5 Fr catheter can securely fit through the lumen of a 5-Fr sheath. The *outer* diameter of a sheath is typically 1.5 to 2 Fr larger than the inner diameter (▶ **Table 2.1**).

Often, a dilator and sheath come attached together in a combined device (▶ **Fig. 2.2**). The dilator fits securely in the lumen of the sheath, with the tapered dilator tip projecting beyond the end of the sheath. A dilator-sheath can be passed over the guidewire during insertion. The central dilator is removed along with the guidewire, leaving the sheath behind in the vessel lumen.

The sequence of needle, guidewire, dilator, and sheath is the basis for vascular access using the Seldinger technique. For initial access, the **micro-access kit** (often referred to by the brand name Micropuncture, Cook Medical) is very popular (▶ **Fig. 2.2**). First,

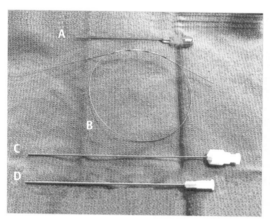

Fig. 2.2 The access kit that is commonly used to access blood vessels includes the **(A)** 21 gauge micropuncture needle; **(B)** 0.018 inch Cope Mandril guidewire; **(C)** 3 Fr inner transitional dilator separate from its **(D)** 4 Fr outer sheath. The sheath and inner dilator come as a single unit (sometimes called the introducer-sheath). Once the dilator-sheath unit is inserted over the wire into the blood vessel, the inner dilator is removed, leaving the 4 Fr sheath in place within the lumen.

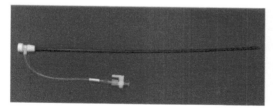

Fig. 2.3 Example of a sheath; a sheath is parked within the blood vessel and allows for convenient, frequent insertions and exchanges of instruments. A side-port allows for flushing of the sheath.

Table 2.1 Sizing nomenclature of common IR tools

Tool	What the size refers to
Access/hypodermic needles	Outer diameter (in gauge)
Guidewires	Outer diameter ("Oh-one-eight wire" = 0.018 inch)
Dilators	Outer diameter (in French)
Catheters	Outer diameter (in French)
Sheaths	Inner diameter (in French)

a 21-gauge needle is used to puncture the vessel. An 0.018-inch guidewire called a **microwire** is passed through the needle and into the vessel lumen. The microwire is a short guidewire that is used only during access. The needle is pulled out and removed over the wire. A dilator-sheath combination, called an **introducer-sheath,** is advanced over the microwire into the vessel. The introducer-sheath is composed of a dilator within a 4 or 5 Fr sheath. Since most tools in IR are used over a 0.035 wire system, the microwire needs to be exchanged for the larger guidewire. When the microwire and inner dilator are removed, a 0.035-inch guidewire can then be passed through the microaccess sheath. With the larger guidewire in place, the sheath can be exchanged for a larger one over the 0.035 wire. With an appropriately sized sheath secured in place, the operator can proceed with the case. Do not be surprised if you see some attendings use an 18- or 19-gauge access needle and jump straight to 0.035- or a 0.038-inch wire for initial access. The end goal is to get a 0.035 system in place.

Navigating the Vasculature

Surgeries, including complex ones like a Whipple, often have a predetermined set of steps that surgeons try not to deviate from. IR procedures are different in that they begin with the end-goal in mind, but the intervening steps and tools used can vary from case to case. An excellent interventionalist has a strong knowledge of the tools at their disposal, and uses those tools creatively to troubleshoot the problems that invariably arise. Equally important is to know when *not* to use a particular tool, particularly when the circumstances make it unsafe to do so.

Guidewires and catheters are the main tools used to navigate through the vasculature, making it possible to access nearly any vessel in the body. A general rule when using catheters is that they should only be advanced in the vessel over a wire. Advancing a catheter without a wire can cause a perforation or dissection as the open tip traumatizes the vessel. The guidewire is used to traverse blood vessels, penetrate deeper into smaller vessels, and course around bends and turns. Once the guidewire has been carefully navigated into the target vessel, the catheter is advanced over the wire into a secure position within the branch. There are *many* different types of guidewires and catheters, each with their own characteristics. With a specific goal in mind, the right guidewire-catheter combination can be selected based on their individual characteristics.

Stiff wires, also known as "working wires," provide the structural support over which catheters and other tools are advanced. They are also used to maintain access. Most guidewires have a central core that is tightly wrapped by a coiled wire. A guidewire's stiffness is a function of the central core's composition and thickness (▶ Table 2.2 and ▶ Table 2.3). The central core and coil wrapping are welded together at the back end

Table 2.2 Guidewire properties

Guidewire property	Importance
Length	Typical guidewires → 145–180 cm long Access guidewires (microwires) → short Exchange guidewires → very long
Stiffness (determined by the inner core's properties)	"Working wires" → stiff "Traversing wires" → floppy
Outer coating	Hydrophilic wires Nonhydrophilic wires

Table 2.3 Common guidewires and their properties

	Diameter (inch)	Stiffness	Tip	Coating	Use
Cope Mandril (Cook Medical)	0.018	++	Floppy	Nonhydrophilic	Access wire
Bentson (Cook Medical)	0.035	++	Very floppy	Nonhydrophilic	Traversing or working wire
Rosen (Cook Medical)	0.035	+++	Curved	Nonhydrophilic	Working wire
Amplatz (Boston Scientific)	0.035	++++	Floppy	Nonhydrophilic	Working wire
Lunderquist (Cook Medical)	0.035	+++++	Stiff	Nonhydrophilic	Working wire
Glidewire (Terumo Medical)	0.018 or 0.035	++	Straight or curved	Hydrophilic	Traversing wire
V18 (Boston Scientific)	0.018	+++	Floppy	Hydrophilic tip	Working wire

of the wire, referred to as the stiff end. The central core tapers at the front-end of the wire. The guidewire tip's floppiness is a function of how quickly the central core at the front-end tapers. Most guidewires have floppy tips that allow it to navigate around bends, curves, and plaque within a vessel, without causing trauma to the tunica intima. The shape of the tip may be straight, curved, or J-shaped. J-shaped wires vary in the radius of curvature. Selection of the appropriate guidewire requires consideration of the tip location, the tortuosity of the wire course from the access point to the tip, and the stiffness and trackability of the tools the operator plans to advance over the wire.

Guidewires are typically around 145 cm in length. Length is important in that when a catheter is being slid off for an exchange, the guidewire needs to be long enough to maintain position within the target vessel but also have enough length *outside* the body to be able to slide a catheter on or off. A longer guidewire in the range of 180 to 300 cm is considered "**exchange length**," and is used when longer catheters are used.

Like guidewires, there are a variety of catheters at our disposal, which are characterized by their tip, size, and material. Early in the procedure, a catheter is used for angiography to delineate vascular anatomy, either for diagnostic purposes or to assist in navigation. Larger vessels like the aorta necessitate a higher flow rate in order to fully opacify the large lumen. As such, the ideal catheter needs to provide a high flow rate and be able to inject contrast in the center of the lumen. This is accomplished with flush catheters, which have curled or recurved tips and robust construction, allowing high-volume contrast injections (i.e., aortography). The tips have multiple sideholes, which allow contrast material to be dispersed diffusely.

Procedures that involve navigation into branch vessels require curved-tip, **selective catheters** (▶Fig. 2.4). Selective catheters are useful when targeting branches of main vessels. Selective catheters may vary considerably with respect to shape and function. The catheters can have slightly angled, curved, J-shaped, or reverse curved tips. The target vessel's angle of origin off the parent vessel dictates the most appropriate tip shape. For example, subtly angled tips may be appropriate when navigating through the carotid and subclavian arteries. Curved, J-shaped, or reverse curved catheter tips may be more useful when attempting to cross the aortic bifurcation, or when selectively catheterizing a visceral or renal artery origin. Other tip configurations can be used based on the anatomy of the branch vessel of interest. A plethora of tip shapes are available, usually named after their shape or the individual who created it.

Sometimes, a catheter can be used to select a vessel of interest without a wire already into the branch. This is typically accomplished by slowly retracting the catheter until the tip pops into the ostium. At this point, a soft tipped guidewire can be advanced into the branch while keeping the catheter in place. Use of a soft tip reduces the risk of arterial spasm or dissection.

If distal branches need to be selected, a **microcatheter system** is typically used. A microwire/microcatheter combination is advanced through the catheter (parked at the branch vessel origin) and into the branch vessel (▶Fig. 2.5). Microcatheters may be straight or shaped, and are typically between 2 and 3 Fr. They are able to access narrow vessels without causing vessel spasm.

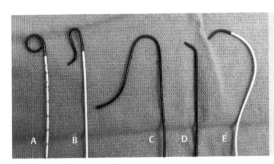

Fig. 2.4 Choosing the right catheter is important when selecting vessels and navigating the vasculature. Some common catheters you may encounter include (A) pigtail flush catheter, (B) Sos catheter, (C) Simmons catheter, (D) Berenstein catheter, and (E) Cobra catheter.

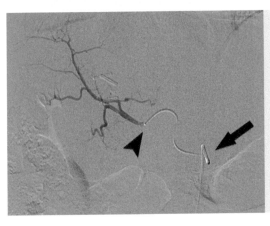

Fig. 2.5 The microcatheter-microwire system is used to navigate smaller caliber vessels. In this digital subtraction angiography image, the selective catheter is parked in the celiac axis (*arrow*), with the microcatheter advanced into the right hepatic artery (*arrowhead*).

Small and tortuous, stenotic, or occluded vessels may pose problems for a regular guidewire. Special **hydrophilic guidewires**, such as the Glidewire, and hydrophilic catheters (Glidecath) maintain a slippery surface when wet due to their polytetrafluoroethylene coating (PTFE). The tips of the wires are often curved, with the direction of the tip able to be "steered" with the aid of a torque device, which is tightened down onto the back end of the wire. **Tip deflecting wires** are also available to help advance catheters past difficult angles. Their tip can be angulated while inside the catheter by manipulation of a specially designed handle. These characteristics allow the guidewire/catheter to more easily navigate through complex anatomy. Once the catheter/guidewire has reached the region of interest in the vasculature, the intervention can be carried out.

Balloon Angioplasty

Vessel stenosis or occlusion can occur secondary to a number of pathologic conditions including atherosclerosis, fibromuscular dysplasia, or external compression. Reopening a stenotic blood vessel is usually accomplished with balloon angioplasty and also stent placement in some cases.

Balloon angioplasty involves treating a vessel by expanding a balloon within the lesion and exerting outward radial pressure to fracture the lesion. For atherosclerosis, the mechanism of an effective angioplasty is controlled intimal injury, with the repair response leading to increased luminal cross-sectional area.

Balloons are integrated into the tip of a catheter, allowing them to be advanced across the lesion over a wire before being inflated. They come in different sizes and lengths, and vary by the amount of radial pressure they exert (▶ Fig. 2.6). The **insufflator** is a handheld pump that fills the balloon with dilute contrast.

At each end of the balloon, there are two radio-opaque markers which indicate the balloon length. The balloon between these markers is referred to as the "working length," which is the part of the balloon that delivers maximal radial pressure to lesion being treated. These radio-opaque markers are essential in positioning the balloon's working length within the target lesion. The balloon inflates from outside in, with the

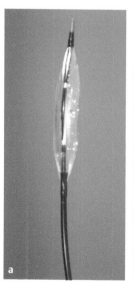
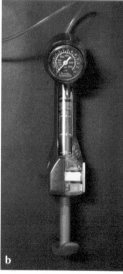

Fig. 2.6 (a) Example of an inflated balloon used in angioplasty. Balloon angioplasty is performed by positioning the deflated balloon at the target lesion and using a **(b)** pump (insufflator) to inflate the balloon.

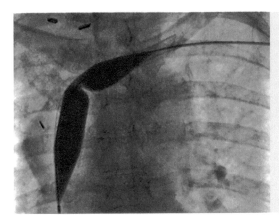

Fig. 2.7 Example of a waist. This represents the portion of the obstruction/lesion still resistant to the radial force exerted by the balloon. (This image is provided courtesy of Joshua Pinter, MD, University of Pittsburgh Medical Center.)

central portion of the balloon inflating last. A "waist" in the middle of the balloon represents a portion of the lesion that is resistant to the radial force (▶ **Fig. 2.7**). A successfully treated lesion should have no waist.

Before balloons are deployed in vessels, they have to be selected and sized appropriately, which will depend on the target vessel, the nature of the lesion being treated, lesion length, and location within the vessel (i.e., mid-vessel versus ostial).

An ideal angioplasty balloon will cover the entire length of the lesion with some room to spare, be 5 to 10% greater than the normal lumen diameter, and exert enough radial pressure to increase the intraluminal surface area. Some lesions are heavily calcified and/or composed of tough fibrous tissue, which may require a large amount of radial pressure to give way. This often requires balloons that are capable of withstanding high amounts of pressure without bursting.

Nominal pressure refers to the amount of pressure (in atmospheres) required for the balloon to assume its listed diameter. **Burst pressure** refers to how much pressure the balloon can safely withstand without bursting. Think of the burst pressure as a soft upper limit for insufflation. You can go higher but any additional pressure past the burst pressure will increase the chance of balloon rupture.

Another important characteristic of balloons is the ability to expand in response to applied pressure. Balloons can be compliant, semicompliant, or noncompliant. Each has its unique applications. **Compliant balloons** mold to the vasculature contour as they are inflated without putting excessive pressure at any single point along the length of the balloon. They are ideal for occluding flow or fully expanding/molding stent-grafts against the vessel wall.

In contrast to compliant balloons, **noncompliant balloons** experience a smaller increase in diameter per unit of pressure increase. As pressure and rigidity increase, noncompliant balloons do not conform as readily to the contours of the vessel. As a result, more force is exerted against lesions at a given inflation pressure. This property makes noncompliant balloons ideal for angioplasty of heavily calcified lesions. **Cutting balloons** are a type of noncompliant balloon with microsurgical blades mounted longitudinally on the outer surface. When the balloon is expanded, the blades score the lesion to facilitate dilation at a lower pressure.

Semicompliant balloons are the most common used for angioplasty. The compliance of these balloons falls in between that of compliant and noncompliant balloons. They continue to expand with increasing pressure but at much lower rate. They are used primarily to angioplasty the "run-of-the-mill" atherosclerotic lesions.

Once inflated, balloons are held in place for between 30 seconds and 2 minutes. If over-inflated, balloons can rupture. Balloon rupture is less problematic than vessel rupture, so it is preferable to be initially conservative and err on the side of undersizing the balloon.

Stenting

Stents are scaffolds that are placed within vessels or ducts to maintain the luminal surface area. There are several different types of stents you will encounter, including biliary, nephroureteral, and vascular stents. The function of a stent is to maintain the diameter of a stenotic lumen after plasty and resist external compression.

The two main subcategories of stents include self-expanding and balloon expandable stents. **Self-expanding stents** are typically made of a nickel–titanium alloy called nitinol. They are compressible and held within a stent delivery system (▶**Fig. 2.8**). The stent and stent delivery system can be delivered through a sheath to the lesion. Once deployed, self-expanding stents will tend to return to their original shape even after being compressed. Because of this property, they are often the stent of choice for vessels subject to compression or tortuous vessels. One disadvantage is that some self-expanding stents can shorten during deployment, which can add a layer of difficulty in accurate placement.

Balloon-expandable stents are mounted on balloon catheters. When delivered to the target lesion, the balloon is inflated to facilitate stent expansion. These will not expand on their own. Once they are deformed, they stay deformed. However, these stents exert a much higher radial force than self-expanding stents, and typically do not shorten when deployed. They are preferred in nontortuous vessels that are not externally compressible.

Variations to the above include drug-eluting and drug-coated stents. They are coated in specific medications that prevent neointimal hyperplasia, a significant cause of long-term restenosis. Commonly used drugs include paclitaxel and sirolimus. While they are most commonly used in the coronary arteries, their use is increasing in the peripheral vasculature. The major disadvantage is their high cost.

Most stents are open along their lengths (like wire fences), serving as scaffolds inside the vessel. Blood flowing through can still contact the vessel wall through the stent interstices. **Stent grafts** are metallic stents, either self-expanding or balloon expandable, which are covered by a fabric graft material (typically PTFE) (▶**Fig. 2.9**). Blood flowing through a stent graft does not contact the vessel wall; the covering serves as the effective vessel wall, thereby creating a new flow conduit. This makes stent grafts an excellent choice when a portion of the vessel needs to be excluded from the circulation. You will often see stent grafts used to treat vessel ruptures and aneurysms.

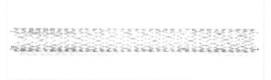

Fig. 2.8 Example of a self-expanding vascular stent; placement of a stent augments the lumen and increases the luminal surface area.

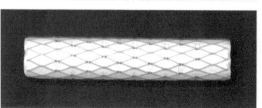

Fig. 2.9 Example of a covered stent; covered stents are commonly placed over vascular defects (such as an arterial injury) to cover the defect and reroute blood through the stent.

Embolization

Embolization is a technique used to cause blockage of flow within a vessel. Various embolic agents including coils, plugs, particles, and sclerosants are delivered through catheters to carry out the occlusion. Each agent has its own unique applications, and comes with advantages and disadvantages. The specific agent to be deployed depends on the reason for embolization, the target vessel, and operator preference.

Metallic coils are the workhorse of embolization, and can stop bleeding or redirect blood flow in several different scenarios (▶ Fig. 2.10). Constructed of various metals, including titanium, tungsten, platinum, nitinol, or stainless steel, coils can conform or expand to fit almost any vessel. The coil itself typically does not completely occlude the vessel, but instead slows flow enough to activate the body's intrinsic clotting mechanism. Dacron fibers are often woven into coils to activate and accelerate thrombogenesis. Coils are available in a variety of shapes and sizes. Their wire diameter ranges from 0.010- to 0.035-inch, which determines the softness of the coil and the catheter through which it can be delivered. Additionally, coils are defined by their deployed diameter and shape (for example, 6 mm helical), and by their length (e.g., 14 cm). The length is a measurement of the coil if it was completely straightened out, and is simply meant to provide a framework for the operator to determine the approximate deployed length. The ideal coil size is selected based on the vessel characteristics.

Pushable coils are loaded into the catheter, and are either pushed from behind using a wire or flushed through the catheter with saline. A drawback is that once these coils are deployed, their positioning cannot be adjusted. Newer generations of coils are detachable. The operator may reposition or completely remove the coil if unsatisfied with positioning after deployment within the vessel. They can then be completely detached through a variety of mechanisms once the coil is perfectly positioned. This advantage in precision makes them higher priced compared to standard coils. The degree of control and the mechanism of detachment vary by model and manufacturer. Other specialty coils, such as hydrocoils, are not only detachable but are also expansile, meaning that they thicken once exposed to blood in the vessel. This reduces microchannels present within the coil pack and decreases the rate of vessel recanalization.

Coils are advantageous due to their utility in a wide range of vessel sizes. They are effective in high-flow arteries but equally effective in slower-flow, lower-pressure veins. They are not absorbed by the body and keep vessels occluded long-term. The major drawback of coils is that once they are placed, it is nearly impossible for a repeat treatment distal to that point.

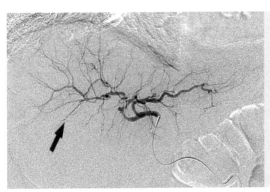

Fig. 2.10 Digital subtraction angiography image of a coil (*arrow*) placed within a bleeding branch of the hepatic artery; achieving hemostasis. (This image is provided courtesy of Matthew Evan Krosin, MD, University of Pittsburgh Medical Center.)

Similar to coils, **vascular plugs** are disc-shaped or cork-like baskets woven together with nitinol wires that promote vessel occlusion and activation of the intrinsic clotting cascade (▶ **Fig. 2.11**). Plugs have evolved over the years, taking inspiration from devices that were first used in closing cardiac septal defects. Plugs have the advantage of a lower risk of migration following placement, even when placed in large vessels with high flow rates. Plugs are detachable, just like some of the more expensive coils, allowing for precise positioning. A single plug can be used to block a large-caliber vessel, where even multiple stacked coils might be insufficient. Disadvantages of plugs include higher cost, lower rates of complete initial occlusion, unpredictable occlusion times following deployment, and difficulty in deployment within tortuous or distal vessels due to the larger delivery catheters required. Newer plugs are more thrombogenic and smaller, helping to mitigate some of these drawbacks. Use in splenic trauma is the most common emergent application. Other uses include treatment of vascular malformations and plug-assisted gastric variceal embolization (PARTO).

Particles are microscopic spheres or polygons with diameters between 40 and 1300 microns (▶ **Fig. 2.12**). Particles are constructed from a variety of different materials including tris-acryl gelatin (TAGM) and polyvinyl alcohol (PVA). Particles are almost always mixed with contrast and flushed through a catheter, where they lodge distally in the arteries of the target organ, causing inflammation and subsequent thrombosis.

A major advantage of particles is that they can reach the intricate networks of arteries too small and too distal for a catheter to reach. A catch is that the particles must be deployed upstream from the target, and once the particles leave the catheter, there is no control over their destination. The site of administration must be carefully considered and executed to avoid particles traveling to unintended areas, a complication referred to as "nontarget embolization." In emergent bronchial and uterine hemorrhage, particles are the most commonly used agents. Other uses include treatment of tumors in various organs.

Gelfoam is a biologic substance derived from dermal gelatin, a hemostatic agent used in surgery. Gelfoam also has a long-standing track record as an effective embolic agent. Small pieces are mixed with contrast and injected into the target vessel. Gelfoam produces partial vessel occlusion and promotes intrinsic thrombus formation. The unique advantage of Gelfoam is its temporary effect. After a few weeks, the Gelfoam will resorb, and treated vessels may recanalize. Gelfoam is thus an excellent choice for achieving hemostasis and allowing for eventual restoration of flow to healed tissues.

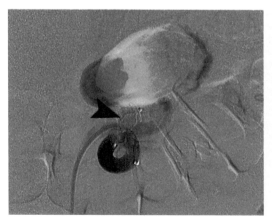

Fig. 2.11 Digital subtraction angiography image of a successful deployment of a vascular plug (*arrowhead*) within the proximal splenic artery in a patient with traumatic splenic injury. (This image is provided courtesy of Matthew Evan Krosin, MD, University of Pittsburgh Medical Center.)

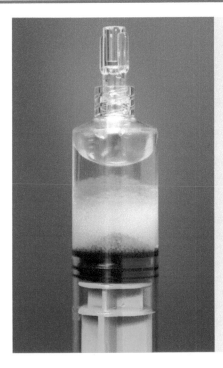

Fig. 2.12 Particles are often made of tris-acryl gelatin or polyvinyl alcohol. They are mixed with contrast and flushed through a catheter where they lodge distally in the arteries of the target organ, causing inflammation and subsequent thrombosis.

Other advantages include low cost, ease of use, and extensive track record demonstrating efficacy. Disadvantages, aside from its temporary effect, are minimal. A common use is for emergent pelvic trauma.

Liquid embolic agents can be of great utility in certain circumstances. Two popular agents are *n*-butyl-2-cyanoacrylate (*n*-BCA, also called glue, and marketed under the trade name Trufill) and ethyl vinyl alcohol (EVOH, trade name Onyx). The embolic agent is injected through a catheter or microcatheter and flow carries it to the desired site of embolization. The anions in blood cause the mixture to polymerize and form intravascular casts.

A major advantage of these agents is that they do not rely on the intrinsic coagulation cascade. Glue rapidly forms solid casts, which quickly block flow. Disadvantages include a high degree of experience required for use, risk of adherence to the delivery catheter (making the catheter difficult to remove from the vessel), and nontarget embolization.

These agents are not typically used in emergency settings, although in certain situations can be considered. For example, glue or EVOH can effectively embolize arterial hemorrhages from distal vessels within the chest and abdominal wall, although its use is mostly reserved for cases where coagulopathy prevents effective use of other agents. These agents also have a number of nonemergent applications, particularly in the treatment of vascular malformations.

Sclerosants are agents such as sodium tetradecyl sulfate, polidocanol, and ethanol which damage the endothelial and medial cells within a vessel wall, leading to scarring, vessel destruction, platelet activation, and coagulation cascade activation. Sclerosants are typically used in veins or to treat lymphovascular malformations. The use of sclerosants in emergency situations is limited.

Closure Devices

Once the procedure is complete, the guidewire, catheter, and sheath need to be removed and the hole in the vessel needs to be closed. Venotomy sites can usually be closed with simple manual compression for a few minutes. Arteriotomy sites can also be managed with manual compression, though the compression time necessary for hemostasis is greater, ranging from 10 minutes to as long as an hour in coagulopathic patients. Closure devices are frequently used for arteriotomies to close the access site and reduce the amount of manual compression time. Selection of a closure device is largely based on provider preference, as many types are capable of achieving adequate hemostasis. Devices add a layer of convenience to both provider and patient, as they enable patients to ambulate after an arterial procedure sooner.

A Perclose closure device (Abbott Vascular, Santa Clara, CA) is introduced over a guidewire through the arterial access site. Once positioned inside the artery, a foot with suture material is deployed off the distal end of the device within the artery lumen. Two needles (both part of the closure device) can then be advanced through the artery wall on opposite sides of the site. These needles capture the suture ends off the foot of the device. The needles are then retracted back through the artery wall with the suture ends in tow. The suture ends are then fastened to seal off the arterial access site.

The AngioSeal closure device (Terumo Interventional Systems, Tokyo, Japan) creates a mechanical seal, sandwiching the arterial puncture site between a copolymer anchor and collagen sponge. This seal is held securely in place by a suture that connects the anchor and sponge. The anchor, sponge, and suture are all naturally absorbed over time.

The Mynx closure device (Cordis, Milpitas, CA) initially achieves hemostasis by the introduction and deployment of an intra-arterial balloon. Once the balloon is inflated, it is retracted back toward the deep surface of the arteriotomy. Subsequently, a polyethylene glycol sealant is delivered to the superficial surface of the arteriotomy. The balloon is then deflated and removed with the sealant left in place. The sealant is naturally absorbed over time.

The Starclose closure device (Abbott Vascular, Santa Clara, CA) deploys a nitinol clip to seal off the arterial access site. The clip is introduced on the superficial surface of the artery and mechanically seals off the arteriotomy.

2.2 Nonvascular Procedures

Nonvascular procedures involve draining fluid collections, sampling of tissue, intervening on the urinary or biliary systems, and injecting material for therapeutic purposes. In all cases, the first step is access to the target using the Seldinger or Trocar technique. From there, a number of different tools are available to complete the procedure.

Despite some similarities between vascular and nonvascular procedures, the tools and techniques used in nonvascular access are more variable. For vascular access, the target access site is relatively superficial, and there are usually no critical structures between it and the skin. For nonvascular procedures, the target can be much deeper in the body, sometimes requiring different tools and techniques.

Drainage Procedures

Drainage catheters can be inserted in the body to aspirate fluid collections if the total volume is small, or left in place for continuous drainage for larger collections. The Seldinger technique for nonvascular access is similar to that used for vascular access. The major difference is that a longer needle and introducer system may be required.

The same Micropuncture kit used in vascular access can be used for nonvascular access. However, the introducer sheath in most kits is only 7 cm in length, limiting its use to more superficial targets.

For deeper targets, common access needles include **Accustick** (Boston Scientific, Natick, MA) and **Chiba** (Cook Medical, Bloomington, IN) which are 18 to 22 gauge, and between 10 and 20 cm in length (▶ **Fig. 2.1**). Using these needles, the sequence is as follows:

1. Using image guidance, the needle is advanced into the target.
2. An 0.018 microwire is passed through the needle into the collection.
3. The needle is exchanged over the wire for a coaxial introducer sheath (consisting of a stiffener, an inner dilator, and an outer sheath).
4. The microwire is removed and exchanged for a 0.035 wire.

An example of an alternative method to the above is the **Yueh catheter** (Cook Medical, Bloomington, IN), or similar device, which is a coaxial system consisting of a hollow needle within a 4 or 5 Fr catheter (ranging from 5 to 20 cm in length) (▶ **Fig. 2.13**). The system is advanced into the target in a similar fashion to the other access needles, but after removal of the needle an 0.035 wire can be directly passed through the catheter. This skips the intermediate steps of using 0.018 wire and introducer sheath to size up to an 0.035 system.

Having an 0.035-inch guidewire in place is critical as it allows for a robust scaffold that is less likely to bend or kink in the deep tissues as tools are slid over it. With the 0.035 guidewire in place, the drainage catheter is ready to be inserted over the wire and into the target.

To provide additional support and rigidity to the catheter as it is being advanced over the guidewire, most drainage catheters come with a stiffening inner cannula. Some catheters may even have two stiffening cannulas (one rigid, one flexible). Once the catheter and inner cannula assembly are advanced up to the collection, the stiffening cannula is pinned, and just the catheter advanced into the collection.

The **trocar technique** is an alternative to the Seldinger technique. The idea is to reach the target directly without doing over the wire exchanges. To insert the drainage catheter into a fluid collection with the trocar technique, the catheter is first loaded onto a stiffening cannula. Within the cannula resides a sharp stylet. There is no guidewire or predilated tract that leads the catheter to the collection. Instead, the sharp stylet will create a tract as the assembly is advanced, allowing for penetration through tissue and into the collection. The stiffening cannula provides rigidity and support for the catheter while it passes through tissue.

The trocar technique starts with a skin nick at the chosen insertion site. The unit is inserted through the skin nick and advanced until the tip is within the target. Then the

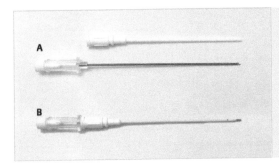

A

B

Fig. 2.13 Yueh catheters consist of a hollow needle within a 5 Fr catheter. **(A)** Once the tip has reached the target, the needle can be removed leaving the 5 Fr catheter behind. An 0.035-inch wire can then be advanced through the 5 Fr catheter. **(B)** Appearance of the Yueh catheter assembled together as a unit.

catheter is advanced off the stylet and stiffener, into the collection. Once the catheter is in, a stopcock and drainage bag can be attached to the external portion. The catheter should also be secured to the body by sutures.

The advantage of this technique is the ability to advance a relatively large catheter (8–16 Fr) directly into the target, without the need for guidewires or separate dilators. In general, the trocar technique is best suited for more superficial and larger targets, without nearby vital structures to worry about, and when real-time ultrasound guidance can be used.

Drainage catheters vary in shape and size, depending on their intended use. Many drainage catheter tips can be locked into a pigtail configuration by pulling back on a string on the external portion of the catheter. Locking a catheter reduces the likelihood that it will migrate or be displaced.

Standard, locking **pigtail catheters** are used to drain collections. These catheters have sideholes at their tip, which facilitates drainage. The size of the pigtail is chosen based on the size of the collection that needs drainage. A 25 mm pigtail works for any "average" collection, while a 10 mm pigtail is often used for smaller collections. Two common pigtail catheter variants you may encounter include the Dawson-Mueller and the Multipurpose Drainage Catheter (Cook Medical). They are similar, but the Multipurpose Drainage Catheter has a 25 mm pigtail and more sideholes.

While the pigtail drainage catheter will work for most simple collections, larger diameter catheters with more sideholes are necessary for complex or viscous collections. One example of such a catheter is the Gordon large-bore drainage catheter (Cook Medical).

Biliary drainage catheters vary in stiffness and length but all share the same feature; in addition to having sideholes at the tip, they also have sideholes along the length of the catheter, which maximizes drainage along its course (▶ **Fig. 2.14**). The tip can be locked into a pigtail configuration after being advanced through the common bile duct and into the duodenum. This allows bile to enter the drain above the level of obstruction and exit the drain at the pigtail; hence, the tube can be capped and function as as an internalized stent.

Nephrostomy drainage catheters have locking tips that terminate in the renal pelvis. Nephroureterostomy drains (also called a nephroureterostomy *stent*) are long catheters that terminate in the bladder. They have an externalized portion outside the patient along with *two* pigtails that are formed within the body; one pigtail is formed in the renal pelvis and the second formed within the bladder. Urine in the kidney enters the proximal pigtail and the ureteral portion of the catheter carries urine down to into the bladder.

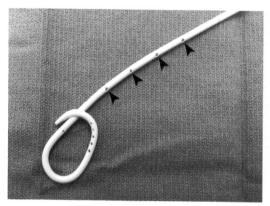

Fig. 2.14 Example of a 12 Fr internal–external biliary drainage catheter. Once advanced into the duodenum, the string can be pulled from the outside, locking the catheter tip into a pigtail configuration. Note the sideholes not only at the catheter tip, but also along the length of the catheter (*arrowheads*).

Biopsy Procedures

Biopsy procedures are similar to other procedures that require nonvascular access. The concept is the same; CT or ultrasound is used to guide needle placement into the target (the lesion to be biopsied), while ensuring there are no vital structures along the way. There are two main techniques to reach the target lesion: the coaxial technique and the tandem technique.

The **coaxial technique** involves inserting an initial larger-diameter needle to the edge of the lesion. A thinner and longer needle is then slid into the larger needle, and advanced into the lesion. The major advantage of the coaxial technique is that only one puncture is made.

The **tandem technique** uses an initial reference needle placed into the lesion, with the biopsy needle then placed in tandem, using the reference needle's depth and trajectory as a guide.

In either technique, once the target lesion is reached you are ready to obtain a biopsy sample. There are two ways to obtain a sample: fine-needle biopsy and core biopsy. The major difference between the two is the size and quality of the tissue sample obtained.

Fine-needle biopsies provide cells from the lesion for cytology. The needles used range between 20 and 25 gauge, with a variety of tip shapes, all of which are constructed to provide a cutting edge. The most common way to perform a fine-needle biopsy is via a **fine needle aspiration** (FNA). FNA is performed by attaching a 10-mL syringe to the needle and pulling back on the needle to apply suction. The cutting needle tip is moved back-and-forth to shear and agitate the tissue, all the while applying suction. Blood and cells from the tissue should begin filling the syringe.

The fine-needle nonaspiration technique is less commonly used, and involves simply stabbing the lesion and making multiple back-and-forth passes in the lesion. No syringe is attached to the needle and no suction is applied. After making multiple passes in the lesion, blood and cells from the tissue fill the needle by capillary action.

If an actual chunk of tissue is required, a **core biopsy** can be obtained with a larger gauge biopsy needle (14–20 gauge) (▸ Fig. 2.15). Core biopsy needles have a long inner needle with a trough at the end. An outer needle sits further back, ready to be deployed. This outer needle is spring-activated. When deployed, it quickly slides over the inner needle and over the trough (▸ Fig. 2.16). When the inner needle is in the lesion, the target tissue is embedded in the trough. The spring-activated outer needle sliding over the trough traps a chunk of the tissue. The length of the trough determines the throw length (which determines how much tissue is obtained). Core needle biopsy devices can be repeatedly used to obtain multiple samples.

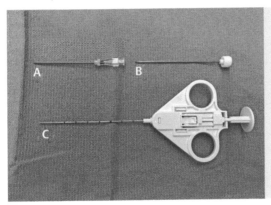

Fig. 2.15 Biopsy device along with the **(A)** introducer needle and **(B)** stylet. Introducer needle/stylet unit is advanced to the edge of the target lesion. The **(C)** biopsy needle's inner needle (with a trough at the tip) is advanced through the introducer needle and embedded in the lesion. Spring activation forces the biopsy needle's outer needle to snap over the inner needle, capturing the tissue within the trough.

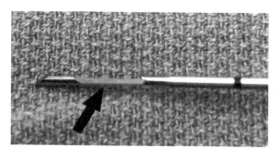

Fig. 2.16 Biopsy needles have an inner needle with a trough (*arrow*) at its tip, along with an outer needle that sits further back, ready to be deployed.

Suggested Readings

[1] Kaufman JA, Lee MJ. Vascular and Interventional Radiology: The Requisites. 2nd ed. Amsterdam: Elsevier; 2014

[2] Harrigan MR, Deveikis JP. Handbook of cerebrovascular disease and neurointerventional technique. 2nd ed. Totowa, NJ: Humana Press; 2013

[3] Zhu X, Tam MD, Pierce G, et al. Utility of the Amplatzer Vascular Plug in splenic artery embolization: a comparison study with conventional coil technique. Cardiovasc Intervent Radiol. 2011; 34(3):522–531

[4] Lopera JE. The Amplatzer Vascular Plug: review of evolution and current applications. Semin Intervent Radiol. 2015; 32(4):356–369

[5] Das R, Champaneria R, Daniels JP, Belli A-M. Comparison of embolic agents used in uterine artery embolisation: a systematic review and meta-analysis. Cardiovasc Intervent Radiol. 2014; 37(5): 1179–1190

[6] Bauer JR, Ray CE, Jr. Transcatheter arterial embolization in the trauma patient: a review. Semin Intervent Radiol. 2004; 21(1):11–22

[7] Vaidya S, Tozer KR, Chen J. An overview of embolic agents. Semin Intervent Radiol. 2008; 25(3): 204–215

3 Vascular Access

Suraj Prakash, Lisa Liu, Aaron M. Fischman, and Gregory E. Guy

Gaining access to a vessel is the first step for the majority of IR procedures, and is often a starting point for students or residents to get early hands on experience. Those who have been in practice for some time can gain access effortlessly in the vast majority of cases, however there is still a step by step process that should be followed in every case.

Most procedures will have a preferred site of vascular access, which is usually at the neck, groin, or the extremity. Before starting, the proposed access site should be inspected to make sure there are no contraindications to needle puncture. Areas with ongoing skin infection, recent surgical incision, or dense scarring should be avoided if possible. Although the target vessel can be found by palpation and use of landmarks, the standard of care is ultrasound guidance, which allows you to maintain visualization of your needle as it enters the target vessel. Use of image guidance substantially reduces the risk of complications related to access. Ultrasound can be used to ensure the target vessel is patent before the patient is prepped and draped. The IR technologist will often do this for you, but it's a good idea to practice doing it yourself. If the vessel of choice is inaccessible due to chronic occlusion or the presence of thrombus, check the contralateral side (▶ **Fig. 3.1**).

Prior to puncturing the skin, the access site must be sanitized with an antiseptic solution and the surrounding area draped. From this point on you'll need to have a sterile gown and gloves on. With this done, you can now give lidocaine using a hypodermic needle near the anticipated area of needle puncture.

Obtaining vascular access properly requires two-handed coordination. You'll take the ultrasound probe in one hand, and your needle in the other. Some choose to have a syringe attached to the needle for the initial puncture, but it is a matter of personal preference. In either case, the probe is held perpendicular to the skin and the needle near parallel to it, with the bevel facing up. The goal is to advance the needle in the same plane as the probe, watching the needle tip the whole time. If you are uncertain of whether what you are seeing is the needle tip, a gentle rocking motion of the probe will show the tip come in and out of the field of view. The tendency will be to want to

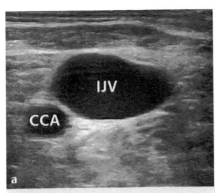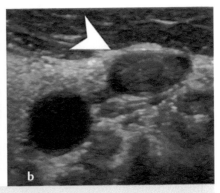

Fig. 3.1 **(a)** Normal relationship between right internal jugular vein (IJV) and the more medial right common carotid artery (CCA). **(b)** Preprocedure ultrasound evaluation of the right IJV revealed an occlusive thrombus within the vein (*arrow*).

look down at the needle but try to keep your eyes on the ultrasound screen. It will become more natural as you get the feel for this maneuver with practice.

Ideally, you will watch your needle tip enter the vessel as you advance it. Other clues to help guide you include the appearance of a vessel wall "tenting" before the needle pokes through, as well as the tactile feedback of the puncture (▶Fig. 3.2). There should be blood return through the needle once inside the vessel lumen. In an artery the blood return will be pulsatile, while in a vein it will trickle out of the needle. If you have a syringe on the needle, you can try aspirating; with the needle in a vein you will draw back purple-colored venous blood but will meet resistance if the needle is extraluminal.

Once the needle is inside the vessel, the remaining steps of vascular access follow the Seldinger technique, as described in Chapter 2. When advancing a guidewire through the needle, there should not be significant resistance. This can indicate attempted passage of the guidewire into the subintimal space or outside of the vessel lumen completely. Once the guidewire is in a #11 blade scalpel may be used to create a small nick in skin where the guidewire enters. The point of this is to ensure that the subsequent tools can be passed without getting caught on skin, which would require extra force. Care should be taken to not cut the vessel or guidewire with the blade when making a skin nick. Alternatively, some people prefer to make this skin nick as the first step, just before needle puncture.

With the guidewire in place and skin nick made, a dilator sheath can be slid over the wire and into the vessel. After the dilator sheath is hubbed at the skin, the inner dilator and guidewire are both removed, leaving just the sheath in place. Vascular access to the vessel is now secure and further tools (specialty catheters, guidewires, etc.) can be inserted.

3.1 Venous Access

Most IR procedures involving the venous system start with internal jugular or femoral venous access. Both the access site and the laterality are important to consider. For example, the right internal jugular vein (IJV) has a straighter course to the heart and minimizes

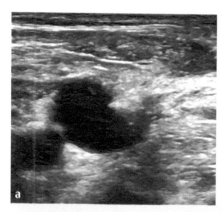
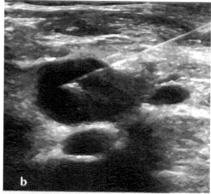

Fig. 3.2 Example of ultrasound-guided internal jugular vein (IJV) access. (a) Advancement of the needle tip into the exterior wall of the vein "tents" the vessel inward. (b) Additional advancement of the needle or sometimes a quick, short jab with the needle will allow the needle tip to enter the IJ lumen. Visualizing the needle tip in the IJ can help confirm proper positioning before moving forward with the procedure. (These images are provided courtesy of Avinash Medsinge, MD and Pattana Wangaryattawanich, MD, University of Pittsburgh Medical Center.)

bends in the catheter, which is desirable for certain procedures. When attempting IJV access, ultrasound should be used to first identify the common carotid artery. The IJV should be lateral and anterior to the artery; however, this is variable (▶ **Fig. 3.1**). It should also be compressible and increase in diameter with the Valsalva maneuver.

If the IJV is occluded, the contralateral side or the external jugular vein may be used alternatively and subclavian vein access considered if the jugular veins are inaccessible. Ultrasound guidance for **subclavian access** can sometimes be challenging due to the clavicle lying directly above the vein. **Femoral vein access** is relatively straightforward using ultrasound, with the femoral vein typically residing medial to the artery ("venous toward the penis").

The risk of complications with venous access is less significant due to lower intraluminal pressure and thinner vessel walls. Nevertheless, occasional complications do occur and may include symptomatic thrombosis at the puncture site, venous perforation, and injury to adjacent structures. Complications specific to IJV access include pneumothorax and hemothorax, however these are rare. Hematomas can occur with venous access, usually in coagulopathic patients.

Ultrasound guidance and preferential use of the IJV have almost completely eliminated the risk of pneumothorax. Though pneumothoraces are a greater concern during subclavian vein access, it is important to be conscientious of your needle trajectory with IJ access, keeping the needle about 1 cm above the clavicle and in constant view by ultrasound if possible.

3.2 Arterial Access

Arterial access sites are limited, with most procedures performed via the femoral artery, radial artery, or brachial artery. Pedal or antegrade arterial access in the lower leg can also be obtained for certain peripheral vascular procedures.

Prior to attempting arterial access, the distal pulse strength and capillary refill should be checked as a precaution in case an occlusive or embolic complication occurs as a result of the procedure. Blood pressure measurement and perfusion of the digits are particularly important to check prior to upper extremity arterial access.

Common femoral artery (CFA) access is the most common for arterial interventions. However, arterial patency may preclude CFA access. For example, if a patient has severe aortoiliac disease and requires mesenteric artery interrogation, brachial or radial artery access may be necessary. For lower extremity arterial intervention such as recanalization of tibial or femoropopliteal occlusion, antegrade femoral access with or without pedal access can be used. The dorsalis pedis and posterior tibial artery are both options for the latter.

The target for a femoral artery stick is the arterial segment overlying the femoral head (▶ **Fig. 3.3**). The bony landmark offers rigid support to compress and tamponade the femoral artery when needed. Just inferior to the inguinal ligament, a radiopaque object such as a hemostat should be placed with the tip at the approximate location of the midfemoral head, and an anteroposterior (AP) fluoroscopic spot image taken to confirm placement. The femoral artery should be accessed in this approximate location after successfully palpating the artery just proximal and distal to the desired access site. The femoral bifurcation also needs to be lower than this point, verified using ultrasound.

The brachial artery is readily visible with ultrasound, however its depth and a lack of underlying support diminishes the potential effectiveness of manual compression.

For the past 20 years, support in the interventional cardiology community has steadily shifted toward **transradial access (TRA)** as the preferred approach for coronary interventions. Recently, the use of TRA in IR has also gained traction, though widespread implementation has been limited by operator familiarity and training, as well as equipment availability, such as appropriate catheter length and shape. Radial access has some notable benefits compared to femoral access. The advantages of radial access include more effective postprocedure hemostasis, immediate ambulation postprocedure, and increased patient comfort. It is also helpful when intervening on obese patients, for whom femoral access is a challenge.

Vasospasm is of particular concern for transradial access, and several strategies are employed to reduce this risk. This includes the use of special hydrophilic sheaths and injection of an antispasmodic solution consisting of heparin, nitroglycerin, and verapamil. After completion of the procedure, a radial compression device is wrapped around the wrist to achieve nonocclusive "patent" hemostasis, which minimizes risk of radial artery occlusion (▶ Fig. 3.4). The band can be removed 75 to 90 minutes after application.

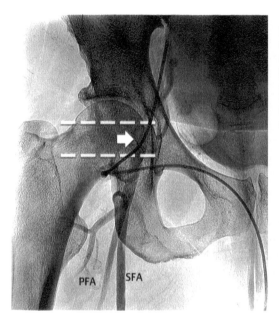

Fig. 3.3 The ideal location for a common femoral artery (CFA) arteriotomy should be where the CFA crosses over the middle third of the femoral head. The femoral head provides a firm "back-wall" to compress against when necessary to achieve hemostasis.

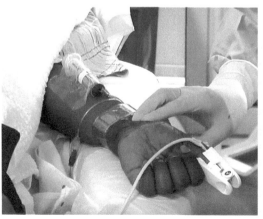

Fig. 3.4 A compression device is used to tamponade the radial artery arteriotomy site after radial access. Patients tend to be more comfortable after radial access as compared to femoral artery access.

The most common complication related to arterial access is **hematoma** formation. Risk factors include an uncorrected coagulopathy, poor compression at the arteriotomy site, improper closure device deployment, and uncontrolled hypertension. The risk can be reduced by reversing heparin at the end of the procedure with protamine sulfate, and administration of fresh frozen plasma (FFP) for any patient with an INR greater than 1.5.

The signs, symptoms, and complications of hematoma formation are location dependent. Femoral hematomas are most commonly associated with groin and thigh pain, whereas brachial artery hematomas may be associated with median nerve compression. With the latter, permanent neurological deficits can occur if the compartment is not promptly decompressed. Regular postprocedure peripheral neurological examinations are a must for these patients. Neurologic damage from a femoral hematoma is less common, but they can still be quite painful. Radial hematomas are far less symptomatic as they are usually detected early, and can be managed expectantly. Hemodynamic instability as a result of arterial access hematoma is extremely rare.

Pseudoaneurysms are sometimes confused for hematomas. Iatrogenic pseudoaneurysms occur when an arterial puncture site fails to seal, allowing blood to pool outside the vessel, contained by the adventitia, neighboring tissues, or fascia. Risk factors for pseudoaneurysm formation include the use of large catheters and sheaths, anticoagulant or antiplatelet medications, and improper arterial puncture site (superficial femoral artery, external iliac artery, etc.).

Pseudoaneurysms typically present as a painful, pulsatile mass. They are considered unstable since they lack the integrity of an intact wall to contain the blood flowing into and out of the pseudoaneurysm. Untreated, pseudoaneurysms can rupture, resulting in hemorrhage and ischemic tissue damage. The typical ultrasound appearance of a pseudoaneurysm is that of turbulent blood flow, which appears as a "yin-yang sign" on color flow, with an arterialized "to-and-fro" pattern on pulsed Doppler (▶ **Fig. 3.5**). Several options exist for the treatment of pseudoaneurysms. In IR, the most commonly employed is the ultrasound-directed injection of thrombin into the pseudoaneurysm sac to precipitate immediate thrombosis. A more conservative alternative is ultrasound probe compression at the pseudoaneurysm neck. In refractory cases, a stent-graft across the neck or open surgical repair may be necessary.

An **arterial dissection** occurs when there is a tear in the tunica intima (usually due to guidewire trauma), resulting in a false lumen between the tunica intima and tunica media. Dissections are preventable in many cases with proper technique. If a guidewire meets

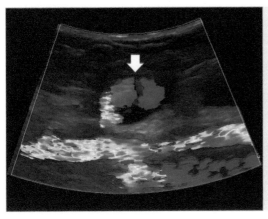

Fig. 3.5 Example of an ultrasound image showing the yin-yang sign seen with a pseudoaneurysm (*arrow*). The to-and-fro movement of blood through the pseudoaneurysm will result in blood moving toward and away from the probe, creating the characteristic red and blue appearance. This pseudoaneurysm occurred after common femoral artery access. (This image is provided courtesy of Scott Beasley, MD, University of Pittsburgh Medical Center.)

resistance while obtaining access, it should be pulled out and the access needle repositioned to ensure that it is squarely within the lumen of the artery. Sometimes a catheter or sheath may also result in dissection, when it is forcibly advanced against resistance.

Transradial access presents a theoretical risk of stroke since access to the descending aorta requires traversing the origins of the great vessels, possibly leading to dissection. However, retrospective studies have shown no such association.

Suspected arterial dissection can be confirmed with imaging showing blood on both sides of the intimal flap. Left untreated, an arterial dissection can propagate along the length of the artery and into branch vessels. If enough blood accumulates within the false lumen, compression or occlusion of the true lumen can lead to arterial thrombosis and ischemic damage. Treatment of iatrogenic dissection typically involves endovascular or surgical repair. Some arterial dissections may resolve spontaneously, particularly those that originate in a direction opposite to the direction of arterial blood flow.

An **arteriovenous fistula** (**AVF**) is a physical connection between the artery and vein. Iatrogenic AVFs can form if both the artery and vein are punctured during access. If small, the AVF may be asymptomatic and spontaneously close. If larger, signs and symptoms include a palpable thrill, continuous bruit, pain, and local swelling. Severe cases can result in high-output cardiac failure and/or distal ischemia. AVFs are diagnosed with duplex ultrasound, which will show a pulsatile waveform in the involved vein, continuous flow during diastole in the artery. Endovascular intervention with stent placement or surgical repair is curative for severe AVFs which do not resolve on their own.

 Distal ischemia is most commonly seen when arterial access is attempted at an atherosclerotic segment of the artery. Disruption of the plaque and resulting atheroembolism can result in downstream ischemia. Patients with a history of atherosclerosis are considered at risk for these complications, and imaging should be reviewed prior to the procedure to ensure the access site is clear of any atherosclerotic burden. Embolization of atherosclerotic material from the origins of the great vessels can occur during upper extremity access; care should be taken when traversing these segments to prevent stroke.

In the case of upper extremity intervention (and especially with transradial access), arterial spasm can also lead to distal ischemia in patients with poor collateral circulation from the ulnar artery. While the best strategy is prevention with the use of antispasmodic solution during the procedure, intra-arterial papaverine infusion can be considered if vasospasm-induced ischemia does occur.

Prior to proceeding with radial artery access, the adequacy of collateral circulation to the hand via ulnopalmar arterial arches needs to be determined. The Barbeau test, a modified Allen's test, may be used to assess ulnopalmar patency. In this test, with the proximal radial artery compressed, a pulse oximeter assesses the radial pulse waveform distally along the radial artery. If the waveform is flattened upon compression and the original waveform does not return within 2 minutes (Barbeau grade D), the ulnopalmar patency is inadequate to safely utilize radial artery access. Only a small minority (< 2%) have Barbeau grade D.

Suggested Readings

[1] Barbeau GR, Arsenault F, Dugas L, Simard S, Larivière MM. Evaluation of the ulnopalmar arterial arches with pulse oximetry and plethysmography: comparison with the Allen's test in 1010 patients. Am Heart J. 2004; 147(3):489–493

[2] Beyer AT, Ng R, Singh A, et al. Topical nitroglycerin and lidocaine to dilate the radial artery prior to transradial cardiac catheterization: a randomized, placebo-controlled, double-blind clinical trial: the PRE-DILATE Study. Int J Cardiol. 2013; 168(3):2575–2578

[3] Boyer N, Beyer A, Gupta V, et al. The effects of intra-arterial vasodilators on radial artery size and spasm: implications for contemporary use of trans-radial access for coronary angiography and percutaneous coronary intervention. Cardiovasc Revasc Med. 2013; 14(6):321–324

[4] Fischman AM, Swinburne NC, Patel RS. A technical guide describing the use of transradial access technique for endovascular interventions. Tech Vasc Interv Radiol. 2015; 18(2):58–65

[5] Kaufman JA, Lee MJ. Vascular and Interventional Radiology: The Requisites. 2nd ed. Amsterdam: Elsevier; 2014

[6] Patel A, Naides AI, Patel R, Fischman A. Transradial intervention: basics. J Vasc Interv Radiol. 2015; 26(5):722

[7] Ratib K, Mamas MA, Routledge HC, Ludman PF, Fraser D, Nolan J. Influence of access site choice on incidence of neurologic complications after percutaneous coronary intervention. Am Heart J. 2013; 165(3):317–324

[8] Romagnoli E, Biondi-Zoccai G, Sciahbasi A, et al. Radial versus femoral randomized investigation in ST-segment elevation acute coronary syndrome: the RIFLE-STEACS (Radial Versus Femoral Randomized Investigation in ST-Elevation Acute Coronary Syndrome) study. J Am Coll Cardiol. 2012; 60(24): 2481–2489

4 Lines, Tubes, and Drains

Devdutta Warhadpande and Gregory J. Woodhead

Familiarity with lines and drains is a must for IR trainees. These procedures, while considered bread and butter by many, have the potential to create headaches if not approached with diligence. Take some time to learn about the different types of equipment, the indications for each, and the complications which may arise.

4.1 Central Venous Access

While many different specialties can place central lines, those placed by IR have greater technical success and are associated with fewer complications. The use of imaging guidance decreases the risk of procedural complications, and adhering to sterile technique in the controlled environment of the IR suite reduces the risk of infection.

Practices vary a great deal from hospital to hospital, both by the preferences of referring physicians and the policies of the IR department. The guidelines presented in this chapter should be taken with a grain of salt, as they may vary depending on your practice setting.

Referrals for central venous access are common in IR. Given the volume of requests, many centers will allow these procedures to be scheduled without a formal consultation. Central line placement is relatively straightforward and does not require an extensive work-up (**Procedure Box 4.1**). However, there are some important preprocedural steps that must not be overlooked.

Procedure Box 4.1: Central Lines

Peripherally inserted central catheters (PICCs) can be placed bedside without fluoroscopic guidance, however, the malposition rate is higher as a result. After accessing a peripheral vein, a peel-away introducer is inserted. The wire is positioned at the junction of the SVC and right atrium under fluoroscopy, and clamped with a hemostat at the hub of the introducer. The catheter is then cut to the appropriate length and inserted through the introducer. The introducer is peeled away, leaving the catheter in place. The hub can then be secured to the skin.

Tunneled catheters and ports placed by IR are typically inserted via the IJV, using ultrasound guidance. Ideal IJ access for tunneled catheters and ports is just above the clavicle. The desired catheter course includes a gentle curve of the catheter from the skin insertion site to the termination in the right atrium. Depending on the line type, the catheter is either cut to the desired length, or a predetermined length is used. Over the wire, a peel-away introducer is inserted. For a tunneled catheter, a skin nick is created approximately 2 to 3 fingerbreadths below the clavicle, through which the catheter is tunneled. After placing the cuff beneath the skin at the skin nick site, the tip of the catheter is inserted all the way into the sheath, which can then be peeled away. After ensuring the tip is in the correct location, the catheter is flushed with heparin solution and secured to the skin with suture.

When a port is placed, a subcutaneous pocket is created at the distal end of the tunnel where the port will reside. The pocket will need to be made just big enough to fit the reservoir, and no greater, as ports can flip if not snug in the pocket. The catheter portion is placed in the same way as a tunneled catheter. The catheter is cut to length, attached to the reservoir, flushed, and then inserted under the skin, after which the skin can be closed with absorbable sutures.

The first consideration is the indication for access and the expected length of time the catheter will be in place. Catheters and ports vary considerably, by number of lumens, caliber, power injectability, and maximum flow rates. It is important to always verify the correct catheter is chosen to meet the clinical need. Not uncommonly, an inappropriate type of line will be requested by the ordering service.

In patients with a history of multiple line placements, review the prior imaging to assess vein patency and history of access complications. Patients who have had prior central lines will often have occluded or thrombosed veins, and will require scrutiny when choosing an appropriate access site.

It should also be determined whether a reason exists for a line to *not* be placed in a specific location. This is especially important when placing PICCs or subclavian vein lines in patients with renal insufficiency, when there may be an anticipated need for dialysis access creation. These types of lines should be avoided in patients who may eventually require a fistula, but if one is absolutely necessary, it should go *contralateral* to the arm selected for fistula creation. A fistula is most commonly placed in the nondominant extremity, so a PICC/subclavian line should be inserted into the dominant arm.

Venous access is broadly divided into four types: PICC, nontunneled central line, tunneled central line, and implantable ports.

A **PICC** is placed via a peripheral vein (basilic, cephalic, or brachial). Indications for a PICC include a long-term need for intravenous antibiotics, total parenteral nutrition (TPN), fluids, and other medications. In many hospitals, these can be placed on the floor by a team of specially trained nurses and physician extenders. IR is typically consulted for challenging cases, including patients with history of prior occlusions, failure of bedside placement, those requiring sedation, and neonates/infants. A PICC can remain in place for a duration of weeks to months.

Nontunneled central lines are commonly placed in the internal jugular (IJ), subclavian, or femoral veins for access in emergent situations. These temporary lines are at increased risk for dislodgement and infection the longer they remain in. When long-term central access is necessary, IR may be consulted for **tunneled central line** placement. Tunneling increases the lifespan of a central line by securing it in place and decreasing the risk of a catheter-related infection. Most tunneled catheters have a cuff that resides in the subcutaneous tunnel, which promotes tissue ingrowth, securing the line in place and limiting migration of bacteria from the skin entry site to the venotomy (▶ **Fig. 4.1**).

You may encounter several named tunneled central catheters, including the Hickman catheter, Groshong catheter, and Broviac catheter. These are all *small-bore* single or

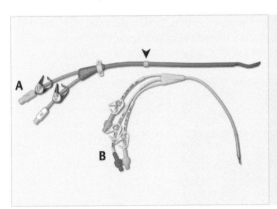

Fig. 4.1 **(A)** Tunneled dialysis catheter. The catheter is sutured to the skin at the hub using the two holes. The cuff (*arrowhead*) is designed to be tucked into the subcutaneous tunnel where it promotes scar formation, securing the catheter within the tunnel. **(B)** Nontunneled trialysis catheter. Note the lack of a cuff. Both devices are large-caliber catheters which allow for the high-flow rates necessary for dialysis.

multilumen catheters used for central access. While they are very similar in functionality, the key difference is that a Groshong catheter has a three-way valve at its tip that prevents back-bleeding into the catheter as well as prevents air from escaping into the blood. The Hickman catheters need to be flushed with heparin after use, while normal saline flushes suffice for the Groshong catheters. Broviac catheters are also very similar to Hickman catheters. A PowerLine (Bard Access Systems, Salt Lake City, UT) is another type of tunneled catheter which appears similar to a PICC, and is frequently mistaken for one, but is inserted in the chest and has a cuff. The word "power" implies that the line is power injectable, which indicates the catheter can tolerate flow rates necessary for large volume injections, such as those required for intravenous contrast during CT scans.

Large-bore tunneled central catheters are necessary for dialysis access and apheresis, which require higher-flow rates (▶ **Fig. 4.1**).

A **port**, also known as "mediport" or "port-a-cath," is a completely subcutaneous central venous access device, which consists of a reservoir inserted into the subcutaneous tissues of the chest wall connected to a tunneled catheter (▶ **Fig. 4.2**). The reservoir is accessed with the use of a needle when the patient requires blood draws, medication, or fluid administration. These are ideal for cancer patients who require central access for frequent outpatient chemotherapy sessions. Ports vary in size, number of lumens, and flow capabilities, but all function in a similar fashion. Given the lack of any exposed components, these devices carry the lowest risk of infection. Tunneled catheters can be left in place for months, while some ports are left in for years.

Aside from PICCs, the hierarchy of vein preference for central venous catheter placement is as follows: right internal jugular > left internal jugular > right external jugular > left external jugular > right subclavian vein > left subclavian. The right internal jugular vein (IJV) is preferred given the straight path down towards the heart. While the subclavian vein has been demonstrated to yield lower rates of infection for nontunneled catheters, this approach carries additional risks during placement, including pneumothorax and the inability to compress any potential bleeding due to the overlying bony clavicle (particularly dangerous if the subclavian artery is inadvertently traumatized). Catheters placed via the subclavian vein are also susceptible to "pinch-off syndrome," which is when the catheter becomes pinched and occluded as it crosses over the first rib. This condition can eventually lead to catheter fracture, allowing the free tip to travel into the heart. Lower extremity veins, such as femoral or greater saphenous, can be utilized, however these are generally considered higher risk sites for infection, and as such are rarely utilized for long-term access. If all suitable veins are unavailable for use, translumbar, transhepatic, and transrenal access is an option, though these are rarely used.

For all central catheters, it is generally recommended to place the line such that the tip terminates in the lower SVC, near the cavoatrial junction. The tip of a tunneled catheter or port can migrate upward by 3 to 4 cm when the patient is standing upright (particularly in women, where breast tissue can pull the catheter hub downward, and thus the tip upward).

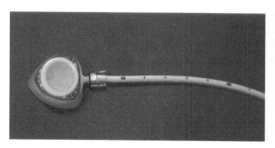

Fig. 4.2 The port reservoir resides within a chest wall subcutaneous pocket and can be accessed with a needle.

When the catheter is being placed, the tip should be in the upper to mid part of the right atrium while the patient is in the supine position to account for this migration. Catheter tips placed too high in the SVC are at risk for tip migration (into the contralateral brachiocephalic vein, jugular vein, or azygos vein), as well as greater rate of thrombosis and catheter dysfunction. Catheter tips placed too low in the right atrium can precipitate arrhythmias.

Line Complications

IR generally does not maintain involvement in the care of patients after a line is placed, unless there are complications. Immediate complications are those encountered during the procedure, and are uncommon due to the use of image guidance. Late complications typically involve malfunction of the catheter in some way or another.

The risk of **pneumothorax** is greatest when accessing the subclavian vein, and lowest with ultrasound-guided internal jugular access. A pneumothorax may be recognized during fluoroscopy or on a postinsertion chest radiograph, and only rarely are they large enough for the patient to become symptomatic. If small and incidentally noted, close observation is often sufficient. Larger pneumothoraces may require chest tube placement.

If not recognized by the pulsatility of blood return during the initial access steps, an inadvertent **arterial puncture** is quickly recognized under fluoroscopy when the guidewire courses along the aortic arch (left of the vertebral bodies). As long as only the guidewire is inserted, the needle and guidewire can simply be taken out and pressure held over the arteriotomy before reattempting. If an arterial puncture goes unrecognized and a sheath/dilator is inserted into the artery, this becomes a more serious problem. Depending on the size and location of the inadvertent arterial access, consideration of most appropriate repair should include both endovascular and open surgical options.

Although rare, an **air embolism** can be fatal. This usually occurs after the peel-away sheath's inner dilator is removed, before the catheter is inserted. Some sheaths have a one-way valve that prevents air from entering, but a good practice is to simply cover the sheath with a finger whenever the dilator is out so air doesn't get sucked in. In the rare event it occurs, the patient may become short of breath, hypotensive, tachycardic, confused, or experience chest pain. If suspected, place the patient in the left lateral decubitus position and provide 100% oxygen. Severe cases may require hyperbaric oxygen therapy or extracorporeal oxygenation (ECMO) until the air has resolved.

Until you have put in many lines and become proficient, one of the challenges of the procedure is ensuring that the catheter runs smoothly in its course. When the catheter bends at an acute angle, it can kink and malfunction. For tunneled catheters, this can be minimized by making sure that the subcutaneous tunnel is an adequate distance lateral to the vein, and that the venotomy where the catheter courses downward is made just about a centimeter above the clavicle. Kinks may be correctable using fluoroscopic manipulation to straighten or reposition the catheter, but sometimes it is just easier to remove it and place a new line. In the rare event of a fracture, as can happen with pinch-off syndrome, the distal fragment may embolize to the heart. An embolized catheter tip should be retrieved if possible. In some cases the risk of retrieval is greater than the risk of leaving the fragment in place. These patients need to be referred to a center experienced in difficult retrievals, and counseled on the risks of removal versus simply leaving it alone before an attempt is made.

Infection is a problem which becomes more common the longer the line has been in place. A catheter serves as a nidus for infection, and if left untreated can lead to sepsis. The reported incidence of infected catheters varies widely in the literature. A **catheter-related bloodstream infection (CRBSI)** should be suspected in the setting of fevers, chills, hypotension, and erythema or purulence around the site of line insertion. Fever is the most sensitive clinical sign. Purulence around the venous line insertion site has a high specificity, but poor sensitivity. CRBSI is diagnosed with blood cultures, ideally two blood samples from the central line and one from a peripheral intravenous. If the culture comes back positive for microbial growth that is not explained by another infectious source (concurrent pneumonia, urinary tract infection, etc.), the diagnosis of CRBSI can be made.

Catheter removal is necessary when a line infection is the presumed cause of severe sepsis, hemodynamic instability, or infective endocarditis. Erythema or purulence around the catheter insertion site, even in the absence of culture confirmation, is an indication to remove a catheter.

In cases of suspected CRBSI, empiric vancomycin and piperacillin–tazobactam are started after blood cultures are drawn. Antibiotics are deescalated based on the results of blood cultures and sensitivities. Blood cultures are also drawn daily until they are cleared and the patient is afebrile.

Catheter salvage may be attempted in select cases. Antimicrobial lock therapy is a method of instilling a high-concentration antibiotics into the catheter lumen and is done in tandem with systemic antibiotics. The patient must not have any purulence or other signs of infection at the exit/tunnel site, otherwise this strategy will not be helpful. Certain microbes including *Staphylococcus aureus* and *Candida* are also a relative contraindication. If cultures remain positive for more than or equal to 72 hours after attempted salvage therapy, the catheter must be removed.

Exchanging catheters over a guidewire at a venous insertion site is a relatively common practice in cases of uncomplicated CRBSI. If the tip of the removed catheter tip shows evidence of phlebitis, thrombus, or purulence, then exchange is inappropriate and a new catheter must be inserted at a different site.

Sometimes a line will malfunction due to a layering of material that accumulates around the catheter. A fibrin sheath can form at the catheter tip, which may impair blood return (common) or cause difficulty flushing (less common). The fibrin sheath acts as a ball valve, which interferes with aspiration. One solution is to infuse tissue plasminogen activator (tPA) into the device, in an attempt to disrupt thrombus at the tip. If this fails, the device can be injected under fluoroscopy, which will often reveal contrast flowing retrograde along the catheter, confirming a fibrin sheath (▶ **Fig. 4.3**). There are three options for fibrin sheath management for tunneled dialysis catheters: (1) catheter exchange, (2) catheter exchange and fibrin sheath maceration with a compliant balloon, or (3) fibrin sheath

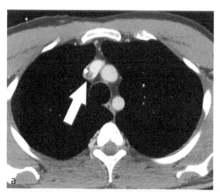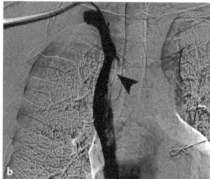

Fig. 4.3 **(a)** Contrast-enhanced CT of the chest showing the catheter tip within the SVC with a surrounding filling defect (*arrow*). **(b)** Contrast was injected and subsequent venogram identifies the filling defect along the catheter tip (*arrowhead*) due to a fibrin sheath.

stripping. Several maneuvers can be performed to strip the fibrin sheath. For example, a snare can be inserted from the groin and the sheath stripped off the catheter from below.

4.2 Enteric Access

Percutaneous enteric access is one of the most common nonvascular procedures performed by IR (**Procedure Box 4.2**). While enteric tubes can also be placed surgically or endoscopically, the use of fluoroscopic-guided techniques is safer and has a high technical success rate.

The most common indication for enteric access is nutritional support for patients unable to have oral intake, which may be the result of neurological insult, swallowing dysfunction, or malignancy. Tube feeds are generally considered whenever there is an expectation that the patient will go more than a week without eating. Another common indication is for decompression of the upper GI tract, which can be helpful for management of ileus or bowel obstruction.

Procedure Box 4.2: Enteric Tube Placement ⓘ

Percutaneous insertion of feeding tubes (gastrostomy and gastrojejunostomy tubes) can be accomplished quickly and with relatively low risk in most patients. Prior to the procedure, history of prior abdominal surgeries should be assessed. Preprocedural CT evaluation is recommended if no recent imaging is available to evaluate the anatomy and identify any intervening structures to be avoided during tube insertion. A fasting period of 6 to 8 hours is necessary for the procedure.

A NG tube is placed and the stomach insufflated with air to bring it in close approximation with the anterior abdominal wall. Intravenous glucagon can be used to close the pylorus and prevent the air from escaping the stomach. Gastropexy using T-fasteners is often performed to fasten the stomach to the anterior abdominal wall, which prevents inadvertent misplacement of the G-tube into the peritoneal cavity. Each T-fastener is inserted into the stomach under fluoroscopic visualization, with the injection of contrast through each needle confirming intraluminal positioning before deploying the fastener.

The most commonly employed method for enteric tube placement in IR is the "push technique." A needle is used to puncture the stomach under fluoroscopic guidance, with definitive position confirmed through the aspiration of gastric air through the needle and opacification of the gastric rugae with contrast injection. A wire is advanced into the stomach or small bowel, depending on the type of tube being placed. The tract is dilated with sequentially larger dilators or a multistep dilator to a size slightly larger than the desired tube diameter, and the tube is then placed through a peel-away introducer. After the tube is advanced into the stomach or small bowel, contrast is injected through each lumen of the catheter under fluoroscopy, confirming appropriate placement. Balloon-retention style tubes require the balloon to be inflated under fluoroscopy to ensure it is positioned with the stomach and not the pylorus or small bowel, which could cause gastric outlet obstruction.

A variation of this technique, known as the "pull method," involves grabbing the percutaneously inserted wire in the stomach using an orally inserted snare. The wire is pulled up and out through the mouth. The gastrostomy tube is connected to wire at this end before being pulled back down through the mouth, into the stomach, and out the anterior abdominal wall. A mushroom type retention piece on the luminal end of the tube keeps it in the stomach, while tension is applied to the outside end of the tube, bringing it snug up again the stomach wall. A bumper slides on over the tube and up against the skin to keep it in place. This method is ideal for patients known to pull on their tubes. The reported technical success rate of percutaneous G-tube placement is greater than 99%.

In most cases, the initial type of access is with a tube passing through the nasal or oral cavity into the stomach (nasogastric/orogastric [NG/OG]) or small intestine (naso-jejunal/orojejunal [NJ/OJ]). These tubes have the advantage of being able to be placed blindly at the bedside, though they have a limited lifespan and are often quite uncomfortable for awake patients. The lumen of these tubes is relatively small, so they typically only last a few weeks before clogging. If access is expected to be short term (i.e., days to weeks), this is a good option for the patient. On the other hand, if it is clear that the patient will need long-term nutritional support, an NG tube may be a temporizing measure until percutaneous access can be obtained. Likewise, an NG tube will usually suffice for decompression in the setting of an ileus or mechanical bowel obstruction. The use of a percutaneous tube for decompression is appropriate when there is a chronic problem such as severe gastroparesis.

Options for percutaneous enteric access include the following:

1. **Gastrostomy** (G-tube): The tube enters the stomach through the abdominal wall and the tip resides within the stomach.
2. **Gastrojejunostomy** (GJ-tube): The tube enters the stomach through the abdominal wall and is advanced so the tip resides within the jejunum.
3. **Jejunostomy** (J-tube) or **cecostomy**: The tube enters the bowel directly through the abdominal wall.

G-tubes are a good option for patients with normal anatomy and normal small bowel motility. GJ-tubes are preferable for those with severe reflux or gastric outlet obstruction, and can be single or double lumen. With a double lumen, the gastric portion can be used to decompress the stomach while the jejunal portion is used for feeding. The advantage of a GJ- over a G-tube is that tip of the tube terminates beyond the ligament of Treitz, minimizing the risk of aspiration. If a patient is having reflux or aspiration with G-tube feeds, the patient can be brought back to convert the tube to a GJ, provided the tract has had time to mature (typically about 1 week, but possibly up to 4). A jejunostomy is an option for patients who have any of the above indications, but have had a prior gastrectomy. Jejunostomy tubes are sometimes also requested in patients who have had a biliary–jejunal anastomosis (e.g., Roux-en-Y gastric bypass or a Whipple procedure) as a means of decompressing a dilated afferent jejunal limb or to provide access to the biliary tree for interventions. Cecostomy tubes are the least common, but may be requested when there is a need for colonic decompression, or sometimes for access to deliver antegrade enemas in patients with chronic constipation.

When reviewing a request for enteric tube placement, it is important to look at any prior imaging. While abdominal radiography may provide some insight, cross-sectional imaging is ideal. For G-tubes, the most important factors to consider are the presence of interposed hepatic parenchyma or colon that could interfere with gastric puncture. This alone is not prohibitive; during the procedure, the stomach is insufflated, which will often have the effect of pushing the liver and colon out of the way, creating a window for access. A decompressive rectal catheter can sometimes help collapse the colon to provide a window. In very challenging cases, rectal contrast can be given at the time of the procedure to delineate the colonic lumen.

Known or suspected gastric tumors, varices, large-volume ascites, and active peptic ulcer disease are all relative contraindications to percutaneous gastrostomy tube placement. Significant bleeding is uncommon, but when it occurs, the culprit is often the superior epigastric artery. Because the superior epigastric runs within the rectus sheath, access lateral to the muscle or along the midline is advised. Smaller gastric arteries along the outer surface of the stomach may also be injured occasionally. Regardless, the procedure is considered moderate risk for bleeding, and as such, uncorrectable coagulopathy is considered an absolute contraindication.

Serious complications from percutaneous gastrostomy tube placement are rare. Peritonitis can occur due to inadvertent infusion of feeding solution into the peritoneal cavity, or if a loop of bowel is perforated during the procedure. It is critical to recognize peritonitis early in these patients. Feeds should be stopped and antibiotics introduced. Pneumoperitoneum more than 48 hours after the procedure is considered indicative of leakage. Other complications include infection of the ostomy, accidental dislodgement, and malfunction of the tube.

Local wound care is important after percutaneous enteric tube placement. Adequate cleansing of the site and regular dressing changes can help prevent cellulitis and unnecessary antibiotic therapy.

After a fresh enteric tube placement, the general rule is to hold gastric feeds for the first 24 hours (the duration may vary by institution). After this, if there are no signs of peritonitis, trickle tube feedings can commence. Residuals are typically measured every 6 hours, while gradually increasing the feeds until the goal rate is reached and tolerated.

Tubes that become dislodged can often be replaced with a tube of the same size at the bedside, provided that a mature tract has formed (typically within 4–6 weeks). Newly placed gastrostomy tubes can have the tract start to close within hours after being pulled out. A common practice is to place a Foley catheter into the gastrostomy as a temporizing measure to keep it from closing up completely. These patients should be brought back to IR to get the tube replaced as soon as possible.

Tube clogging is the most common complication that trainees will encounter, and it is usually due to inappropriate medication delivery through the tube. It can be prevented by ensuring any contents inserted into the tube have been adequately ground. When a tube is clogged, warm water or a high-pressure syringe can often help clear the obstruction. If this does not work, a mixture of pancrelipase, bicarbonate, and 5 mL of water can be injected into the tube to break up the clogged material. A carbonated soft drink into the tube can have the same effect (much cheaper too!).

4.3 Transcatheter Fluid Drainage

Drainage of fluid collections is another common source of referrals (**Procedure Box 4.3**). Upon receiving a consult for a drain placement, the work-up seeks to answer two questions: (1) Is drainage indicated? and (2) is drainage technically feasible?

The cause of most fluid collections can be suspected based on the location in the body, the clinical story, and the imaging characteristics. **Abscesses** most commonly occur in the setting of recent surgery or associated with infection along the bowel. They present nonspecifically with fevers and persistent or uptrending leukocytosis. Pain may or may not be present. Contrast-enhanced CT will identify an abscess as a nonenhancing fluid collection surrounded by an enhancing rim (▶ **Fig. 4.4**). IR will sometimes be asked to drain a hematoma confused for an abscess, however, sterile hematomas should not be drained. If the hematoma becomes infected, management can become quite difficult.

If the imaging and the clinical story are not suggestive of an infected collection, other etiologies are then considered. While large abscesses should be drained, other sterile collections do not necessarily require it.

Percutaneous drainage of fluid collections has almost completely replaced open surgical techniques due to a lower rate of complications and excellent clinical results. For superficial collections, ultrasound is preferred due to the lack of ionizing radiation and the ability to use real-time imaging. For deeper collections or larger patients, CT guidance may be used. Although the shortest route to the target collection is preferred, this is not always possible (e.g., due to intervening bowel loops or other structures).

Once the imaging modality is chosen, the next step is to position the patient and identify the length and course required for needle puncture. An appropriate needle length is selected and inserted under ultrasound or CT guidance until it is within the collection. Aspiration of a small sample of the fluid is performed to confirm positioning and assess viscosity.

If drain placement is deemed necessary, the drain caliber is tailored to the type of collection being drained. Smaller bore size catheters (8 Fr) are sufficient to drain serous or serosanguinous fluids, but a larger bore size catheter (10 Fr or larger) is often needed for purulent or more viscous fluids. Side-hole locations should also be considered. Biliary drainage catheters can be used in certain locations, such as when there is a long, longitudinally oriented collection (such as subphrenic location).

For loculated fluid collections, a longer needle may be utilized to gain access deep into the collection and facilitate disruption of the loculations using the needle or a wire. Either the trocar or the Seldinger technique is used. A stiff guidewire can prevent kinking and ensures that the catheter doesn't stray in its course to the target. Always visualize the wire coiled in the collection before attempting to advance the drain.

A series of sequentially larger-gauge dilators are used to dilate the tract (ideally up to 1-Fr size larger than the intended drain) and the catheter is then placed and coiled within the collection.

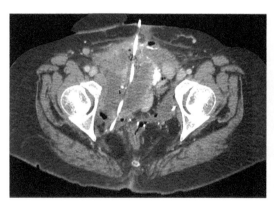

Fig. 4.4 A postoperative patient developed an intra-abdominal abscess requiring placement of a drainage catheter. The abscess was elongated and complex, so a biliary drainage catheter was inserted to account for the shape and allow for adequate drainage along the length of the abscess.

When drainage of a collection is indicated, the interventionalist must then determine whether it is technically possible or not. Technical feasibility requires a safe trajectory from the skin to the collection, without intervening bowel loops or neurovascular structures, as well as an adequate sized collection. Small collections are not amenable to drain placement because pigtail loops cannot form in collections less than 3 cm. Aspiration is an option for small collections if a fluid sample is requested, but it is your responsibility to let the referring service know that a drain will not be left in place.

Superficial collections can be drained with ultrasound guidance, while deeper collections are most commonly approached with CT guidance. Once placed, these drains should ideally be followed by IR to ensure adequate drain function and patency. IR should also be involved in deciding when the drain can be removed.

Drain output should be monitored daily. When drainage decreases to less than 10 to 15 mL/d, the tube should be checked for patency using a saline flush; if the tube can be flushed and the contents aspirated are of similar volume to the amount instilled, the drain can be removed, provided there has also been a clinical response. For tubes that cannot be flushed, or in those for which the volume aspirated is significantly less than the amount instilled during flushing, this suggests obstruction or malposition of the tube. In these cases, reassessment of the collection using cross-sectional imaging or a fluoroscopic drain injection should be performed prior to removal.

Intrathoracic Fluid Collections

The most common type of fluid collection in the chest is a **pleural effusion**, which may be the result of pneumonia, congestive heart failure (CHF), malignancy, or a number of other inciting processes. When a patient has a clinically significant pleural effusion (i.e., patient is hypoxemic, requiring increasing oxygen, or persistently febrile despite antibiotics), the first step is to determine if the effusion is transudative or exudative using Light's criteria. A diagnostic thoracentesis can be done to obtain pleural fluid for laboratory studies. While IR can easily perform this procedure, it is typically simple enough for the clinical service to do at the bedside with ultrasound guidance.

IR is more likely to become involved in the setting of an exudative effusion that requires drainage *or* if there is a large transudative effusion requiring long-term drainage. Most transudative effusions are amenable to percutaneous drainage with a pigtail catheter or a tunneled catheter, such as a PleurX (Becton, Dickinson and Company, Franklin Lakes, NJ).

Inpatients with pleural drains should be followed daily. Changes in the amount of pleural fluid can be monitored with both chest X-ray and measurements of the drain output. In the best case scenario, the effusion will resolve radiographically and the patient will improve clinically. At this point, the drain can be removed. When removing pleural tubes, the hole should be covered with an occlusive dressing (Vaseline gauze covering the hole, 4 × 4s and silk tape) to avoid a pneumothorax.

The situation is not always that simple, however. Exudative effusions can pose several challenges. Parapneumonic effusions that are severe enough to warrant a referral to IR have the tendency to become loculated, which can make percutaneous drainage difficult. If not treated appropriately, exudative effusions can become encased by a fibrinous rind. At that point, percutaneous drainage may be impossible.

For loculated effusions, a mixture of tPA and DNase can be instilled through the pigtail drain to attempt to break up the loculations. This process is repeated twice a day, sometimes for a few days. IR staff may be in charge of this, but in some hospitals it is the pulmonary consult or another service that handles the injections and determines when to stop. Successful lysis of the loculations will increase the drain output and show improvement of the chest X-ray appearance. If it is not successful and a rind forms around the effusion, the patient will need surgical decortication and drainage via a video-assisted thoracoscopy.

It would be helpful for you to have an understanding of how a Pleur-Evac device (Teleflex Medical, Morrisville, NC) works and what information it can provide. Rounding on patients with pleural drains usually boils down to what the Pleur-Evac is telling you.

PleurX catheters are long-term, tunneled pleural drains intended for patients with malignant effusions. The tendency is for these effusions to rapidly recur if a temporary drain is used and removed. These long-term catheters optimize patient comfort by allowing the patient to go home with a capped drain in place. Patients will drain the fluid themselves at regular intervals, either dictated by the speed of fluid recovery or the redevelopment of symptoms. Some patients will require home health visits, during which a nurse can periodically uncap the catheter and drain the pleural fluid.

Although less common, trauma to the thoracic duct can result in **chylothorax**, which is usually iatrogenic in the setting of cardiothoracic surgery. Chylothorax is usually detected after a thoracic surgery when the indwelling chest tubes start draining milky white fluid. A fluid chemistry and positive finding for chylomicrons in the fluid is typically confirmatory.

Management of chylothorax is initially conservative, as many thoracic duct leaks close spontaneously. The patient can be put on a low-fat diet with medium-chain triglycerides. If the chyle output exceeds 1 L/d despite conservative management, interventional or surgical treatment is warranted. Surgery for chylothorax is a thoracic duct ligation. IR can perform a less-invasive **thoracic duct embolization** (TDE).

TDE begins with lymphangiography. Small needles are inserted into lymph nodes in each groin and lipiodol slowly injected, opacifying the pelvic lymphatics. Spot images are obtained serially until the cisterna chyli (dilated sac at the caudal end of the thoracic duct) is opacified. While the viscosity and mild sclerosant effect of lipiodol may close the leak itself, typically percutaneous access into the cisterna is attempted using a needle. A microcatheter can then be inserted into the thoracic duct to attempt to identify a specific site of leakage. Even if none is identified, the thoracic duct may be occluded using coils and liquid embolic material. Additional advanced techniques exist, including those for retrograde access from the venous drainage end of the thoracic duct, and for treatment of lymphatic leakage involving other areas, including the peritoneal cavity. Those who have persistent chyle leakage may require surgery.

Intra-abdominal Fluid Collections

Abscesses are the most common intra-abdominal collection and usually form in the postoperative setting or in association with an intra-abdominal infection. Abscesses can form practically anywhere in the abdomen.

Pyogenic liver abscesses form when an intra-abdominal infection (diverticulitis, appendicitis, etc.) results in localized thrombophlebitis, which can lead to septic emboli passing into the portal venous system and seeding the liver.

Patients typically present with fevers, leukocytosis, and upper abdominal pain, which usually prompts a CT study. In addition to starting antibiotics, pyogenic liver abscesses should be drained percutaneously if possible. The ideal percutaneous course into a hepatic abscess should avoid traversal of any large central vessels, as seeding of the systemic circulation can occur if large vessels are violated. The abscess should also be entered via normal liver to avoid leakage.

A perihepatic collection that may be confused for an abscess is a **biloma**. A biloma is a collection of bile outside the biliary tree and can be intra- or extrahepatic. Bilomas form after either iatrogenic or traumatic biliary tree injury. Iatrogenic injury may occur during hepatobiliary surgery, a transcatheter arterial chemoembolization (TACE), percutaneous biliary drainage, or an endoscopic retrograde cholangiopancreatography (ERCP). Bilomas usually cause no symptoms but have the potential to lead to chemical peritonitis.

Asymptomatic bilomas may be detected on routine CT scans, usually suspected based on their location, lower attenuation appearance, and the clinical history.

Bilomas should be drained. Percutaneous drainage is a good option since most of these collections are readily accessible under ultrasound or CT guidance. If there is an associated biliary tree injury, this will also need to be managed (discussed in Chapter 6).

Splenic abscesses are relatively uncommon, but can be seen in immunosuppressed patients and intravenous drug users. The infection usually originates elsewhere and travels to the spleen hematogenously. Infection can also occur after trauma or splenic infarction. A number of splenic lesions can mimic abscesses, so it's important to ensure that the history fits, and additional imaging is obtained if necessary. Treatment with antibiotics and percutaneous drainage can be successful, but splenectomy may be indicated for some patients, especially for multifocal abscesses.

Most **perienteric abscesses** occur after perforated diverticulitis or appendicitis. These patients may require definitive surgery with a sigmoid colectomy/appendectomy, however early drainage of the abscess often leads to safer and more successful surgery. Patients with Crohn's disease are another group that is prone to the development of intra-abdominal abscesses.

Fluid collections in the pancreas are usually associated with sequelae of pancreatitis, and may be either sterile or infected. **Pancreatic pseudocysts** are walled-off collections of amylase/pancreatic juices surrounded by a rim of fibrous/granulation tissue. They usually form weeks after a bout of acute pancreatitis. Many pseudocysts cause no symptoms and are only detected on routine follow-up imaging after episodes of pancreatitis. Usually pseudocysts resolve on their own, but may become problematic due to mass effect or superimposed infection.

A pseudocyst in a patient who has no clinical signs of an infection should be left alone, as percutaneous access can introduce bacteria into the collection and result in a previously sterile pseudocyst becoming infected. If, however, there is a high likelihood that the pseudocyst is already infected, drainage is indicated. While some pancreatic collections are accessed endoscopically (i.e., cyst-gastrostomy), percutaneous drainage is a reasonable approach in many cases. Pancreatic collections often drain copiously, and patients should be counseled that long-term drainage is the norm for this condition. The possibility of permanent drain placement should be raised. Fluid from infected pseudocysts should be sent for amylase and lipase, in addition to culture, to confirm the diagnosis.

Pancreatic necrosis is a very serious complication of pancreatitis and can usually be diagnosed by CT. These patients are very sick with significant lab abnormalities. Like pseudocysts, sterile necrotic collections should be left alone (▶**Fig. 4.5**). If an infected collection is suspected, IR may be asked to perform a percutaneous aspiration to obtain a sample for culture. A concern many clinicians have is that the percutaneous

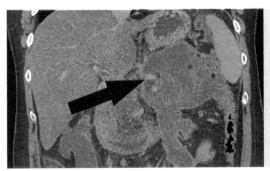

Fig. 4.5 Acute pancreatitis in this patient resulted in a large walled-off peripancreatic necrotic collection (*arrow*). The collection tracks inferiorly into the lower abdomen. This was a sterile collection and did not require drainage.

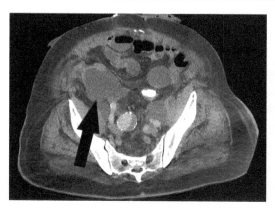

Fig. 4.6 This patient developed a urinoma following a cystoprostatectomy for bladder cancer. A fluid collection can be seen in the right lower quadrant where the ureter inserts into the ileal conduit.

pancreatic necrosis sampling will inadvertently introduce bacteria into a previously sterile collection and cause an infection. Therefore, strict sterile technique is particularly important when performing these cases.

Infected necrotic collections should be evacuated. While open necrosectomy was performed in the past, endoscopic cyst gastrostomy and necrosectomy are now favored. IR's role in necrosectomies is limited, though there may be some occasions where we're asked to provide percutaneous access to the collection. After access creation, the tract is dilated so that a laparoscope can be inserted into the collection, and the necrotic debris removed.

Urinomas are found most commonly after iatrogenic injury to the collecting system, which allows urine to leak from the defect and form a discrete collection (▶ **Fig. 4.6**). Patients with urinomas are often asymptomatic, with the collection discovered only incidentally on cross-sectional imaging. Some patients can become symptomatic secondary to pain, mass effect, or infection.

Small sterile urinomas can be managed conservatively, while larger collections more often require intervention. The first and most critical step is urinary diversion with a nephrostomy tube. The drain allows the urothelium to heal. Sometimes urinary diversion is sufficient to deal with the urinoma. In other cases, when it is causing symptoms or appears to be infected, percutaneous drainage is indicated and generally straightforward. Samples should be sent for a creatinine level and culture.

Rarely, urinary diversion and drainage are insufficient to address the problem. In these cases, surgical repair may be considered for those patients who are candidates. Ureteral embolization can also be considered to permanently occlude the ureter. This is usually reserved for terminal patients who have a short life expectancy.

Pelvic Fluid Collections

The most common infections within the abdominal cavity may also lead to abscess formation in the pelvis. Ruptured diverticulitis or appendicitis can result in infection spreading into the pouch of Douglas in females or rectovesical pouch in males, which is the most dependent portion of the peritoneal cavity.

In general, percutaneous access to deep pelvic abscesses can be very difficult due to the bony pelvic girdle. Alternative approaches include transgluteal, transrectal, and transvaginal access. Transgluteal access should be performed with caution to avoid hitting the sciatic nerve. The needle path should course as close to the sacrum/coccyx as possible, and should stay clear of the ischial tuberosity. Traversing the piriformis muscle is particularly painful for patients, so this should be avoided as well if possible. Transrectal and transvaginal access is ideal for abscesses in the pelvic cul-de-sac, and is relatively straightforward with appropriate equipment.

Tubo-ovarian abscesses (TOAs) can form as a complication of pelvic inflammatory disease. The predominant symptoms are pelvic pain and vaginal discharge, though fever and leukocytosis are also common. When a TOA ruptures, the patient will have peritoneal signs on abdominal examination and can rapidly develop sepsis. In most cases, TOA is suspected when a patient with pelvic inflammatory disease fails to respond to antibiotics. These patients will get a transvaginal ultrasound, which in the case of a TOA will show a multilocated collection that obscures the normal adnexal anatomy. CT is more commonly ordered when abdominal pathology is on the differential.

Findings of a ruptured TOA are an indication for urgent surgical management. For unruptured TOA, antibiotic therapy alone is usually sufficient as long as the patient is hemodynamically stable and the abscess is relatively small. Large abscesses and those patients who fail initial antibiotic therapy are candidates for transcatheter drainage.

Prostatic abscesses are a relatively rare complication of bacterial prostatitis, and are most often seen in immunocompromised and diabetic patients. The presentation is similar to that of acute prostatitis; patients will have perineal or suprapubic pain, dysuria, fever, and chills. Treatment for acute bacterial prostatitis with antibiotics is usually successful. Those who do not improve should be suspected to have a prostatic abscess and warrant evaluation with a transrectal ultrasound (TRUS). A TRUS will readily identify a complex collection within the prostate.

Prostatic abscesses can be drained from a transrectal or perineal approach. Instrumentation of the urethra increases the risk of bacterial translocation into the bloodstream and is avoided if possible.

Suggested Readings

[1]   Mermel LA, Allon M, Bouza E, et al. Clinical practice guidelines for the diagnosis and management of intravascular catheter-related infection: 2009 update by the Infectious Diseases Society of America. Clin Infect Dis. 2009; 49(1):1–45

[2]   National Healthcare Safety Network. Bloodstream Infection Event (Central Line-Associated Bloodstream Infection and Non-Central Line-Associated Bloodstream Infection). http://www.cdc.gov/nhsn/PDFs/pscManual/4PSC_CLABScurrent.pdf; access date: 8/14/2017

5 Emergency IR

Matthew Evan Krosin, L. C. Alexander Skidmore, and Rakesh Navuluri

Management of bleeds accounts for the vast majority of IR emergencies. Bleeding can occur essentially anywhere in the body, including the GI tract, solid abdominal organs, retroperitoneum, and superficial soft tissues. Embolization is a minimally invasive and versatile tool for addressing hemorrhage in emergencies.

5.1 Massive Hemoptysis

Hemoptysis ranges in severity from blood-tinged sputum to gross hemorrhage. Massive hemoptysis can be life threatening, usually as a result of asphyxia rather than hemorrhagic shock. Massive hemoptysis is defined as greater than 500 mL of blood coughed up in a 24-hour span or a rate of 100 mL/h. Most cases of hemoptysis originate from the bronchial arteries, though it can also, rarely, originate from the lower-pressure pulmonary arterial system (▶ **Fig. 5.1**).

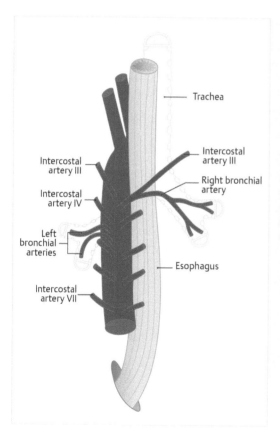

Fig. 5.1 Posterior view of the thoracic aorta showing the most common bronchial artery anatomy, with a single right bronchial artery arising from the intercostobronchial trunk, and two left bronchial arteries arising directly from the aorta. Origins are typically between T3 and T5. (Source: 6 Bronchial Arteries (Rami Bronchiales). In: Wacker F, Lippert H, Pabst R, eds. Arterial Variations in Humans: Key Reference for Radiologists and Surgeons. 1st Edition. Thieme; 2017.)

Approach to Massive Hemoptysis

When a patient presents with suspected hemoptysis, one of the first steps is deciding whether it is true hemoptysis or if the source of bleeding originates from the oropharynx or GI tract (▶ **Fig. 5.2**). Physical examination alone does not usually allow differentiation between hemoptysis and hematemesis, but bleeding from the oropharynx or nasal passages may be more obvious. Consideration of patient risk factors including history of smoking, cystic fibrosis (CF), or vasculitis can help sway your suspicion toward hemoptysis when the diagnosis is uncertain.

If the bleeding is thought to be hemoptysis, the underlying cause and laterality are then determined. The most common causes of hemoptysis include infections, lung malignancies, and diseases associated with bronchiectasis such as CF.

An initial chest X-ray may help in localizing the bleed to either the right or left lung, but the majority of these patients will undergo a chest CT as well. Neoplasms, cavitary lesions, pulmonary infarcts, and bronchiectasis may be evident on CT.

Bronchoscopy is usually performed following patient stabilization. The minimum goal is to establish which lung (and possibly which lobe) is bleeding. If the laterality is determined, the patient should be positioned lying with the affected lung down. This prevents blood from spilling into the contralateral lung. Although not essential, CTA can help confirm the source of the bleed, and should be considered on a case-by-case basis, either before or after bronchoscopy. In addition to active bleeding, CTA can identify the number and location of the bronchial arteries and any variant arterial anatomy, which is useful information to have when evaluating for an intervention.

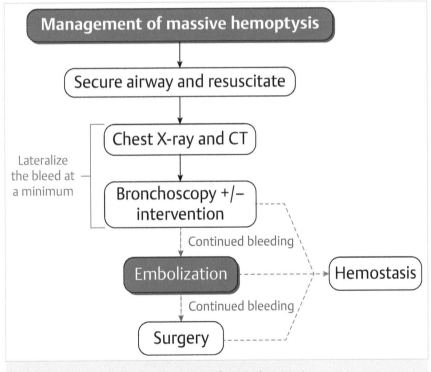

Fig. 5.2 Simplified algorithm for management of massive hemoptysis.

Management of Hemoptysis

Prior to any diagnostics or intervention, patients with massive hemoptysis require fluid resuscitation. Intubation is often required to protect the airway.

As many cases of hemorrhage occur peripherally in the lung, bronchoscopy is primarily a diagnostic procedure, though some bronchoscopic treatments exist. Interventions include laser coagulation, electrocautery, and local hemostatic agents (e.g., epinephrine, thrombin, etc.). In the case of unilateral hemorrhage, a bronchial blocker is sometimes used by the bronchoscopist as a temporizing measure. This involves inflating a balloon within a bronchus of the bleeding lung to prevent spillage of blood into the unaffected airways.

Conventional angiography with embolization has become first-line therapy for severe cases of hemoptysis, since bronchoscopy has limited therapeutic potential, and emergent intrathoracic surgery is associated with high perioperative mortality (**Procedure Box 5.1, Procedure Box 5.2**). Surgery (wedge resection/lobectomy/pneumonectomy) is reserved for patients who fail more conservative options.

Patients treated with bronchial artery embolization are monitored closely in a critical care setting. Extubation should be considered only when the risk of rebleeding is low. Trending hemoglobin is not that useful, as small-volume hemorrhages can still cause asphyxia without a significant effect on the hematocrit values. In cases where an underlying diagnosis remains elusive, bronchoscopy is often repeated after embolization to better evaluate the airways. Rebleeding is not an uncommon problem, particularly in CF patients.

Procedure Box 5.1: Bronchial Artery Embolization

A bronchial angiogram involves catheterizing the bronchial artery origins; these are usually found in the midthoracic aorta, near the mainstem bronchi. On all bronchial arteriograms, careful and deliberate attention should be paid to identify any medullary arteries communicating with the anterior spinal artery, particularly the **artery of Adamkiewicz** (great anterior radiculomedullary artery), which typically arises from an intercostal artery between T9 and T12 and provides the largest supply to the anterior spinal cord. Medullary arteries demonstrate a characteristic pattern, with an upward course followed by a hairpin loop prior to entering the anterior spinal artery. Inadvertent embolization of a spinal artery may result in severe neurological deficits, including paraplegia. Bronchial arteries with a large spinal branch can be treated, but a microcatheter needs to be positioned beyond this branch, with meticulous attention to avoid reflux.

In patients with necrotizing pneumonia or bronchiectasis due to CF, collateral arteries may grow toward the site of insult to perfuse and repair. These novel collaterals may arise from multiple systemic arteries, including the internal mammary, thyrocervical, intercostal, lateral thoracic, and phrenic arteries. These "parasitized arteries" are prone to hemorrhage. Evaluation of a preangiogram CTA can be useful to identify parasitized arteries which may require angiographic interrogation and possible embolization.

Angiographic findings such as abnormally tortuous or hypertrophied vessels, hypervascular lung parenchyma, pseudoaneurysms, or contrast extravasation into airways all indicate sources of hemoptysis. Particles used for embolization are typically 500 to 700 µm in size (larger than most spinal arteries) and are considered front-line embolic agents for hemoptysis. Particles embolize distally within the targeted arterial tree, wedging in the small arteries associated with the underlying tumor, infection, etc. Use of particles allows for repeat intervention should hemoptysis recur. Coils are less desirable since reintervention in the same vessel beyond a deployed coil may be difficult or impossible.

Procedure Box 5.2: Pulmonary Artery Embolization ⓘ

The indications, technique, and potential complications of pulmonary artery embolization vary considerably compared to those of bronchial artery embolization. In pulmonary artery embolization, the common femoral vein is accessed and the pulmonary outflow tract is selected with a special curved pigtail catheter, such as a Van Aman or Grollman. Once the right or left pulmonary artery is selected, pulmonary angiography is performed. Most frequently, the target for pulmonary artery embolization is a pulmonary arteriovenous malformations (AVM). Pulmonary artery pseudoaneurysms may also be implicated, particularly in the setting of previous Swan–Ganz catheter placement or mycobacterial infection.

In contrast to bronchial artery embolization, coils and vascular plugs are the preferred embolic agents for pulmonary artery embolizations. Pulmonary AVMs create right to left shunts by bypassing the intervening pulmonary alveolar capillary network. If particles or glue are deployed into an AVM, these agents are small enough to pass directly into the pulmonary venous outflow due to the lack of intervening capillaries. Nontarget embolization in the systemic circulation can cause devastating complications such as stroke, visceral infarction, and limb ischemia. Embolic agents should be carefully selected for embolization of AVMs in order to prevent migration through the malformation into the pulmonary veins.

Surgery plays an adjunctive role for certain patients after embolization. If the cause of the hemoptysis is due to a mass lesion or mycetoma, wedge resection and lobectomy are viable options, provided the patient is a surgical candidate. When recurrent hemoptysis is due to diffuse pulmonary disease (CF, sarcoidosis, vasculitis), lung transplant remains an option of last resort.

5.2 Upper GI Bleeding

Bleeding from the GI tract proximal to the ligament of Treitz is considered upper GI bleeding (UGIB), whereas bleeding distal to it is considered lower GI bleeding (LGIB). Although UGIB can result in serious hospitalizations, they are less frequently encountered by the IR. Upper endoscopy (EGD) is usually successful in managing UGIB. Endovascular intervention is, however, an important tool for *refractory* UGIB.

Both arterial and venous forms of UGIB can occur; the latter typically a consequence of gastroesophageal varices (discussed separately in Chapter 6).

Peptic ulcers are the most common cause of UGIB. Bleeding occurs when ulcers penetrate beyond the mucosa into the submucosa, causing inflammation, necrosis, and eventual rupture of an artery. *Helicobacter pylori* infection, NSAID use, and hemorrhagic gastritis are also common culprits. Other causes of UGIB are listed in ▶ **Table 5.1**.

Table 5.1 Arterial causes of upper GI bleeding

• Peptic ulcers (gastric or duodenal)	• Gastric cancer
• Mallory–Weiss tear	• Angiodysplasia
• Gastritis/duodenitis/esophagitis	• Hemobilia (iatrogenic)
• Dieulafoy's lesion	• Aortoduodenal fistula

Work-up of an UGIB

Hematemesis and/or melena are the most common presenting symptoms of UGIB. Hematochezia is more likely to come from a lower GI bleed, but can be seen due to a bleed from above with rapid transit through the GI tract. Patients with these brisk bleeds are more likely to be hemodynamically unstable and require emergent intervention. If the presence of UGIB is uncertain, gastric fluid can be lavaged via nasogastric (NG) tube and tested on a stool guaiac strip, although this will miss bleeding that occurs within the proximal duodenum.

Certain clues can help direct the clinician toward a cause of the bleed. Peptic ulcers cause epigastric pain and early satiety, and may present with a history of NSAID use or prior ulcer disease. Mallory–Weiss tears should be suspected when nonbloody emesis precedes hematemesis in an alcoholic patient. Hemorrhagic gastritis produces coffee-ground hematemesis, usually in an ICU patient or someone with a history of chronic steroid use.

Hypotension and hemodynamic shock are imminent threats to life in cases of GI bleeding. Medical management to support blood pressure should always take priority over further diagnostic work-up (▶ **Fig. 5.3**).

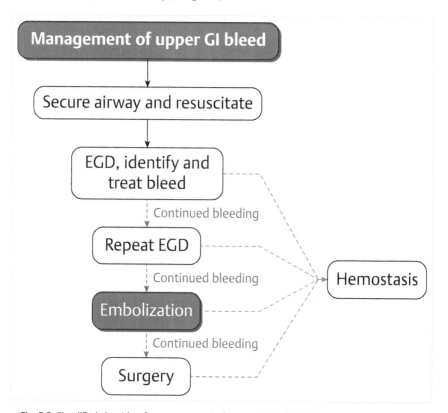

Fig. 5.3 Simplified algorithm for management of upper GI bleeds. EGD, esophagogastroduodenoscopy.

Almost all patients with UGIB initially go to endoscopy due to its ability to localize bleeding and provide rapid targeted therapy. Options for therapy during endoscopy include clipping, banding, thermocoagulation, and vasoconstrictor/sclerosant injection. Clip placement, even when unable to stop a bleed, can serve as a radiopaque marker useful for localization during subsequent angiography. The source of the bleed can sometimes go unidentified, and rebleeding after treatment occurs in nearly a quarter of the patients after endoscopic intervention. Despite this, almost all patients who rebleed should undergo repeat EGD prior to an attempt at endovascular intervention. The exception is hepatobiliary bleeding, since it is outside the reach of endoscopy.

If endoscopy fails to reveal a source of the bleeding, CTA can be performed for localization. CTA offers high-resolution, cross-sectional imaging of the GI tract and its arterial supply. It also has a high sensitivity, detecting bleeds as slow as 0.3 mL/min (compared to 0.5 mL/min by conventional angiography). Hyperdense contrast material that layers within the bowel lumen on arterial phase and increases on delayed phase is indicative of active bleeding. Radionuclide scintigraphy, also known as a tagged red blood cell (RBC) scan, is rarely used in cases of UGIB. Both CTA and scintigraphy are less commonly used for diagnosis of a suspected UGIB, since endoscopy is usually effective at identifying a source.

Management of UGIBs

The airway should always be secured and hemodynamics controlled before taking a patient to endoscopy or angiography for intervention.

In preparation for endoscopy, the patient should be made NPO and placed on an intravenous proton pump inhibitor (PPI), such as pantoprazole. PPIs promote clot formation within the GI tract and reduce rates of rebleeding.

Endoscopic tools may achieve hemostasis by physical, chemical, or thermal means. Physical occlusion of a vessel is performed using metallic clips or rubber bands. Chemical injection of vasoconstrictors, such as epinephrine, are typically more effective when used in conjunction with other therapies. Thermocoagulation works similar to electrocautery.

Patients with UGIB present to IR either because attempts at endoscopic hemostasis have failed, or because the patient is too unstable for evaluation by endoscopy. Cases of suspected or known hemobilia will often proceed directly to endovascular intervention as well. Many IRs prefer for the patient to have a CTA prior to the procedure. It doesn't always identify the location of the bleed, but when it does, the embolization procedure has a much greater chance of being successful. Embolization of UGIBs generally have a high success rate, and can be repeated if the initial study is negative or in cases of rebleeding. (**Procedure Box 5.3**).

Surgery is reserved for those who have failed both endoscopic and endovascular management. Roughly a quarter of UGIB cases that are treated by IR will go on to eventually require surgery. The operative procedure depends on the cause of UGIB, and ranges from ligation of bleeding arteries to resection of a portion of the stomach or duodenum. Patients with uncontrolled hemobilia may undergo liver resection in extreme cases.

After obtaining femoral or radial artery access, selective catheterization of the celiac artery is generally the first step. The key branches to the stomach include the left and right gastric and right gastroepiploic arteries (▶ **Fig. 5.4**). Additionally, a key branch supplying the duodenum is the gastroduodenal artery (GDA), which usually arises from the common hepatic artery and gives off the superior pancreaticoduodenal artery (PDA).

After evaluation of the celiac axis, the superior mesenteric artery (SMA) is then investigated. Its key branch to the proximal small bowel is the inferior PDA. The superior and inferior PDAs form the pancreaticoduodenal arcade, which allows for collateral flow between the celiac and SMA. This is a useful redundancy in case of an occlusion, but can cause problems with recurrent bleeding after embolization. Bleeding that continues following embolization as a result of one of these collaterals is often referred to as a "back door" bleed. Understanding the vascular anatomy in this region is essential in planning an embolization.

The direct angiographic sign of active UGIB is contrast extravasation and pooling within the stomach or proximal bowel (▶ **Fig. 5.5**). Indirect signs suggesting a vascular abnormality include pseudoaneurysm, vessel spasm, or early filling of the venous outflow. A contrast "blush" or area of unexpected hypervascularity could represent an inflammatory process or neoplasm as the underlying cause.

Once a bleed is identified, the goal is to selectively decrease perfusion to the site of arterial injury via embolization, allowing for thrombosis or endogenous vessel repair to occur. Coils, Gelfoam, glue, and particles can all be used to treat UGIB. Coils are used most commonly because they are inexpensive and can be deployed with precision. Bleeds arising from a well-developed collateral pathway require coil embolization proximal *and* distal to the injury. Particles may be used if the bleed originates from an inaccessible distal branch, or if a bleeding tumor needs to be devascularized. In general, permanent embolic agents can be used with minimal concern for gut ischemia when treating UGIBs due to the excellent collateral blood supply. Gelfoam, as a more temporary agent, is often used in combination with coils, but rarely in isolation. It degrades over time, which allows vessels to recanalize within weeks. The risk of bowel ischemia and nontarget embolization are higher when using particles and glue, often when patients have diminished collateral blood flow as a result of prior surgery.

In some cases, empiric embolization of a gastric artery or the GDA may be considered if the angiogram is negative, but a clear source of bleeding was localized to the territories supplied by those arteries on endoscopy.

5.3 Lower GI Bleeding

As with UGIBs, LGIBs can come from both arterial and venous sources. Venous bleeding is usually associated with mesenteric variceal hemorrhage or hemorrhoids. This distinction is important whenever fielding a LGIB consult, as the interventions IR offers for venous hemorrhage is decidedly different often more limited. This section will focus on arterial causes of LGIB.

LGIB can be subdivided into those arising from small intestine and those arising from colon or rectum. Bleeding from the small intestine is often more complex to manage, given the wider variety of contributing pathologies and the anatomy that is often inaccessible by endoscopy.

AVMs, malignancies, diverticuli, ulcers, trauma, and forms of enteritis such as Crohn's disease can all be responsible for a small bowel LGIB (▶ **Fig. 5.6**). Bleeding from

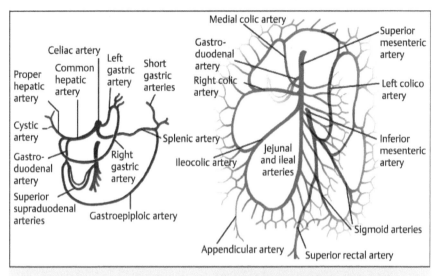

Fig. 5.4 Diagram of the arterial supply to the visceral organs and relationship to adjacent structures. Key branches include the left gastric, right gastric, left gastroepiploic, and right gastroepiploic arteries.

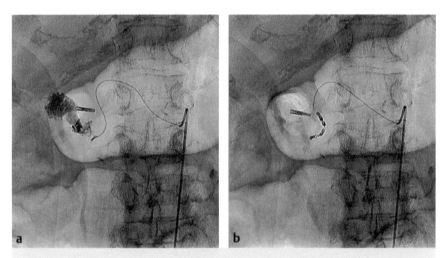

Fig. 5.5 (a) A catheter is parked in the celiac axis with a microcatheter in the gastroduodenal artery (GDA). An angiogram demonstrates active contrast extravasation from the GDA. (b) Coil embolization was performed.

the large intestine occurs most commonly due to diverticuli and angiodysplasia (tiny, usually age-related AVMs). Less common causes include tumors, colitis, and recent interventions (e.g., polypectomy) (▶Table 5.2).

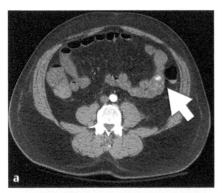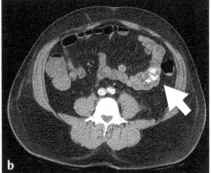

Fig. 5.6 **(a)** Multiphasic CT demonstrates arterial phase contrast pooling within the lumen of the midjejunum. **(b)** Additional contrast is seen pooling on venous phase imaging, indicating active extravasation. The bleeding was due to a jejunal arteriovenous malformation. (These images are provided courtesy of Matthew Evan Krosin, MD, University of Pittsburgh Medical Center.)

Table 5.2 Arterial causes of lower GI bleeding

Small intestine (jejunum and ileum)	Large intestine (colon and rectum)
• Enteritis	• Diverticuli
• Ulcer	• Angiodysplasia
• Tumor	• Tumor
• Arteriovenous malformation (AVM)	• Colitis
• Trauma	• Postprocedural (polypectomy, biopsy)
• Diverticulum (less common)	
• Aortoenteric fistula (rare)	

Work-up of a Lower GI Bleeding

Hematochezia is the typical presentation of a LGIB, though it can also be seen with a brisk UGIB. Melena is uncommon in LGIB, as bleeding distal to the ligament of Treitz does not mix with the gastric and pancreatic juices that cause oxidation and darkening of the blood. However, melena *can* be seen with a proximal LGIB or when there is exceptionally slow transit time.

As with UGIBs, resuscitation should be carried out simultaneously with the initial work-up for a LGIB. A colonoscopy is almost always indicated, but the timing depends on the urgency of the case (▶ **Fig. 5.7**). Patients who are stable after resuscitation are generally admitted and given a bowel prep prior to colonoscopy. Hemodynamic instability and ongoing bleeding may require only an abbreviated prep, and many endoscopists are hesitant to perform the procedure without a prep. LGIB patients are generally more stable than UGIB patients; severe hematochezia and instability should arouse suspicion for an UGIB. These patients get an EGD or NG tube aspiration to rule out a bleed from above prior to colonoscopy.

Colonoscopy does not always successfully identify a source of hemorrhage due to technical difficulty and/or the presence of stool in a suboptimally prepped colon. When endoscopy is unsuccessful and the patient is hemodynamically stable, a CTA may be done to help localize the bleed. CTA can determine bleeding location, underlying pathology, and vascular anatomy.

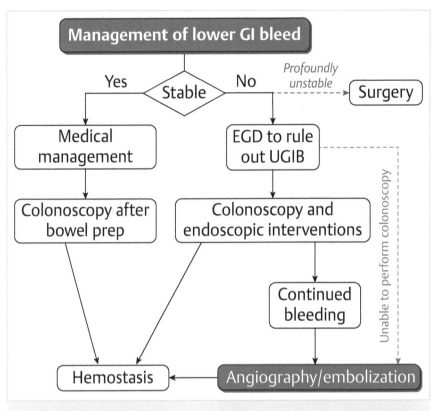

Fig. 5.7 Simplified algorithm for management of lower GI bleeds. EGD, esophagogastroduode-noscopy; UGIB, upper GI bleed.

Radionuclide scintigraphy (tagged RBC scan) is another diagnostic tool available for LGIB. It is the most sensitive, detecting bleeds as slow as 0.1 mL/min. The study involves labeling the patient's own red blood cells with the radiotracer technetium-99m. The radiolabeled cells are injected back into the bloodstream, and the patient is placed under a gamma camera. Images are then acquired every few minutes for about 30 to 90 minutes. Newly appearing radiotracer moving into the bowel indicates a site of active bleeding. This study has longer prep time, lower resolution, and lack of cross-sectional localization. Thet advantages over CTA are increased sensitivity and avoidance of iodinated contrast.

SPECT-CT is a hybrid study, producing cross-sectional CT images that show the three-dimensional position of the radiotracer with greater resolution. It offers the best sensitivity of all of the GIB imaging studies. Drawbacks include its limited availability at smaller institutions, and inability to distinguish arterial from venous bleeding.

Management of Lower GI Bleedings

Acute LGIBs will stop spontaneously in many patients, highlighting the importance of appropriate medical management. Hemodynamic monitoring and fluid resuscitation are initial priorities.

Compared to UGIB patients, LGIB patients have higher hemoglobin levels, need fewer transfusions, and are less likely to decompensate. That being said, the cases seen by IR are more likely to be severe and should be approached with caution.

The advantage of colonoscopy as a first-line test is that it can be both diagnostic and therapeutic. Active bleeding and a visible nonbleeding vessel are indications for treatment. Clips, argon plasma or thermal coagulation, and epinephrine are therapies available for use during colonoscopy. Whether spontaneous or through intervention, bleeding will cease in the majority of cases. However, rebleeding does occur in a minority of patients, not infrequently during the same admission. The guidelines are not yet clear on the best strategy for management of early rebleeding, but if the patient is stable, it is reasonable to perform another colonoscopy, especially when the bowel has already been prepped.

At most institutions, colonoscopy is considered the preferred initial diagnostic and therapeutic option. More aggressive measures are appropriate if the patient is too unstable for colonoscopy. If there are significant resuscitation needs and even an expedited bowel prep cannot be completed, a surgical consultation is usually indicated. If not already done, an UGIB needs to be ruled out.

Surgical management for unstable LGIB is typically accomplished with bowel resection. The data are relatively sparse, but some studies have shown higher mortality associated with surgical management. Guidelines from the American College of Gastroenterology recommend surgery only when all other options have been exhausted. However, given the morbidity and mortality associated with open surgery, angiography and embolization is a minimally invasive option often considered for unstable patients prior to surgical intervention. (**Procedure Box 5.4**).

Procedure Box 5.4: Lower Gastrointestinal Bleed Embolization

After obtaining arterial access, an aortogram is first performed to map the SMA and inferior mesenteric artery (IMA) origins. The SMA and IMA are then sequentially catheterized and injected with contrast, with the initial branch chosen based on the site of most likely hemorrhage. In certain cases where the SMA and IMA are unrevealing, pelvic angiography of the internal iliac arteries can also be performed, as these vessels supply the middle and inferior rectal arteries. If a bleed is visualized, more selective angiograms are performed using a microcatheter advanced into smaller branch vessels. If no bleed is identified but suspicion remains high, provocative maneuvers such as selectively injecting anticoagulants, vasodilators, or fibrinolytics may be considered, however, precautions should be taken, including having blood products in the room and surgery on standby.

As with UGIB, direct angiographic findings of LGIB include active extravasation or pooling of contrast in the bowel. Indirect findings include pseudoaneurysms, early filling of a draining vein from an AVM/angiodysplasia, vasospasm in the setting of an injured vessel, an abruptly truncated vessel, and hyperemia in the setting of tumor.

Multiple embolic agents can be used to control or stop flow to a bleeding territory. Coils are the most commonly used agent for treating LGIB. The goal is for coils to be deployed as close to the bleed as possible without threatening adjacent healthy blood supply. The potential for blocking access distal to the coil, known as "jailing" the bleed, makes precision critical during coil deployment. Some coils are "detachable" or "partially retrievable" and offer more control. Particles, glue, and Gelfoam can also be effective but are used less often, as they are more difficult to control and carry a higher risk of causing bowel ischemia.

Similar to UGIBs, a CTA can be extremely useful prior to angiography to expedite the search for the bleed and decrease contrast volume required for investigation and treatment. The goal of this procedure is first and foremost to identify the bleed, and secondarily, attempt hemostasis with embolization. Even if embolization is not possible, localizing the bleed may make the difference between a hemicolectomy and a total colectomy for the patient (▶ **Fig. 5.8**).

Another indication for angiography is for rebleeding when the initial colonoscopy was unsuccessful in identifying the source of the bleed. As these cases are less urgent, a tagged RBC scan beforehand should be considered. Active bleeding on the tagged RBC scan can be followed immediately by angiography to attempt treatment.

Following intervention, LGIB patients are monitored in an appropriate inpatient unit. Hemoglobin is trended and stool monitored for evidence of rebleeding. Those who were successfully embolized will eventually need a colonoscopy for further evaluation of the underlying problem.

The arterial supply to the lower GI tract is less redundant than that of the upper GI tract, which increases the risk of bowel ischemia after embolization. Use of particles and glue increase this risk, as they occlude distal vessels beyond where collateral flow can prevent ischemia. Patients should be monitored for bowel ischemia after all LGIB embolization procedures. Peritoneal signs or an uptrending serum lactate may warrant further imaging.

5.4 Abdominal Trauma and Solid Organ Bleeds

In addition to GI bleeding, emergencies involving the solid organs are also a common reason for consultation of IR. The approach and management are similar for each of these. Injuries involving other intra-abdominal organs, including the bowel and mesentery, are potentially treated by IR, but are less common and will not be discussed.

Approach to Traumatic Bleeds

IR emergencies involving the solid abdominal organs are most commonly due to trauma. The liver and the spleen are in close proximity to the ribs, well vascularized, and anatomically fixed by ligaments. This makes them highly susceptible to shearing forces, which can result in contusion and laceration. Traumatic injuries involving the kidneys can also occur, but are less frequent. High-energy mechanisms such as motor vehicle collisions and falls from height are more likely to cause solid organ injury than low-impact injuries.

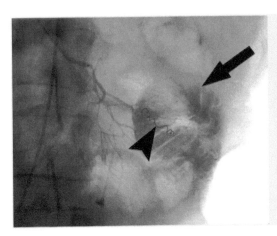

Fig. 5.8 This patient presented with severe lower GI bleeding from a jejunal branch of the superior mesenteric artery. Contrast is seen opacifying the bowel lumen, indicating active bleeding (*arrow*). Coil embolization improved the patient's hemodynamics and allowed for definitive treatment with a short segment bowel resection (*arrowhead*). (This image is provided courtesy of Matthew Evan Krosin, MD, University of Pittsburgh Medical Center.)

While trauma accounts for most IR-managed intra-abdominal emergencies, neoplastic processes such as a ruptured hepatocellular carcinoma or renal angiomyolipoma are circumstances where IR also plays a role. Management in such cases, however, follows many of the same rules as for trauma.

Work-up of Trauma Patients

Patients with traumatic intra-abdominal injury present either directly from the field or as transfers from community hospitals to larger, better-equipped trauma centers. Initial evaluation starts in the trauma bay where a primary survey evaluates the ABCs–airway, breathing, and circulation (▶ **Fig. 5.9**). Usually, multiple things are happening at once: vitals are being obtained, someone is evaluating the airway, another person is

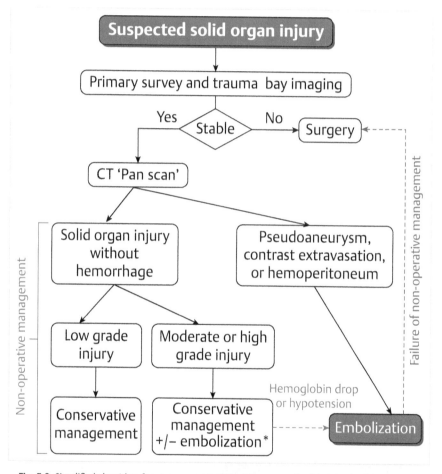

Fig. 5.9 Simplified algorithm for management of blunt trauma and solid abdominal organ injury. *Management is variable for *stable* patients with moderate-to-high-grade solid organ injuries. Some surgeons elect to operate (especially with splenic trauma), however, there is an increasing trend toward managing these stable patients nonoperatively (conservative management + embolization). For stable patients who are being managed conservatively, any hemoglobin drop or decompensation is an indication for IR embolization.

attempting to get peripheral intravenous access, and the trauma team is running through the primary and secondary survey. A careful abdominal examination is the initial test for signs of intra-abdominal injury.

Imaging in the trauma bay includes chest X-ray, pelvic X-ray, and ultrasound (focused assessment with sonography for trauma [FAST] scan). These are obtained within minutes of the patient being rolled in. A hemo- or pneumothorax merits a chest tube. Pericardial tamponade requires a pericardiocentesis. The FAST scan may show intra-abdominal free fluid, in which case the patient will likely need an exploratory laparotomy (ex-lap).

In managing abdominal trauma, key branch points revolve around the patient's mechanism of injury, hemodynamic stability, trauma bay imaging findings, and concomitant lack of intrathoracic injury.

Patients with *penetrating* trauma to the abdomen (gunshot wound or stabbing) will likely proceed directly to ex-lap, as there is no immediate way of knowing what organs have been violated until an intraoperative evaluation of the viscera can be performed. Patients with *blunt* trauma including a fall from height, motor vehicle crash, or assault are likely to have solid organ injuries, which may or may not be immediately evident.

For hemodynamically unstable patients with positive FAST scans, intra-abdominal hemorrhage is likely, and immediate exploratory laparotomy is indicated. Patients usually proceed directly to the OR, being too unstable for further imaging or less invasive endovascular interventions.

For hemodynamically stable patients with a negative FAST scan, the next step in the work-up is CT of the chest, abdomen, and pelvis. Note that some trauma surgeons send the patient to the CT scanner even if they have a positive FAST scan, provided they are stable enough. Whole body imaging (the trauma "pan-scan") has become routine in trauma centers. The contrast-enhanced scan often includes the chest and upper abdomen during the arterial phase and the upper abdomen and pelvis during the venous phase. Intraperitoneal fluid with density measuring 40 to 60 HU indicates blood, and direct evidence of parenchymal lacerations may be apparent. With this protocol, images of the liver, spleen, and kidneys are included during both contrast phases, increasing the sensitivity for vascular injury.

Vascular injury can be broadly divided into contained or uncontained hemorrhage. In **contained hemorrhage**, a vessel wall has been violated, but the leaking blood is contained by either the surrounding organ parenchyma or the perivascular connective tissue. Pseudoaneurysms are an example of contained hemorrhage. These injuries have fairly well-defined borders that do not change significantly between contrast phases, and are often located in continuity with or adjacent to a major vessel. **Uncontained hemorrhage**, or active extravasation, is more worrisome. This is characterized by ill-defined contrast extravasation which increases in size and density, forms layers, and/or redistributes distantly on subsequent venous phase imaging.

If injury to the renal collecting system is suspected based on the presence of hematuria or high-grade renal injury on initial scans, delayed CT images obtained 10 to 15 minutes after contrast injection can detect urinary system disruption, as contrast has been excreted into the collecting system by this point. Dilute contrast can also be infused through a Foley catheter prior to scanning to evaluate for bladder rupture.

The American Association for the Surgery of Trauma (AAST) has established a CT-based categorization system for solid organ injury (AAST Injury Scale), which can be reviewed independently. A higher grade indicates a more severe injury. While the AAST Injury Scale is a quick and easy surrogate measure of the severity of organ injury, a major downside of the categorization scheme is that it does not take the presence of hemorrhage into consideration, which is often one of the most important imaging findings in determining whether or not the patient gets treated by IR.

Management of Traumatic Solid Organ Injuries

Management options for traumatic solid organ injury include conservative management, embolization, or surgery. Conservative management and embolization are sometimes lumped under the term "nonoperative management."

Conservative management includes adequate resuscitation, close monitoring of
vitals and laboratory results, and serial abdominal examinations.

Hemodynamics, the presence or absence of hemorrhage on CT, and the severity of
organ injury are the most important factors that drive management decisions in
abdominal emergencies.

Consider a patient brought in with blunt force trauma. If the patient is *unstable,*
they will be triaged in the trauma bay and go straight to the OR. If the patient is stable,
they will be sent to the CT scanner for a trauma pan-scan. Imaging may reveal no
intra-abdominal injury whatsoever, a low-grade solid organ injury, or a moderate-to-
high-grade solid organ injury. If the patient becomes hemodynamically unstable at any
point, most surgeons have a low threshold to take them to the OR. If they remain
stable, however, they are candidates for nonoperative management.

The goal with nonoperative management is to avoid surgery. These patients are
treated conservatively but may additionally be sent to IR to undergo embolization,
depending on the CT findings. Contrast extravasation, hemoperitoneum, and pseudoaneurysm formation are features that indicate an increased risk of failure of nonoperative
management. Embolization in these select patients serves as a less invasive option to
avoid surgery and hopefully salvage the organ.

Conservative management is most successful in the setting of a stable patient with
a low-grade solid organ injury and no active hemorrhage. Many are young and otherwise healthy, with robust internal clotting mechanisms, vessels capable of adequate
vasospasm, and good cardiopulmonary reserve. These patients are observed in the hospital and discharged once other injuries are excluded. Conservative management of any
organ is also more favored in children, even those with injuries that may be severe
enough to warrant intervention in adults.

Endovascular management is most useful in stable patients with moderate-to-high
grade organ injuries and CT findings showing contrast extravasation or pseudoaneurysms. Embolization in these patients can increase the chance of success of nonoperative management and spare the patient a surgery. Contained and uncontained
hemorrhage within the liver, spleen, and kidney can all be addressed using similar
endovascular techniques. Management of moderate-to-high-grade injuries varies
slightly by the organ involved.

Even high-grade **splenic injuries** can be managed nonoperatively in some cases,
despite a sometimes frightening imaging appearance. While institutional practices
vary, candidates for embolization include those with CT findings of active extravasation, hemoperitoneum, or vascular injury resulting in AV fistula or pseudoaneurysm
formation. It is also viable in a patient who has a downtrending hemoglobin or recurrent
episodes of hypotension, though remains fluid responsive. In patients with these
findings, conservative management alone tends to result in rebleeding and a delayed
splenectomy (failure of nonoperative management). Splenic artery embolization
decreases this risk (**Procedure Box 5.5**).

Procedure Box 5.5: Splenic Artery Embolization ⓘ

Splenic artery embolization may be performed to treat bleeding or to decrease perfusion and reduce the size of the spleen in the setting of thrombocytopenia due to sequestration. Additionally, it may be performed in some cases of gastric variceal bleeding where a transjugular intrahepatic portosystemic shunt (TIPS) is not possible and a massive spleen is present. There are two strategies for splenic artery embolization: proximal and distal.

Proximal embolization involves accessing the celiac artery and identifying the tortuous splenic artery as it courses toward the left upper quadrant. An angiogram of the spleen is performed, and the extent of injury evaluated. If multiple areas of the spleen are injured and demonstrate pseudoaneurysm formation or active extravasation, an embolic agent such as a plug or pack of coils is placed proximally in the splenic artery (▶ Fig. 5.10). The objective of proximal embolization is to lower the arterial pressure to the spleen while allowing low-volume splenic perfusion via smaller collateral vessels. The vessel should be occluded distal to the origin of the dorsal pancreatic artery to prevent pancreatic ischemia, and to allow collateral splenic perfusion. In addition to the pancreatic arcade, the gastro-epiploic arteries and short gastric arteries also provide collateral perfusion to the spleen, which can prevent splenic necrosis following this technique. The patient's intrinsic clotting cascade is more likely to activate and enhance organ healing under decreased perfusion pressure. A proximal splenic embolization is analogous to blocking a major highway under construction and forcing traffic to divert via smaller side streets. Eventually, traffic reaches the destination, but it does so at a slower rate, so that road construction can occur more easily without being overwhelmed.

Distal splenic embolization can be more challenging to perform and is considered when splenic injury involves only one portion of the organ. A microcatheter is advanced distally into the small branches feeding the injured splenic parenchyma, close to the site of hemorrhage. Gelfoam, particles, or coils can be deployed to devascularize the injured splenic segment; minimizing the degree of vascular occlusion is critical to preserve as much splenic parenchyma as possible. Distal embolization should be performed with caution; splenic infarcts are a potential complication and are seen more frequently with distal embolizations than proximal.

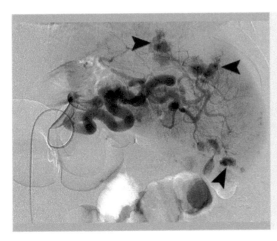

Fig. 5.10 Digital subtraction angiography demonstrates multiple splenic pseudoaneurysms in a trauma patient (*arrowheads*). Since multiple segments of the spleen were involved, this patient was treated with proximal splenic artery embolization. Proximal splenic artery embolization shortens procedure time, reduces radiation dose, and lowers the risk of postoperative complications. (This image is provided courtesy of Matthew Evan Krosin, MD, University of Pittsburgh Medical Center.)

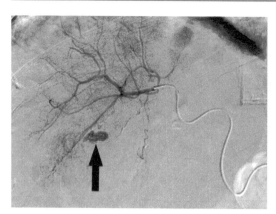

Fig. 5.11 Digital subtraction angiography demonstrated active extravasation from a branch of the right hepatic artery (*arrow*). This was successfully coil embolized. (This image is provided courtesy of Matthew Evan Krosin, MD, University of Pittsburgh Medical Center.)

With **liver trauma**, nonoperative management is the preferred route for stable patients. Open hepatic surgery carries high morbidity and mortality, and is therefore avoided when possible. If active extravasation is seen on CT, embolization is indicated (▶ **Fig. 5.11**). Conservative management is usually sufficient in the absence of active extravasation, though some trauma surgeons may ask for empiric hepatic artery embolization in the setting of high-grade injuries, even without extravasation. Pseudoaneurysms are rare in the acute setting but may be identified on follow-up imaging. Gelfoam, coils, plugs, glue, and particles may all be appropriate for embolization depending on the injury and size of the associated vessels. Ischemia is less of a concern with hepatic artery embolization due to the dual blood supply of the liver, and so treatment can be more aggressive.

In comparison to the other solid organs, **renal injuries** are the most likely to be appropriate for conservative management. The kidney has a tough capsule and is contained within a small space by the perirenal fascia, meaning the potential for large-volume hemorrhage is rather low. Embolization is performed in the setting of renal trauma if there are pseudoaneurysms on CT. The kidneys have minimal collateral blood supply, so embolization should be done selectively and sparingly. An overly aggressive approach may infarct a significant portion of the kidney and lead to renal insufficiency.

Renal injury is much less frequently treated surgically, with the exception of cases involving urinary extravasation or damage to the vascular pedicle. Disrupted perfusion can lead to renal infarction within hours of injury, which is typically not enough time to get the patient to IR for endovascular management. These cases are treated with emergent surgery to attempt salvage of the kidney.

Postprocedure Management

Patients with abdominal organ injury, regardless of treatment undertaken, are monitored in an intensive care unit, with care deescalated as hemodynamics, fluid requirements, pain control, and labs improve. With both splenic embolization and splenectomy patients, immunizations for encapsulated organisms, including *Meningococcus, Pneumococcus* and *Haemophilus,* should be given.

Bile leak is a complication unique to hepatic trauma, so liver injuries should be monitored with serial liver function tests (LFTs). When suspected, a nuclear medicine HIDA scan can be helpful to diagnose and localize the source.

Repeat contrast-enhanced CT imaging is usually performed at 24 to 48 hours to evaluate for early complications, including tissue necrosis, post-traumatic arteriovenous fistula, and delayed organ rupture.

Abscess formation is a noteworthy complication that can occur in the spleen (and sometimes kidney), particularly when *distal* embolization is performed. Patients either fail to improve while hospitalized or are discharged and then return with abdominal pain and systemic signs of infection. Repeat cross-sectional imaging can confirm the diagnosis of abscess. These are generally managed with percutaneous drain placement or splenectomy. Hepatic abscesses are less common due to the dual blood supply.

5.5 Pelvic Trauma

Pelvic trauma can often be life threatening. Fractures or diastasis at the pubic symphysis ("open book pelvis") increase the volume of the pelvic cavity, which has potential to allow multiple liters of blood to accumulate. These patients can exsanguinate rapidly.

Severe pelvic injuries are usually due to motor vehicle accidents but may also occur with falls from height or penetrating trauma. This can result in bleeding from arteries, veins, and the medullary space of fractured bone.

Most patients with significant pelvic trauma have multiple sites of injury and therefore may be bleeding from multiple locations simultaneously. These polytrauma situations complicate care and cause management dilemmas.

Work-up of Traumatic Pelvic Injuries

As with other emergencies, evaluation of patients with pelvic injuries starts with the primary and secondary survey in the trauma bay (▶ **Fig. 5.12**). Applying anteroposterior force to the bilateral iliac crests with the patient supine on a trauma backboard tests for pelvic instability. Sturdiness suggests an intact pelvis, while mobility or deformation under small amounts of force raises concern for pelvic disruption.

Indirect signs of pelvic injury include hematuria, hip dislocations, and suprapubic tenderness. These examination findings raise suspicion for pelvic injury even before imaging is performed.

Large fractures will typically be detected on the trauma bay pelvic X-ray. Radiographs are sensitive for the detection of diastasis (widening) at the pubic symphysis or the sacroiliac joints. Hip dislocations can also be detected.

The FAST scan will often identify concomitant intra-abdominal injury. If the patient is hemodynamically unstable with a positive FAST scan, a trip to the OR is indicated.

Contrast-enhanced CT is the gold standard for diagnostic evaluation of pelvic injury in stable patients. Contrast extravasation indicates active bleeding and the need for more aggressive management. The real benefit of CT for pelvic injury is its negative predictive value, which approaches 100%. Conservative management of pelvic injury can be considered when the CT is negative for bleeding.

Management of Pelvic Injuries

For stable patients without evidence of active arterial extravasation, pelvic injury is managed conservatively. Unstable patients with pelvic injuries are taken to the OR. Many of these patients have simultaneous intra-abdominal injuries that need to be managed operatively. However, surgery is *not* the definitive treatment for pelvic bleeds. Pelvic injuries are notoriously difficult to treat surgically due to extensive pelvic arterial anastomoses. Pelvic vessels can be hard to identify, as they are individually buried within the retroperitoneal space, and operative hemostasis is a challenge due to collateralization.

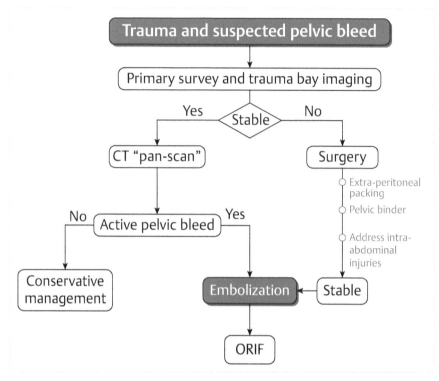

Fig. 5.12 Simplified algorithm for management of traumatic pelvic injuries. ORIF, open reduction internal fixation.

Extraperitoneal packing is one surgical strategy for controlling pelvic hemorrhage. The idea is to pack the potential space where hemorrhage would otherwise freely accumulate. For unstable patients who are taken straight to the OR, extraperitoneal packing can be performed as a bridge to embolization.

For unstable patients with pelvic injuries, pelvic binders can be used to increase intrapelvic pressure and tamponade hemorrhage. The pelvic binder also aids with initial closed reduction of pelvic fractures. The benefit is usually temporary, as bleeding may resume when the binder is removed. Something to keep in mind is that pelvic binders can pose a logistical challenge to the interventional radiologist, since it physically covers the inguinal regions and may need to be cut with shears to allow a window for femoral access.

Patients with pelvic arterial bleeds, stable or unstable, will eventually make their way to IR for an embolization. While institutional criteria vary, patients who undergo embolization for pelvic injuries are those with some combination of active extravasation on CT, hemodynamic instability, and complex pelvic fractures (**Procedure Box 5.6**). In the absence of hematuria or other clinical signs suggesting urethral injury, a Foley is usually inserted to decompress the bladder and remove any contrast that has accumulated within it. This is an important step since a radiopaque distended bladder can obscure pelvic vessels and make angiography difficult.

Patients with pelvic fractures will eventually need open reduction. It is usually done late in the acute course, once other life-threatening injuries are addressed.

Procedure Box 5.6: Pelvic Bleed Embolization ⓘ

Femoral arterial access for pelvic angiography should ideally be established contralateral to the hemorrhage if it appears to be asymmetric. Alternatively, radial access can be utilized. The internal iliac artery is selected and angiography is performed. This vessel provides extensive pelvic arterial anastomoses via up to 11 total branches from its anterior and posterior divisions.

When multiple distal sites of vessel injury or extravasation are identified, nonselective injection of Gelfoam can be performed from the proximal internal iliac artery. If injury seems isolated to anterior branches based on CT and angiographic features, the injection is often delivered to just the anterior division, sparing the posterior branches supplying the lumbar and gluteal musculature, and sacrum.

Gelfoam is most effective in noncoagulopathic patients, as it relies on intrinsic clotting mechanisms. The beauty of Gelfoam in the pelvis is its temporary effect, which allows for eventual vessel recanalization weeks later once healing occurs. This preserves the pelvic arterial anastomoses long term. Glue is an option in cases of severe coagulopathy (where Gelfoam may not be effective), but is more difficult to use and does not allow recanalization. Isolated vascular injuries, as indicated by focal pseudoaneurysms or extravasation, may occasionally be treated at the site of injury using coils delivered by microcatheter.

An important angiographic sign often overlooked is the appearance of an abruptly truncated artery, which may represent a completely transected vessel temporarily occluded by use of a pelvic binder or tamponade from an adjacent expanding hematoma. If unaddressed, these transected vessels are at high risk for delayed rebleeding. Treatment using coils or plugs placed both distal (if possible) and proximal to the site of injury can reduce the risk of delayed or persistent hemorrhage.

5.6 Retroperitoneal and Soft Tissue Bleeds

Retroperitoneal bleeding (RPB) and certain forms of soft tissue bleeding have common features and can occasionally fall under the care of the interventional radiologist. These forms of bleeding are often a challenge to diagnose and have potential to become quite serious.

Rich with vascular structures and several vital organs, the retroperitoneum has many possible sources of bleeding. Attention to the location within the retroperitoneum can be a clue toward identifying a source. Bleeding in the central retroperitoneum (Zone 1) occurs from the abdominal aorta, IVC, celiac axis, SMA, IMA, renal vasculature, pancreas, and duodenum. Bleeding in the lateral retroperitoneum (Zone 2) occurs from the kidneys, adrenals, and proximal ureters. Bleeding below the aortic bifurcation (Zone 3) occurs from the iliac vessels, colon, or distal ureters.

Soft tissue bleeds can occur practically anywhere. A common one to be aware of is a rectus sheath hematoma. Rectus sheath hematomas (RSH) occur within the anterior abdominal wall, below the arcuate line, where the vessels are fixed and therefore susceptible to shearing forces. Despite the tamponade effect of the abdominal fascial layers, hemorrhagic shock can still occur from large extravasation.

In considering nontraumatic RPB and RSH, the root causes can be categorized as spontaneous and iatrogenic. Spontaneous bleeds are usually seen in patients on blood thinners. Increased intra-abdominal pressure, such as with coughing, vomiting, or Valsalva can be a trigger. RPB can also occur from solid organ tumors, arterial aneurysms, or acute necrotizing pancreatitis.

Iatrogenic forms of RPB and RSH occur as a result of surgical, percutaneous, or endo-vascular interventions. Nephrectomy, nephrostomy tube placement, and IVC filter retrieval are examples of procedures that carry the risk of RPB. RSH is most commonly caused by damage to an inferior epigastric artery or occasionally a deep circumflex iliac artery during punctures or incisions into the lower anterior abdominal wall. The classic example is a paracentesis performed blindly without attention given to anatomical landmarks. Ultrasound with color Doppler flow should ideally be used to identify and avoid these potentially dangerous vessels.

Work-up of RPB/RSH

Clinicians should be alert to the risk factors for RPB and RSH mentioned above, as the presentation can vary widely. Large bleeds, especially in an obese patient, may not show symptoms until the point of developing hemodynamic instability (▶ **Fig. 5.13**). Slow but persistent bleeds, as seen with anticoagulated patients, may present with tachycardia, downtrending hemoglobin, flank pain, or ecchymoses.

When seeing a patient with a soft tissue hematoma/RSH, it may be helpful to use a skin marker to draw a circle around the hematoma edges. This allows the team to track hematoma growth/regression. Overlying cutaneous changes should be monitored, as pressure necrosis of the skin can occur secondary to a large underlying hematoma. A focused physical examination should evaluate for mass effect on adjacent structures. For example, an extremity hematoma merits a peripheral vascular and neurological examination, a neck hematoma requires assessment of the airway, etc.

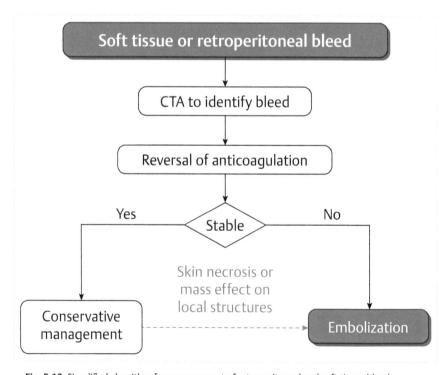

Fig. 5.13 Simplified algorithm for management of retroperitoneal and soft tissue bleeds.

If the hematoma is large enough, noncontrast CT may show a soft tissue mass or blood density collection (▶ **Fig. 5.14**). CTA can identify a hyperdense blush when there is active bleeding. Delayed phases may demonstrate hyperdense contrast layering within a hematoma, adding further evidence of ongoing bleeding. (▶ **Fig. 5.15**).

Finally, when seeing a consult for a soft tissue hematoma/RPB, always be aware that venous bleeding is quite common. This is important to keep in mind, as venous bleeding into these areas is rarely manageable with endovascular techniques.

Management of RPB/RSH

Rectus sheath hematomas are usually self-limited due to the presence of fascial layers, and are therefore managed conservatively in the majority of cases. In the setting of hemodynamic stability, conservative management and reversal of anticoagulation should always be attempted. Many soft tissue bleeds resolve on their own once the patient's coagulation status is normalized. Depending on the anticoagulant being used, this may involve passively waiting, or administering reversal agents if immediate results are necessary.

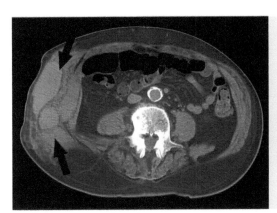

Fig. 5.14 Unenhanced axial CT demonstrates a hematoma in the right lateral abdominal wall. Size, acute appearance, and hemodynamic instability prompted angiography to confirm and treat active bleeding. (This image is provided courtesy of Matthew Evan Krosin, MD, University of Pittsburgh Medical Center.)

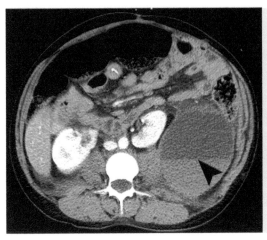

Fig. 5.15 Arterial phase contrast-enhanced axial CT demonstrates a fluid–fluid level in the left retroperitoneal space (*arrowhead*). The layering of densities indicates recent or ongoing hemorrhage. The patient had a supratherapeutic international normalized ratio. (This image is provided courtesy of Matthew Evan Krosin, MD, University of Pittsburgh Medical Center.)

Patients with soft tissue hematomas that develop persistent hemodynamic instability require escalation of care. In addition, exam findings such as skin necrosis or evidence of mass effect on surrounding structures are also indications for further intervention.

Endovascular therapy has replaced surgery as the primary treatment option (**Procedure Box 5.7**). A surgical incision into the hematoma and subsequent decompression tends to release the tamponade effect, resulting in rebleeding. The one exception to this rule is if the hematoma is in the neck and there is concern for imminent airway compromise. Surgery and anesthesia teams need to be involved immediately to secure the airway and surgically evacuate the hematoma.

As with soft tissue hematomas, hemodynamically unstable patients with RP bleeds from an arterial source require intervention. While endovascular treatment is preferred, surgery is sometimes necessary. IR has the advantage of being able to easily access retroperitoneal anatomy that is often difficult to surgically explore.

Surgical exploration is rarely indicated in cases of spontaneous RP bleeds. Patients sent for surgery are those that fail endovascular embolization, anyone with abdominal compartment syndrome, or those who require surgery for other reasons.

Postprocedural Management

In cases of spontaneous RPB and RSH that undergo embolization, technical success (angiographic evidence of hemostasis) is very high. The few cases that do have rebleeding are thought to be caused by new spontaneous bleeds.

Normalizing hemoglobin and coagulation panel values are reassuring signs in the follow-up of these patients, however clinical signs of rebleeding can again be ambiguous. Patients who have suspected rebleeding typically are appropriate to undergo repeat embolization. Surgery is recommended in the rare case of embolization refractory bleeding, superinfected hematoma, or abdominal compartment syndrome.

Procedure Box 5.7: Retroperitoneal and Soft Tissue Bleeds ⓘ

Endovascular investigation of a retroperitoneal bleed begins with DSA of the aorta to map the major arterial takeoffs; this may be skipped if CTA provides an adequate roadmap. Interrogation of the major retroperitoneal branches is performed, often starting with the most common source of bleeding, the lumbar arteries. Intercostal, inferior phrenic, renal, adrenal, mesenteric, and iliac arteries may also be interrogated (▶ **Fig. 5.16**). Once a bleed is identified, coils are used for larger or more proximal feeding vessels. Gelfoam is often used as an adjunct for embolization of distal or small vessels, given the rich collateral supply in the retroperitoneum.

Cases of RSH that persist despite conservative therapy or result in hemodynamic instability should proceed to angiography and embolization of the bleeding inferior epigastric or deep circumflex iliac artery, both of which arise from the distal external iliac artery at the level of the inguinal ligament. Iliac arteriography is performed to identify the branch origins, which are then selected with a base catheter. Arteriography and embolization is then typically performed through a microcatheter if an abnormality is identified. Similar to the treatment of retroperitoneal bleeds, Gelfoam is preferred for embolization of distal or small vessels than cannot be reached with a microcatheter; coils can be deployed proximal and distal to sites of bleeding to prevent continued bleeding through collateral pathways in injuries affecting larger segments of these vessels.

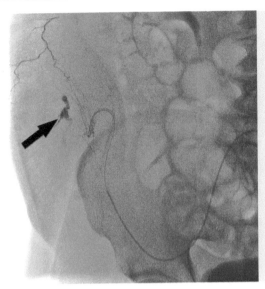

Fig. 5.16 Digital subtraction angiography demonstrates contrast extravasation in the distribution of the right deep circumflex artery (*arrow*), the cause of an abdominal wall hemorrhage. N-BCA, a glue, was slowly infused, achieving hemostasis. (This image is provided courtesy of Matthew Evan Krosin, MD, University of Pittsburgh Medical Center.)

5.7 Obstetric Emergencies

Obstetric emergencies involve postpartum hemorrhage secondary to either uterine atony or placental implantation abnormalities. Patients experiencing intractable post-partum hemorrhage unresponsive to fluids, drugs, and manual maneuvers may undergo uterine artery embolization with Gelfoam or particles to stop the hemorrhage. This intervention is important, as it can potentially avoid hysterectomy when preservation of the uterus and future fertility are a key focus.

Placental implantation abnormalities (placenta increta/accreta/percreta) are often diagnosed on prenatal imaging and can be managed prophylactically by IR. This involves placing occlusion balloons within the anterior divisions of the bilateral internal iliac arteries prior to planned C-section and/or hysterectomy. With the balloons in place, the obstetrician or interventional radiologist can inflate and occlude the hypertrophied uterine arteries if bleeding is uncontrollable during the surgery, and even blindly inject a Gelfoam slurry to control bleeding if necessary.

5.8 Orthopaedic Emergencies

Orthopaedic emergencies will occasionally benefit from IR intervention when there is vascular injury. Most commonly, a fractured bone may lacerate an adjacent vessel. Management of these injuries is similar to peripheral vascular interventions using stent-grafts and coils.

In addition to vascular injury, IR may be involved with patients suffering from bone metastasis. Certain cancers such as renal cell, breast, lung, and melanoma create hyper-vascular bone metastasis. When a pathological fracture occurs, orthopaedists perform surgeries to fixate the bone, and will often request preoperative embolization to limit intraoperative blood loss. Embolization of tumors in bone can be performed with a variety of embolic agents, and postprocedural management relies on orthopaedic comanagement.

Suggested Readings

[1] Chimpiri AR, Natarajan B. Visceral arteriography in trauma. Semin Intervent Radiol. 2009; 26(3): 207–214

[2] Ierardi AM, Duka E, Lu, cchina N, et al. The role of interventional radiology in abdominopelvic trauma. Br J Radiol. 2016; 89(1061):20150866

[3] Khalil A, Fedida B, Parrot A, Haddad S, Fartoukh M, Carette MF. Severe hemoptysis: from diagnosis to embolization. Diagn Interv Imaging. 2015; 96(7–8):775–788

[4] Lopera JE. Embolization in trauma: principles and techniques. Semin Intervent Radiol. 2010; 27(1): 14–28

[5] Navuluri R, Kang L, Patel J, Van Ha T. Acute lower gastrointestinal bleeding. Semin Intervent Radiol. 2012; 29(3):178–186

[6] Navuluri R, Patel J, Kang L. Role of interventional radiology in the emergent management of acute upper gastrointestinal bleeding. Semin Intervent Radiol. 2012; 29(3):169–177

[7] Newsome J, Martin JG, Bercu Z, Shah J, Shekhani H, Peters G. Postpartum Hemorrhage. Tech Vasc Interv Radiol. 2017; 20(4):266–273

[8] Scemama U, Dabadie A, Varoquaux A, et al. Pelvic trauma and vascular emergencies. Diagn Interv Imaging. 2015; 96(7–8):717–729

6 Hepatobiliary

Orrie Close, Alexandria S. Jo, Patrick Grierson, and Bill Saliba Majdalany

Interventional radiologists care for patients with both acute and chronic hepatobiliary diseases. Patients with acute hepatobiliary disease most commonly present with right upper quadrant (RUQ) pain, and are diagnosed with a combination of labs and imaging. Patients with chronic disease may be asymptomatic, and only diagnosed after incidental imaging findings demonstrate morphological changes in the liver. In either case, identifying the pattern of liver function tests (LFTs) is often a good first step when approaching disease of the hepatobiliary system.

Abnormal LFTs should be interpreted in conjunction with the patient's history and physical exam. This should narrow the differential prior to obtaining imaging. It is not necessary for you to understand the full differential and work-up, but a basic understanding of certain LFT patterns is useful.

Elevated transaminases are often an indication of hepatocyte damage, and the degree of elevation is an important distinction. Numbers in the thousands are seen with viral hepatitis, drug-related or ischemic damage. Numbers in the hundreds may be due to chronic hepatitis, other infections, or hepatic congestion related to heart failure. Mild elevations might be seen with alcoholic liver disease. While alanine aminotransferase (ALT) is specific to hepatocytes, aspartate aminotransferase (AST) is less so, and can be elevated in rhabdomyolysis or other muscle disorders.

If liver disease is suspected and labs show a significantly elevated alkaline phosphatase (ALP), cholestasis or biliary obstruction should be considered. As with AST, ALP is nonspecific, and an isolated elevation in ALP can be related to a number of different diseases. However, elevation of ALP in conjunction with elevation in gamma-glutamyl transferase (GGT) increases the specificity for liver disease. A *direct* hyperbilirubinemia suggests that hepatocytes are functioning but that the liver is not able to excrete normally, possibly due to obstruction. *Indirect* hyperbilirubinemia is more consistent with hemolysis or intrinsic hepatocyte dysfunction.

Certain labs can also indicate the overall health of the liver. If the liver is significantly damaged, you may note signs of compromised synthetic function. Elevated prothrombin time (PT)/international normalized ratio (INR) and low albumin can be seen, but other confounding factors such as malnutrition, malabsorption, or warfarin use need to be ruled out to be certain synthetic dysfunction is to blame.

6.1 General Anatomical Principles

The liver consists of three functional lobes: the right, left, and caudate. The middle hepatic vein separates the left and right lobes. The falciform ligament, portal and remaining hepatic veins further subdivide the right and left lobes into eight functional segments, known as the **Couinaud's classification system** (▶Fig. 6.1). Each segment has its own arterial supply, venous and biliary drainage.

The arterial supply to the liver originates from the celiac axis via the common hepatic artery, though this represents only a portion of the blood supply. Greater than 75% comes from the portal vein.

The portal venous system includes veins that drain blood from the GI tract, spleen, and pancreas. The main portal vein is formed by the superior mesenteric and splenic veins. It enters the liver at the porta hepatis, where it bifurcates into the left and right hepatic lobes.

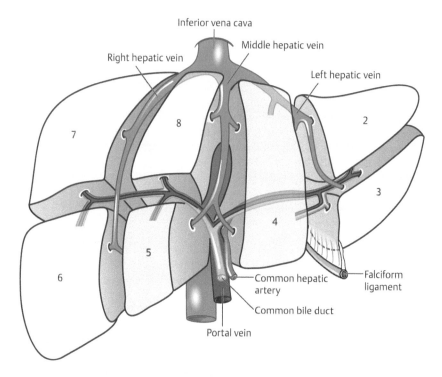

Fig. 6.1 Hepatic anatomy showing the liver segments and their relationship with the hepatic veins, hepatic arteries, and bile ducts. (Source: 9 Normal Anatomy and Variants. In: Beek E, Van Rijn R, eds. Diagnostic Pediatric Ultrasound. 1st Edition. Thieme; 2015.)

The hepatic veins, as part of the systemic circulation, allow passage of blood from the liver parenchyma to the IVC at the confluence of the right, middle, and left hepatic veins (▶ **Fig. 6.1**). The caudate lobe drains directly into the IVC (which is why it is typically spared in disease processes such as Budd–Chiari syndrome). There are a number of anastomoses between the systemic and portal venous systems, which will be important to understand for our discussion of portal hypertension.

The intrahepatic biliary system is comprised of the right and left hepatic ducts, which run in parallel to the portal veins, and join to form the common hepatic duct. The caudate lobe biliary drainage is variable, but typically occurs through ducts that join to both the left and right hepatic ducts. The left and right hepatic ducts join to become the common hepatic duct, which joins the cystic duct extrahepatically to become the common bile duct (CBD).

6.2 Biliary Disease

The normal physiology of the biliary system is neurohormonally regulated, alternating storage and passage of bile during fasting and digestive states, respectively. When this flow is disrupted, it's thought that rising concentrations of cholesterol in the bile induces an inflammatory response along the bile duct epithelial lining. Inflammation is often, but not always, associated with some form of mechanical obstruction within the biliary tree.

Patients with biliary disease present differently depending on a number of factors. The location of the obstruction/inflammation within the biliary tree determines the degree of laboratory derangements and presence or absence of jaundice. Pain is typically a consequence of how rapidly the problem arises and may be absent in chronic cases. The acuity of the problem, and hence the approach to management, is determined by the degree of inflammation and sometimes the presence of a superimposed infectious process. From the IR perspective, biliary disease can be broken down into pathology of the gallbladder, CBD, or hepatic ducts.

Gallbladder Disease

Acute cholecystitis is most often the result of gallstone disease, although it can also occur in patients without stones (acalculous cholecystitis). A stone that obstructs the cystic duct will result in an inflamed gallbladder. Patients classically present with RUQ pain, low-grade fever, nausea, vomiting, and elevated white count. The pain may be colicky at first, but then becomes constant. LFTs are typically normal or only mildly elevated. Significant LFT abnormalities should be a clue that the problem resides elsewhere in the biliary system.

Patients with a presentation suggestive of acute cholecystitis will initially undergo a RUQ ultrasound. Positive findings include a distended gallbladder with cholelithiasis, wall thickening, pericholecystic fluid, and a sonographic Murphy's sign (pain when applying pressure with the ultrasound probe directly over the gallbladder). Wall thickening is the most sensitive sign, but it is not specific. When ultrasound findings are indeterminate, a nuclear medicine HIDA scan can be used. The HIDA scan is the most accurate imaging modality for diagnosing cholecystitis; a positive study will demonstrate lack of radiotracer filling of the gallbladder, which indicates cystic duct obstruction. Contrast-enhanced CT or MRI is more sensitive for the detection of gangrenous cholecystitis, which is a severe complication that results from ischemia of the gallbladder wall.

The combination of a positive physical exam, systemic signs of inflammation, and at least one characteristic imaging finding is required to make a definitive diagnosis of acute cholecystitis.

Once diagnosed, the patient is made NPO, analgesics and antibiotics are administered, and general surgery is consulted. For symptomatic patients who are healthy enough to undergo surgery, laparoscopic cholecystectomy (lap chole) is considered the treatment of choice. In addition to symptomatic relief, prompt surgical management can prevent complications of acute cholecystitis such as gallbladder rupture and sepsis. Surgery should ideally be performed within the first day of hospitalization, as delaying it has been shown to increase the incidence of complications and conversion to open cholecystectomy.

Those who are too sick to undergo surgery may benefit from placement of a **percutaneous cholecystostomy tube (PCT)** by IR (**Procedure Box 6.1**) (▶ **Fig. 6.2**). The purpose of the tube is to drain the infected fluid and decrease gallbladder inflammation. Although it is not as definitive of a treatment as surgery, it can achieve adequate symptom control and reduce the risk of complications, while allowing the inflammatory process to cool down. There are few contraindications to PCT placement, which is fortuitous for very sick patients. Ascites has historically been considered a relative contraindication out of concern that it could prevent tract formation for the tube, but more recently studies have disproven this.

Determining who should undergo surgery versus PCT is not always clear-cut. Recommendations set forth by the Tokyo guidelines, updated most recently in 2018, offer a grading system for management based on a number of patient risk factors (▶Table 6.1).

Grade I (mild) acute cholecystitis patients should undergo a lap chole, provided they are healthy enough to undergo surgery from a comorbidity standpoint. Those who are not healthy enough for surgery are treated conservatively with antibiotics. Surgery is considered if their status changes favorably. Grade II (moderate) patients can undergo a lap chole if they are healthy enough *and* they are treated at an advanced surgical

Procedure Box 6.1: Cholecystostomy Tube ⓘ

Cholecystostomy placement is most commonly performed for drainage of the gallbladder in the setting of acute cholecystitis in nonsurgical candidates. Percutaneous gallbladder access may be obtained through a transhepatic or transperitoneal approach. A transhepatic approach is often preferred because of greater catheter stability, quicker tract maturation, decreased incidence of bile peritonitis, and less chance of bowel injury. Transperitoneal access is typically reserved for patients with diffuse liver disease, uncorrectable coagulopathy, or a pendulous gallbladder positioned far from the liver surface. The gallbladder is usually accessed using a 21- or 22-gauge needle, and intraluminal access confirmed with 5 cc of contrast; a large contrast dose should be avoided as this could potentiate sepsis. Once a guidewire is placed into the gallbladder, the cholecystostomy drain can be advanced over the wire. In select patients and in the hands of an experienced operator, direct gallbladder access using a sharp stylet and trocar technique can also be performed.

Postprocedurally, the catheter should be gently flushed every 24 hours. The catheter tract matures in about 4 to 6 weeks; long-term catheters should be changed every 3 months. The drain can be pulled if there is confirmed resolution of the cholecystitis and evidence of a patent cystic duct, confirmed by a tube cholecystostogram. Sometimes the drain remains in place until the patient goes to the operating room for an interval cholecystectomy and is removed at that time.

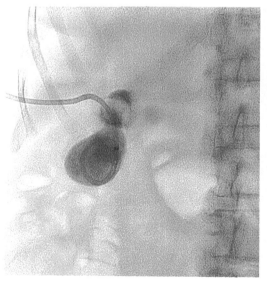

Fig. 6.2 An 8.5-Fr pigtail cholecystostomy tube placed by a transhepatic approach for a patient with acute cholecystitis who was a poor surgical candidate.

Table 6.1 Tokyo guidelines severity grading for acute cholecystitis

Grade	Criteria
I	Healthy patient without organ dysfunction Mild inflammatory changes of the gallbladder
II	WBC > 18,000 Palpable RUQ mass > 72 h of symptoms Cholecystitis complications (gangrenous cholecystitis, abscess formation, biliary peritonitis)
III	Cardiovascular dysfunction, hypotension requires pressors Respiratory failure Acute renal failure Neurological dysfunction Hepatic dysfunction Thrombocytopenia

Abbreviations: RUQ, right upper quadrant pain; WBC, white blood cells.

center. Otherwise, biliary drainage with PCT should be considered when the patient does not respond to initial medical management. When surgery is pursued, the surgeon should be prepared to convert to an open cholecystectomy or perform a subtotal cholecystectomy, if required. Grade III (severe) patients have evidence of organ dysfunction and have historically been considered noncandidates for surgery. The updated guidelines suggest that renal dysfunction and cardiovascular dysfunction are more favorable than the other types of organ failure, and therefore may not preclude surgery if there is appropriate initial medical management and the patient is treated at an advanced surgical center. However, the majority of grade III patients are better off treated with PCT placement.

For those who undergo PCT placement, a cholecystectomy can be performed on an elective basis once inflammation has subsided and the patient is healthy enough for surgery. No randomized controlled trials have yet been performed to determine the ideal timing of cholecystectomy after PCT, but a few observational studies have suggested that early surgery after percutaneous gallbladder drainage is associated with a higher incidence of complications. There is no consensus on optimal timing for surgery after PCT, but that may change as more data become available.

The Tokyo guidelines grading system is validated by a multitude of retrospective studies which have identified factors associated with higher operative risk in acute cholecystitis patients. Even with all of these studies, it is difficult to directly compare outcomes between emergent lap chole and percutaneous drainage (with or without subsequent cholecystectomy), as there is an inherent selection bias for sicker patients receiving the latter. The CHOCOLATE trial is a multicenter prospective study that seeks to sort this out by randomizing management of high-risk acute cholecystitis patients to either lap chole or PCT. When published, the results of this large prospective study may redefine how PCT fits into the treatment algorithm for acute cholecystitis.

Acalculous cholecystitis represents a special circumstance in which PCT may be beneficial. In contrast to calculous cholecystitis, these are usually inpatients who are severely septic with no known source. As part of the sepsis work-up, a RUQ ultrasound might be performed if there is suspicion for a biliary etiology. With acalculous cholecystitis, the gallbladder will show signs of inflammation without identifiable stones. Some of these patients will meet some, but not all, of the diagnostic criteria for acute cholecystitis. If a PCT is placed for one of these patients and he or she improves, it supports acalculous cholecystitis being the source of sepsis. The drained fluid can be cultured for the purpose of tailoring antibiotics.

When gallstones cause repeated bouts of subacute cholecystitis, **chronic cholecystitis** can result. Radiographically, the gallbladder is fibrotic, shrunken, and filled with gallstones. The treatment for chronic cholecystitis is cholecystectomy, especially if a porcelain gallbladder is present (as this can also be seen in gallbladder carcinoma). IR is not typically involved in the care of patients with chronic cholecystitis unless they have an acute flare and have an indication for PCT.

Bile Duct Disease

Cholecystitis affects the gallbladder and cystic duct, while in most circumstances the remainder of the biliary tree remains relatively unaffected, allowing unimpeded flow of bile from the liver to the duodenum. When obstruction and inflammation affect the CBD or hepatic ducts, bile no longer flows freely. It backs up within the liver, causing hepatic dysfunction and increased bile components entering the systemic circulation. In these patients, labs will show a direct bilirubinemia, and the patient may present with scleral icterus, jaundice, and clay-colored stools.

Acute obstruction of the CBD occurs in **choledocholithiasis**. With passage of a gallstone into the CBD resulting in obstruction, the pathophysiology of choledocholithiasis is similar to cholecystitis, stemming from the inflammatory reaction of cholestasis. Patients have RUQ pain, nausea, vomiting, and mild fever, but additionally have bilirubinemia. Lab values may also identify elevated transaminases, ALP, and GGT.

Chronic obstruction of the biliary ampulla or bile ducts can be due to a number of benign etiologies, including anastomotic strictures, or due to malignant etiologies such as pancreatic cancer or cholangiocarcinoma (▶ **Table 6.2**). As these are relatively slow to develop, the patient commonly presents with painless jaundice. When there is complete occlusion of the CBD, the gallbladder becomes distended and may be palpable on exam (Courvoisier's sign).

Biliary obstruction, regardless of the etiology or chronicity, is a risk factor for **ascending cholangitis.** Disruption of the normal flow of bile can permit retrograde migration of bacteria from the small bowel into the biliary tree. Once inside the bile duct, infection can rapidly spread into the bloodstream and result in sepsis. These patients present with jaundice, fever, and RUQ pain (Charcot's triad), as well as a leukocytosis and eventually hypotension.

Table 6.2 Etiologies of bile duct obstruction

Benign	Malignant
Trauma	Primary hepatobiliary neoplasm
Surgery and radiation	Pancreatic neoplasms
Infection	Gallbladder carcinoma
Primary sclerosing cholangitis, pseudocyst, chronic pancreatitis	Regional lymph node enlargement
Ischemia	
Mirizzi's syndrome, gallstones, portal cholangiopathy	

A number of intrahepatic processes (e.g., primary biliary cirrhosis, primary sclerosing cholangitis, drug reactions) may also lead to cholestasis. The mechanism can be due to hepatocyte dysfunction, metabolic disturbance of bile production, or destruction of the intrahepatic bile ducts. The most common symptom associated with intrahepatic cholestasis is pruritus, with jaundice less common than it is with extrahepatic cholestasis. For patients with a cholestatic LFT pattern, making the distinction between an intrahepatic and extrahepatic cause should be determined early since the work-up for each is quite different.

When a patient presents with jaundice, before any imaging is ordered, it is important to rule out emergent problems including acute cholangitis, liver failure, or massive hemolysis. These can be life threatening and require immediate attention.

If there is clinical suspicion for biliary obstruction based on history and labs, the preferred initial imaging modality is ultrasound. A dilated CBD on ultrasound is suggestive of a distal obstruction within the duct, and choledocholithiasis is likely if the presentation is acute. Although ultrasound does not always identify the obstructing stone (frequently the case due to overlying bowel gas), the presence of stones in the gallbladder and the finding of a dilated CBD strongly suggests choledocholithiasis. The absence of stones in the gallbladder implies there may be another cause. If the CBD is nondistended, obstruction may be more proximal in the intrahepatic ducts.

Abdominal CT is also commonly used for initial imaging (▶ **Table 6.3**). CT is quick and is not operator dependent. While not ideal, CT can show dilated ducts and/or calcified stones, as well as exclude alternative diagnoses. CT may be preferred in two scenarios: (1) when there is low suspicion for obstruction and a detailed look at the

Table 6.3 Imaging options for biliary obstructions

Diagnostic tool	Advantages	Disadvantages
RUQ US	Great for evaluating gallbladder pathology, common bile duct, focal liver lesion	Operator-dependent; body habitus and bowel gas can limit evaluation
CT abdomen	Comprehensive cross-sectional anatomy provided; rapid, widely available, and reproducible	Radiation exposure; does not evaluate gallbladder pathology as well as RUQ US; does not adequately evaluate distal biliary tree
MRCP	Provides full delineation of the biliary tree	More expensive, time consuming, and susceptible to motion artifact
ERCP	Provides delineation of the distal biliary tree; can relieve distal obstructions through stenting; can perform sphincterotomy to facilitate stone passage; can biopsy distal lesions	Invasive procedure; risk of pancreatitis, hemorrhage, biliary injury; proximal biliary system can be difficult to opacify
PTC	Provides full delineation of the biliary tree (proximal and distal); can relieve obstruction through stenting; can provide alternate route for biliary drainage	Invasive procedure, traversing liver capsule with risk of hemorrhage; potential patient discomfort if drain is left in place

Abbreviations: ERCP, endoscopic retrograde cholangiopancreatography; MRCP, magnetic resonance cholangiopancreatography; PTC, percutaneous transhepatic cholangiography; RUQ US, right upper quadrant ultrasound.

liver is desirable, or (2) when the presentation strongly suggests malignant obstruction and the scan will be better at delineating the mass. Imaging features of a malignant obstruction include a periductal mass, biliary hyperenhancement, wall thickness greater than 1.5 mm, long segment involvement, and asymmetric wall thickening. A smooth, symmetric, or focal stricture is more likely benign.

If there is a high probability of an obstruction in the CBD based on ultrasound or CT, **endoscopic retrograde cholangiopancreatography (ERCP)** is usually the next step. ERCP is performed by gastroenterology, and is diagnostically valuable in differentiating between choledocholithiasis, biliary stricture, and masses distal in the CBD. It has the advantage of being able to simultaneously diagnose the problem and perform interventions or take tissue samples. The downside is the risk of iatrogenic pancreatitis associated with the procedure. It is also only suitable for those with normal GI anatomy.

Magnetic resonance cholangiopancreatography (MRCP) is an alternative to ERCP. MRCP avoids the use of radiation and contrast, and does not have the same risks of iatrogenic injury as with ERCP. It can delineate the anatomy of the entire biliary tree, including ducts distal to an obstruction (sometimes impossible with ERCP). Disadvantages include susceptibility to artifacts associated with MRI and a reduced sensitivity for detecting small stones or lesions. MRCP is often chosen over ERCP when the patient is too sick to undergo the procedure, and in other circumstances when there is no anticipated need for an intervention.

Management of Biliary Obstruction

Although the utilization of interventional procedures for biliary obstruction has considerable overlap between benign and malignant etiologies, they really ought to be approached differently, in keeping with the unique management goals of each.

The most common, *acute* cause of benign biliary obstruction is choledocholithiasis. In a patient with choledocholithiasis, the goal is symptomatic relief, as well as avoidance of the most serious complications: cholangitis and pancreatitis. Some patients may already have a complication at the initial presentation, requiring more emergent treatment.

Those that present with acute cholangitis require fluids, broad-spectrum antibiotics, and often ICU admission. After the patient's status has improved with medical management, typically a day or two into the admission, ERCP can be performed to attempt to remove the obstructing stone. After cannulating the ampulla of Vater, stones can be removed with the use of a snare or balloon. Removing the stone and allowing the decompression of upstream infected bile is the key to achieving source control (much like drainage of an abscess). When ERCP is unavailable, anatomically unfeasible, or has already been attempted and failed, IR can assist with **percutaneous transhepatic cholangiography (PTC)** and **percutaneous transhepatic biliary drainage (PTBD)** (**Procedure Box 6.2**) (▶ **Fig. 6.3**, ▶ **Fig. 6.4**). PTBD in the context of treating acute cholangitis has success rates that approach ERCP, however, the rate of complications is somewhat higher.

Gallstone pancreatitis has a wide spectrum of clinical severity. Supportive care is appropriate for the initial management of all patients, however, several studies have shown a benefit of urgent ERCP to restore biliary patency in severe cases, when there is rapidly uptrending LFTs in the first 48 hours of admission. The procedure has been shown to be safe, even in the setting of acute pancreatitis. Percutaneous biliary drainage is not helpful for these patients because the problem stems from the physical presence of the obstructing stone, rather than biliary stasis. Once the patient is stable, cholecystectomy is necessary to prevent recurrent pancreatitis.

Procedure Box 6.2: PTC/PTBD   i

Percutaneous access to the biliary tree is performed for diagnostic cholangiography, biliary drain or stent placement, choledochoscopy, cholangioplasty, and treatment of stones. Biliary access can be safely obtained from a right- or left-sided approach. The right lobe ducts are typically accessed from the right mid-axillary line, usually through the lower intercostal spaces. The left ducts are generally accessed from the epigastrium, below the xyphoid process. It is important to avoid potential interposed stomach or bowel with either approach.

After sterile preparation of the abdomen, a 21- or 22-gauge needle is inserted into the liver using ultrasound or fluoroscopic guidance. Ultrasound guidance can often allow for direct access into a biliary branch, while fluoroscopic approaches require the injection of contrast while withdrawing the needle under fluoroscopic guidance until the biliary tree is opacified. Knowledge of fluoroscopic liver anatomy is critical during these pullback injections, as the veins and arteries are often opacified during this technique. When contrast opacifies the biliary tree under fluoroscopy, a cholangiogram is performed in multiple obliquities and the suitability of the initial access site is determined; if the access is too central, the opacified biliary tree can then be targeted more peripherally under fluoroscopic guidance with a second needle.

After performing cholangiography, a wire is advanced through the needle into the central biliary ducts. The needle is removed and replaced with a transitional dilator which can be disassembled to accommodate a catheter and/or larger guidewire. This facilitates crossing an obstruction and placement of a stiff guidewire for subsequent drain placement or intervention. If the obstruction cannot be crossed, a pigtail drain is placed in the central biliary ducts to allow external drainage; after several weeks of external drainage, inflammation often subsides and strictures or obstructions may be easier to cross. Of note, in the setting of cholangitis, overdistension of the biliary tree with contrast and extensive wire manipulation or intervention should be avoided in the initial access procedure, as this may precipitate biliary sepsis. Serious complications of PTC/PTBD include bleeding, bile leak, and pneumothorax. Arterial hemorrhage can be life threatening and is more likely to occur when the access is too central. Minor hemorrhage may be clinically silent, but more severe hemorrhage can be life threatening and needs to be addressed with an emergent hepatic artery embolization.

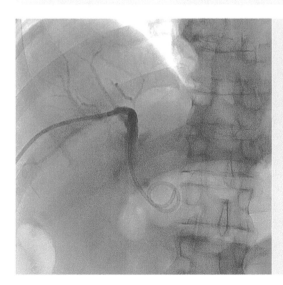

Fig. 6.3 This patient with a choledochojejunal anastomotic stricture required percutaneous placement of an internal–external biliary drainage catheter. An 8.5-Fr biliary catheter was advanced into position with subsequent cholangiogram identifying the catheter loop in the bowel. The catheter side holes span the length of the biliary tree.

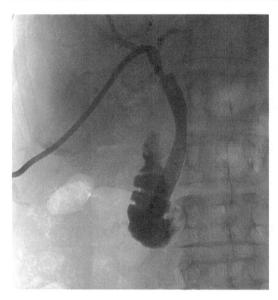

Fig. 6.4 Cholangiogram in a patient with malignant stricture, requiring the placement of a biliary stent. An external drain has been left in place above the stent as a safety for a week to ensure the stent can adequately decompress the biliary tree, after which it will be removed.

In the absence of cholangitis or gallstone pancreatitis, ERCP remains the first-line treatment for uncomplicated choledocholithiasis and has a very high success rate for extracting the stone. When challenges arise, it is typically related to an exceptionally large stone or a stone more proximal in the biliary tree, where navigation of the endoscopic instruments is limited.

For large stones refractory to ERCP, extracorporeal shock wave lithotripsy can be performed, which involves targeting an externally generated sound wave toward the region of the bile duct. The procedure can be quite effective for breaking up large stones, but requires general anesthesia due to the severe pain involved.

If ERCP fails or cannot be performed due to anatomical considerations (i.e., Roux-en-Y anatomy), IR can perform PTC/PTBD and either extract the stone through the percutaneous access site or perform a sphincteroplasty with an angioplasty balloon and push the stone out into the duodenum. In addition, IR can assist the endoscopist by gaining percutaneous access and passing a wire through the CBD into the duodenum where GI can snare it and gain retrograde access to the biliary tree—this is referred to as a "rendezvous procedure."

Anastomotic strictures in postsurgical patients are one of the more common benign biliary strictures treated by IR. ERCP cannot be performed in patients with a duct-to-bowel (choledochojejunal) anastomosis due to the altered anatomy. These patients are managed with plasty of the stricture, and an internal–external drain left in place for a few weeks. The patient is brought back in for a cholangiogram, and if the anastomosis remains patent, the catheter can be removed. Stenting across the anastomotic stricture is considered if balloon dilation fails, although some patients may require surgical revision. Iatrogenic strictures, such as after a cholecystectomy, are also treated quite often percutaneously by IR.

Malignant obstructions generally require tissue diagnosis with either endoscopic ultrasound-guided biopsy or bile duct brushings prior to intervention. Once malignancy is confirmed, the first question is whether the malignancy can be surgically resected, since this could potentially be curative. A discussion of surgical candidacy for pancreaticobiliary malignancies is beyond the scope of this text. In short, if the lesion is unresectable (due to lesion location, involvement of blood vessels, or patient comorbidities), the goal of care is palliative stenting to maintain biliary tree patency.

Stenting can be performed by ERCP or percutaneously by IR (▶ **Fig. 6.4**). Proximal obstructions in the liver or in the hila are more amenable to a percutaneous approach, while distal obstructions are more amenable to ERCP.

For both endoscopic and percutaneous approaches, either plastic or metal stents can be used. Plastic stents tend to become obstructed in the course of several months and require an exchange every 3 months, whereas metal stents (especially covered stents) are less likely to become occluded.

6.3 Chronic Liver Disease and Cirrhosis

One way to understand chronic liver disease is to consider how the liver responds to injury. In acute injury, we expect that once damage is done, the liver heals and the lab abnormalities normalize. This is why asymptomatic patients with incidentally found and mildly abnormal LFTs can be managed with watchful waiting. On the other hand, persistently elevated LFTs (> 6 months) indicate there is ongoing inflammation and necessitates further work-up, even for the asymptomatic patient. The first step is usually a viral hepatitis panel. If this is negative, you would check for less common causes of chronic liver disease such as autoimmune hepatitis, hemochromatosis, or Wilson's disease. If there is a chronic cholestatic pattern, one should also consider primary biliary cirrhosis or primary sclerosing cholangitis. For patients with known risk factors such as long-standing alcohol abuse, hepatitis C, or obesity, a complete serological work-up may be unnecessary.

Liver biopsy for tissue diagnosis remains the cornerstone for diagnosing liver disease. This is particularly important when a patient has liver disease of unknown origin or when a certain liver disease is suspected but needs confirmation. Liver biopsies are also obtained for prognostic and treatment planning purposes when the diagnosis is already known, as with chronic hepatitis. Options for liver biopsies include percutaneous, surgical, or transvenous approaches (**Procedure Box 6.3**).

Procedure Box 6.3: Transvenous Liver Biopsy

Transvenous liver biopsies offer a method of hepatic parenchymal sampling in patients who have intractable coagulopathy (high risk for percutaneous biopsy), with the added benefit of providing portal venous pressure measurement.

A right internal jugular vein approach is preferred for a transvenous liver biopsy as it allows for a better angle into the liver through the inferiorly directed hepatic veins, although this may change in patients with severely shrunken livers in advanced cirrhosis, or in patients who have undergone previous liver transplantation. After obtaining right internal jugular access, one of the hepatic veins (usually the right) is selected and a venogram performed. The right hepatic vein is the posteriormost vein and allows for the biopsy needle to be directed anteriorly into the bulk of the liver parenchyma. Oblique fluoroscopic images are usually obtained to confirm this position.

The biopsy needle is then inserted through a stiff-angled guide cannula into the right hepatic vein, with the cannula directed anteriorly. The biopsy needle is advanced into the liver parenchyma, and biopsies are obtained. This procedure is often accompanied with wedged hepatic vein manometry, which involves placing a catheter distally into a small hepatic vein or inflation of a balloon to temporarily occlude flow, and then connecting the balloon catheter to a pressure monitor; similar to pulmonary wedge pressure measurements, this allows estimation of the portal venous pressure.

Regardless of the hepatic insult, the common pathophysiologic response over time is inflammation that outpaces healing, and resultant fibrosis of the liver parenchyma. We recognize this histologically as **cirrhosis**. The liver compensates for this rather well, and it is not until roughly 80% of the liver is fibrosed that symptoms start to manifest. This is the reason that cirrhosis remains undetected for a long period of time, and is more often an incidental finding.

When symptoms arise, it is due to either: (1) an inability of the liver's synthetic or detoxification function to keep up with the body's demands, or (2) scarring and fibrosis that causes a physical impedance to blood flow into and out of the liver, resulting in portal hypertension.

Symptomatic patients usually undergo imaging studies such as CT or MRI, which may reveal changes in the appearance of the liver or spleen, possibly with the presence of varices, ascites, or perfusional changes (▶ **Fig. 6.5**). Any of these anatomic findings suggests a degree of portal hypertension and requires further evaluation. A relatively new technology is ultrasound or magnetic resonance **elastography.** The technique measures tissue elasticity, which can be used to quantify the fibrotic changes within the liver. Though not widely adopted, its use has been increasing.

Cirrhosis is categorized as being compensated or decompensated. *Compensated* cirrhosis implies that patients have few problems related to their liver dysfunction. They may present with vague symptoms such as weight loss, weakness, or decreased appetite. These patients benefit from routine surveillance for early detection of hepatocellular carcinoma (HCC) and gastroesophageal varices. For HCC surveillance, patients should receive liver ultrasound and alpha-fetoprotein checks every 6 to 12 months.

Patients enter the *decompensated* cirrhosis stage when they become jaundiced, suffer variceal bleeds, ascites, spontaneous bacterial peritonitis, or manifest symptoms of hepatic encephalopathy. A number of scoring/grading systems are available to quantify the level of liver dysfunction. The most commonly used are the model for end-stage liver disease (MELD) score and the Child–Pugh score.

The **MELD** or MELD-Na score takes into account serum bilirubin, serum creatinine, PT/INR, and serum sodium in some cases. Online calculators are readily available and provide a numerical value which corresponds to a 3-month mortality rate (▶ **Table 6.4**). This is also used by the United Network for Organ Sharing (UNOS) for allocation of liver transplants.

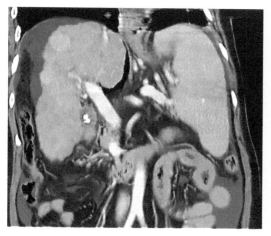

Fig. 6.5 CT image of the abdomen in the coronal plane showing stigmata of cirrhosis: nodular liver contour, splenomegaly, ascites, and an enlarged portal vein. (Source: Herzog C. Differential diagnosis of diseases of the spleen (CT). In: Burgener F, Zaunbauer W, Meyers S, et al., eds. Differential Diagnosis in Computed Tomography. 2nd Edition. Stuttgart: Thieme; 2011.)

Table 6.4 MELD score 3-month mortality

MELD score	3-month mortality
> 40	71%
30–39	53%
20–29	20%
10–19	5–10%
< 9	2%

Abbreviation: MELD, model for end-stage liver disease.

Table 6.5 Child–Pugh score and prognosis

	1 point	2 points	3 points
Total bilirubin	< 2	2–3	> 3
Serum albumin	> 3.5	2.8–3.5	< 2.8
Prothrombin time	< 4	4–6	> 6
Ascites	None	Mild/controlled	Moderate/severe/refractory
Hepatic encephalopathy	None	Grade I–II	Grade III–IV

Child–Pugh A: 5–6 points (2-year survival 85%)
Child–Pugh B: 7–9 points (2-year survival 57%)
Child–Pugh C: 10–15 points (2-year survival 35%)

The **Child–Pugh score** was originally intended to predict operative mortality but is now a prognostic indicator for patients undergoing evaluation for transplant. The score is based on the patient's total bilirubin, serum albumin, PT/INR, degree of ascites, and hepatic encephalopathy (▶ **Table 6.5**).

6.4 Portal Hypertension

Increased intravascular resistance in the cirrhotic liver is a result of both architectural disruption and biochemically mediated vasoconstriction within the hepatic sinusoids. A decrease in vessel diameter increases pressure, resulting in downstream vascular congestion of the portal system. Though cirrhosis is the most common cause of portal hypertension, several other entities can cause it by disrupting flow at different parts of the hepatic vasculature. This includes problems with inflow of portal blood, transit across the hepatic sinusoids, and flow out the hepatic veins (▶ **Table 6.6**).

The hepatic venous pressure gradient (HVPG) is a commonly used clinical parameter for quantifying portal hypertension. The pressure gradient serves as a surrogate for the pressure difference between the systemic and portal systems, and can be measured through a transvenous technique. The portal pressure is obtained by wedging a catheter tip into a hepatic vein. The actual measurement is hepatic sinusoidal pressure, but in a cirrhotic liver the sinusoidal and portal pressures equilibrate, which is why this technique works. The systemic venous pressure is measured free in the hepatic vein, just beyond its interface with the IVC.

A normal pressure gradient is between 1 and 5 mm Hg; pressures exceeding this value define portal hypertension. Keep in mind that a single HVPG measurement is an

Table 6.6 Common causes of portal hypertension

Location	Pathology
Prehepatic	Portal vein thrombosis, pancreatitis
Hepatic/sinusoidal	Cirrhosis, malignancies, infiltrative disorders
Postsinusoidal	Budd–Chiari

approximation. The likelihood is that the gradient fluctuates even when repeating a measurement just minutes later, similar to what you would expect if the same were done measuring your systemic blood pressure with a cuff. However arbitrary it may be, we use the number to help stratify patients and decide when to intervene.

Clinical sequelae of portal hypertension start to develop only when the HVPG is roughly 10 mm Hg or higher, and studies have shown that decreasing the gradient can help reduce the risk of this happening. **Transvenous intrahepatic portosystemic shunt (TIPS)** is a procedure performed by IR with this goal in mind.

The TIPS procedure involves the creation of a channel through the liver parenchyma, connecting the portal vein to a hepatic vein directly, allowing decompression of the portal system. The larger the diameter of the TIPS, the greater the reduction in the pressure gradient. The goal is a reduction to a gradient less than 12 mm Hg, or even lower for non-variceal indications like refractory ascites. This procedure carries with it a significant risk profile, and it is important to fully understand the physiological ramifications before performing it (**Procedure Box 6.4**).

TIPS reduces the amount of blood that travels through the normal anatomical circulation within the liver. Remember that the liver parenchyma receives the majority of its supply from the portal vein. Patients with advanced cirrhosis do not have enough functional reserve to tolerate the shunting of portal blood that occurs after a TIPS (▶ **Table 6.7**). Patients with a MELD score greater than 18 or Child–Pugh grade C disease are usually not candidates for TIPS creation, as this may push these patients into fulminant liver failure (although occasionally it is performed for moribund patients with refractory variceal bleeding with little chance of survival without it). Patients with significant heart failure should also not have TIPS created since the shunt will increase cardiac preload and lead to decompensation. Anyone being considered for TIPS should ideally have an echocardiogram demonstrating right atrial pressure less than 20 mm Hg in order to be considered a candidate.

One of the most common postoperative complications seen is an increase in systemic ammonia, which can cause significant hepatic encephalopathy. The newly created intrahepatic shunt allows blood to go directly from the portal to the systemic circulation, bypassing detoxification by the liver. New or worsening encephalopathy occurs in many patients and manifests within 2 to 3 weeks of shunt creation. Patients older than 65 years, pre-existing hepatic encephalopathy, and large shunt diameter are risk factors for development of post-TIPS encephalopathy. Oral lactulose and/or rifaximin are first line for management of post-TIPS encephalopathy, and are dosed to achieve a target of two to three bowel movements per day. Hepatic encephalopathy that is refractory to medical management may require a TIPS revision with attempted shunt reduction or even occlusion.

A TIPS may also become stenotic or completely occlude on its own, which can be challenging to manage. Patients undergo surveillance with Doppler ultrasound at 4 weeks postprocedure, and then every 6 to 12 months to measure the velocity of blood through the shunt. Velocities less than or equal to 50 cm/s or greater than 250 cm/s are sensitive measures in diagnosing shunt dysfunction. In-stent stenosis or thrombosis warrants venography. Thrombosis can be treated with thrombolysis or thrombectomy, and stenoses with angioplasty; occasionally, re-lining of the shunt with a new stent-graft (particularly if the original shunt was made with a non-covered stent) will be required. Problems with TIPS can also be suspected if there is a recurrence of ascites,

---

Procedure Box 6.4: TIPS

The TIPS procedure is performed to provide an outflow for the overpressurized portal venous system in the setting of cirrhosis, or sometimes hepatic venous outflow obstruction. As ascites expands the potential space between the liver capsule and surrounding tissues, paracentesis is recommended prior to TIPS creation in case the needle inadvertently traverses the liver capsule during the procedure (which could result in life-threatening hemorrhage).

Intravenous antibiotic prophylaxis prior to TIPS creation is recommended. The biliary tree and peritoneum may be colonized with bacteria in cirrhotic patients, which could lead to translocation of bacteria into the bloodstream or seeding of the stent-graft. Many hospitals use general anesthesia when performing TIPS, however, the procedure can be performed under conscious sedation in some patients, particularly in elective cases.

The right internal jugular vein is the preferred access, as there is a relatively straight course into the hepatic veins. Hepatic vein catheterization is performed using a curved catheter and guidewire. The right hepatic vein is preferred as it is usually the posterior-most hepatic vein, which decreases the risk of capsular perforation during needle passes. After advancing the catheter into the right hepatic vein, the catheter is wedged in a venule and a wedged hepatic venogram is performed using CO_2; the low viscosity of CO_2 passes readily through the hepatic sinusoids and fills the portal veins, providing a guide for the direction of needle passage. Another method of increasing popularity is the use of intravascular ultrasound guidance. An ultrasound-tipped catheter can be used to visualize the portal vein. The TIPS needle can then be visualized entering the portal vein. A pre-TIPS portal pressure is also measured.

Multiple commercial TIPS sets are available for parenchymal puncture. The guiding cannula of the TIPS set is advanced over a stiff guidewire into the hepatic vein and directed toward the portal vein (anterior and slightly lateral, in the case of right hepatic vein TIPS). After passing the needle toward the portal vein, the needle or catheter is aspirated using a syringe as it is withdrawn until blood is aspirated. Contrast injection is used to confirm location within the portal vein.

If the portal vein has been accessed in an acceptable location, a wire is then passed, the cannula removed, and a catheter advanced over the wire into the portal system. Pressure measurements are recorded and portal venography is performed to confirm the diagnosis of portal hypertension and to delineate the length of the parenchymal tract. The tract is then predilated with a balloon, allowing a sheath to be advanced through it.

A specially designed stent is used for most TIPS procedures (▶ Fig. 6.6). It has a covered portion (which lies within the intraparenchymal tract), and a 2-cm-long uncovered segment situated in the portal vein. The uncovered portion allows flow to be maintained beyond the stent, into the downstream portal vein. The covered portion extends beyond the tract into the hepatic vein, and sometimes to the level of the IVC. This helps to decrease the risk of stenosis at the hepatic end of the stent.

Following deployment, the stent is expanded using an 8- to 10-mm balloon (▶ Fig. 6.7). Repeat portography is performed and pressure measurements are obtained. A decrease in portal pressure by 50% or portal pressure gradient of less than 12 mm Hg is indicative of a good result.

Table 6.7 Contraindications to TIPS creation

Absolute	Relative
Congestive heart failure	Severe coagulopathy (INR > 3)
Severe pulmonary hypertension (MPWP > 45 mm Hg)	Large liver tumor
Severe tricuspid regurgitation	Thrombocytopenia (platelets < 20,000)
Sepsis	
Liver failure	
Unrelieved biliary obstruction	

Abbreviations: INR, international normalized ratio; MPWP, mean pulmonary wedge pressure; TIPS, transvenous intrahepatic portosystemic shunt.

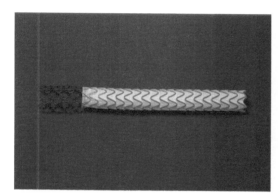

Fig. 6.6 The stent-graft used for transvenous intrahepatic porto-systemic shunt is unique in that it has a covered portion that sits within the newly made tract in the liver, and an uncovered portion within the portal vein.

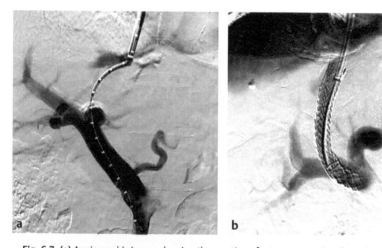

Fig. 6.7 **(a)** Angiographic image showing the creation of a transvenous intrahepatic portosystemic shunt, with a catheter in the hepatic vein, traversing liver parenchyma, and passing into the portal vein. **(b)** A covered stent-graft is placed, maintaining the shunt. The portion of the stent within the new tract is covered, while the portion of the stent that hangs into the portal vein is uncovered.

variceal hemorrhage, or renal dysfunction; these may be a clue that there is a problem with the shunt and warrant further evaluated with an ultrasound. Sometimes a recurrence of symptoms is simply due to a suboptimal reduction in portal pressure. In these cases, a second TIPS can be created in parallel to the first.

6.5 Gastroesophageal Varices and Portosystemic Shunts

When portal hypertension is severe, one physiological consequence is the rerouting of portal blood flow through naturally-occurring collateral pathways that connect the portal and systemic circulation. Normal, low-flow venous communications can become dilated and tortuous as pressure increases, referred to as **varices**. The clinical significance of varices is the potential for rupture, which can cause life-threatening hemorrhage. The goal for managing these patients is to lower the risk of bleeding as much as possible. Taking the time to understand the basic anatomy and physiology of varices will give you a strong foundation to learn about the scope of IR involvement in the care of these patients. Varices can form in several different locations throughout the body, with the esophagus and stomach being the most relevant for IR.

The veins along the upper two-thirds of the esophagus are part of the systemic circulation, draining into the azygous vein and subsequently the SVC. The esophageal veins in the bottom third of the esophagus are part of the portal circulation, draining into the left gastric vein. The upper esophageal veins anastomose with the esophageal veins along the bottom third (▶ **Fig. 6.8**). Portal hypertension in the setting of cirrhosis increases hepatofugal flow of blood (away from the liver) into this pathway, resulting in dilation of the esophageal veins.

Gastric varices are more complicated since the stomach has several different tributaries to the portal vein. The classification can be perplexing considering the number of multiple afferent and efferent vessels, and variation of the drainage pathways. It is extremely important to understand this complexity in order to perform gastric variceal interventions safely. One way to think about them is to classify gastric varices as cardiac or isolated. **Cardiac varices** form from submucosal veins coming off the left gastric vein at the level of the cardia and are continuous with the esophageal veins immediately above. **Isolated varices** are located along the fundus or body, and are supplied by the short gastric, posterior gastric, and gastroepiploic veins. The dominant pathway for reaching the systemic circulation is the gastrorenal shunt, which drains into the left renal vein. A smaller proportion of gastric varices drain into the IVC through a gastrocaval shunt (▶ **Fig. 6.9**). Gastric varices tend to bleed at a lower portal pressure and also have a greater mortality compared to esophageal varices.

Diagnosis of esophageal and gastric varices is made as an incidental finding on cross-sectional imaging, through screening endoscopy specifically looking for varices in a patient with known cirrhosis, or after the patient presents with hematemesis secondary to a variceal bleed.

Management of Varices

In general, management of gastroesophageal varices can be broken down into: (1) primary prophylaxis in patients who have never had a bleed, (2) resuscitation and hemostasis during and immediately after an active variceal bleed, and (3) secondary prophylaxis after a bleed has occurred to prevent recurrence.

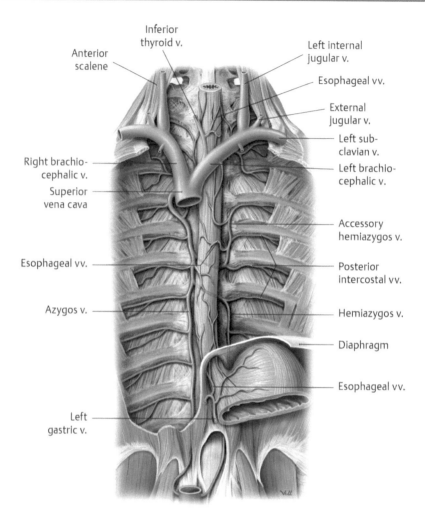

Fig. 6.8 Venous drainage of the esophagus. Note that the distal esophagus is drained by the left gastric vein (part of the portal circulation) while the proximal esophagus is drained by the azygous system (part of systemic circulation). The distal esophageal veins communicate with the more superior esophageal veins. (Source: Gilroy AM, MacPherson BR, Ross LM, eds. Atlas of Anatomy. 2nd ed. Stuttgart: Thieme; 2013:107.)

1. Primary Prophylaxis and Variceal Classification

Patients with newly diagnosed cirrhosis should get an esophagogastroduodenoscopy (EGD) at the time of diagnosis to look for varices (▶ **Fig. 6.10**). Esophageal varices are classified as small (< 5 mm) or large (> 5 mm). The endoscopic appearance of the varix can also identify signs of high risk for bleeding (i.e., red wale marks, "white nipple sign"), and diagnose an active or recent bleed. Gastric varices can be classified based on their location (Sarin classification) and the number of veins feeding or draining the varix. In both esophageal and

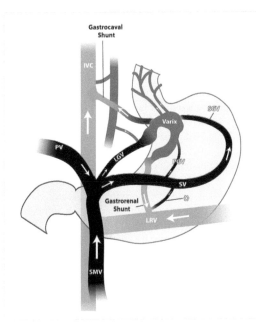

Fig. 6.9 Anatomy of a gastric varix. Portal hypertension forces portal blood flow into the gastric veins, into the varix, which drains out into the left renal vein by way of the gastrorenal shunt. Alternatively, the varix can drain into the IVC by way of the gastrocaval shunt. The arrows in the vessels denote the direction of flow. The gastrorenal shunt is a common target for accessing the varix. (Source: Al-Osaimi A, Caldwell S. Medical and Endoscopic Management of Gastric Varices. Seminars in Interventional Radiology. 2011; 28(03): 273–282.)

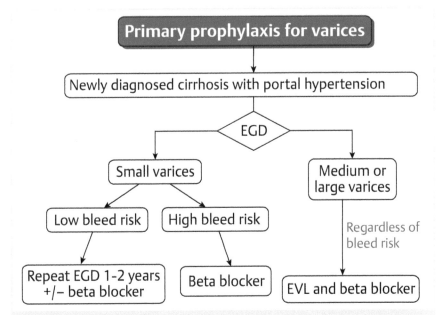

Fig. 6.10 Simplified algorithm for gastroesophageal varices primary prophylaxis. EGD, esophagogastroduodenoscopy; EVL, endoscopic variceal ligation.

gastric varices, the risk of bleeding increases as the size of the varix increases and as the portal hypertension worsens (i.e., increasing pressure gradient).

Patients are risk stratified by varix size, endoscopic high-risk signs, and liver dysfunction. If no varices are found on the initial EGD, no prophylactic treatment is needed. They can return for a repeat surveillance EGD in 2 to 3 years.

Those with small, stable-appearing varices with compensated cirrhosis are considered low risk and are typically put on prophylactic nonselective β-blockers. β-Blockers work by decreasing cardiac output and causing splanchnic vasoconstriction. The latter effect reduces flow in the portal circulation, and in turn decreases pressure within varices.

Some studies have shown a significant reduction in the rate of initial variceal bleeding when patients with small varices are put on a prophylactic β-blocker. However, this is somewhat controversial, as a number of other studies have failed to redemonstrate this decrease in bleeding risk, especially for those with minimal risk factors. Another issue is that β-blockers can cause treatment-limiting side effects in a minority of patients and may need to be discontinued after an initial trial.

If prophylactic treatment is *not* pursued for patients with small varices and compensated cirrhosis (low-risk patients), the recommendation is a repeat EGD in 1-2 years to assess for varix enlargement/development of high-risk signs.

If the small varices have associated endoscopic high-risk signs, the question of whether to start prophylactic nonselective β-blockers is less of an issue. In these cases, β-blockers should definitely be started.

Patients are classified as high risk when varices enlarge, begin to show signs of an imminent bleed, or when liver function deteriorates. High-risk patients are candidates for prophylactic **endoscopic variceal ligation** (EVL), which is an endoscopic technique to stretch a rubber band around the base of the varix. Banding causes the varix to thrombose and eventually slough off. The procedure is typically repeated every 1 to 3 weeks until this happens. Some data support the use of EVL over β-blockers for primary prophylaxis in high-risk patients to prevent a first-time bleed, but it is not straightforward, and the major consensus guidelines suggest that either approach is reasonable.

Neither β-blockers nor EVL actually reduce mortality rate, only reduce the rate of bleeding. Those treated with EVL need to have further surveillance with EGD every 6 to 12 months.

2. Acute Variceal Bleeds

Patients with cirrhosis who present with hematemesis should be assumed to be bleeding secondary to ruptured varices. Management begins with attention to airway, breathing, and circulation, with a low threshold for intubation (▶ Fig. 6.11). These patients can decompensate quickly, and often require ICU-level care.

Splanchnic vasoconstrictive agents, like vasopressin or octreotide, are almost always administered very early to decrease bleeding. Patients are also given prophylactic antibiotics (i.e., norfloxacin), since variceal bleeds cause bacterial gut translocation and subsequent infections.

Once the patient is hemodynamically stable, EGD is performed. Endoscopy will establish the diagnosis of esophageal or gastric varices and allow for intervention.

Bleeding esophageal varices are usually managed with EVL, the same technique used for primary prophylaxis. Sclerotherapy is an older technique that involves injection of a chemical into the varix, causing irritation and thrombosis. It is considered second line since EVL is somewhat safer; however, it is still used as an alternative treatment when EVL is not possible.

Gastric varices at the esophageal junction may be treated with ligation or sclerotherapy, but those within the body or fundus are managed by **endoscopic variceal**

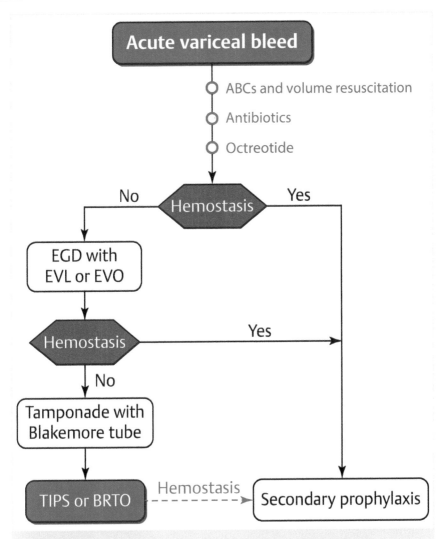

Fig. 6.11 Simplified algorithm for management of acute variceal bleeds. BRTO, balloon-occluded retrograde transvenous obliteration; EGD, esophagogastroduodenoscopy; EVL, endoscopic variceal ligation; EVO, endoscopic variceal obturation; TIPS, transjugular intrahepatic portosystemic shunt.

obturation (EVO). Thicker gastric mucosa in this part of the stomach can make ligation difficult or impossible. EVO involves injection of a superglue-like material into the varix to cause thrombosis.

If patients continue to bleed despite endoscopic therapy, there are several salvage therapeutic measures available. A Sengstaken–Blakemore tube is a balloon-inflatable device that can be inserted into the esophagus as a temporizing measure to tamponade the variceal bleed. EVL or EVO can be reattempted, or otherwise the patient may be brought to IR for an intervention. TIPS can achieve hemostasis in acute variceal bleeds and also reduce the likelihood of a rebleed.

A therapeutic option for acute *gastric* variceal bleeds (but not for esophageal varices) is **balloon-occluded retrograde transvenous obliteration** (**BRTO**). BRTO is an IR procedure used for management of gastric variceal hemorrhage when endoscopic hemostasis fails, provided the anatomy is favorable, and TIPS is not an option.

BRTO involves endovascular delivery of a sclerosant into the varix (**Procedure Box 6.5**). Because a low-resistance pathway is occluded, portal blood flow (and portal pressure) tends to increase after a BRTO. The increase in portal blood flow actually seems to improve liver function and decrease hepatic encephalopathy in some patients after a BRTO. However, the increased portal blood flow also worsens portal hypertension. This is especially important in patients with concomitant esophageal varices as well as gastric varices. The BRTO may take care of the gastric varices but by doing so, esophageal varices may worsen.

Another major complication to keep in mind is acute varix rupture. When the balloon is deployed to occlude the shunt or when the sclerosant is injected into the varix, the increased intravarix pressure may cause the varix to rupture and cause an emergent, possibly life-threatening bleed. In Asia, BRTO has been used for years, and it is gaining traction in the United States.

Transient and self-limited epigastric, chest and back pain, fever, and hematuria are the most common reported complications in the immediate postprocedural setting. A serious complication of BRTO is balloon rupture, allowing systemic dissemination of sclerosant material as it flows downstream into the left renal vein. Rupture of the varix itself can occur during balloon occlusion and injection of the sclerosant, with the potential for massive hemorrhage. These vessels are often very fragile, and wire manipulation should be performed with care to avoid perforation.

Procedure Box 6.5: BRTO

BRTO is a technique used to occlude bleeding gastric varices in the setting of portal hypertension when TIPS is not an option, such as in those who already suffer from hepatic encephalopathy; it may be used regardless of TIPS candidacy for gastric varices in the non-emergent setting. Preprocedural imaging with CTA or MRA is necessary to evaluate for the presence of a gastrorenal/splenorenal shunt, which is frequently identified in these patients.

The procedure is most commonly performed from a right common femoral vein approach; however, the right internal jugular vein can also be utilized. The left renal vein is selected using a catheter and a sheath inserted into the renal vein. Left renal venography is performed and the gastrorenal shunt (typically arising from the cephalad aspect of the midrenal vein) is accessed. A compliant occlusion balloon catheter sized to occlude the draining vein of the gastrorenal shunt is inflated in the shunt, just beyond any important veins that should be spared (such as the left adrenal vein). Balloon occlusion venography can delineate the variceal system and relevant anatomy. The varices are filled with a mixture of sclerosants, contrast or lipiodol, and air (which create a foam consistency and dwells longer in the desired vessels). This is performed using a catheter inserted through or adjacent to the balloon catheter. Sclerosants incite an inflammatory response when exposed to biological tissues. The use of ethanolamine oleate (EO), sodium tetradecyl sulfate (STS), and polidocanol has been described. In the United States, STS is the primary sclerosant used. The sclerosant is administered until the varices are filled but stopped before the material refluxes into the portal venous system. The sclerosant can be contained within the shunt by deploying coils or plugs at the site of the balloon occlusion catheter prior to deflation, or the balloon can be left in place for several hours.

3. Secondary Prophylaxis

Despite the efficacy of many different treatment approaches for variceal bleeding in the acute setting, the risk of a rebleed is high (~ 60%) in the days, weeks, and even years afterward. It is not uncommon for the initial diagnosis of varices to be heralded by an acute bleed, and this type of patient is often a candidate to be started on a β-blocker before discharge from the hospital (▶ **Fig. 6.12**). When used for secondary prophylaxis, β-blockers are typically combined with a nitrate. Together, these medications reduce the rate of rebleeding significantly, but the risk remains rather significant. These medications are also often limited by side effects.

A better strategy is to try to eliminate any varices that are amenable to treatment. The endoscopist can repeat EVL in multiple sessions, with a goal of banding any potentially dangerous varices. Once they are no longer a threat, the patient returns to a surveillance program, with an EGD performed every 6 months and repeat EVL performed as needed. In combination with the use of β-blockers, surveillance and EVL further reduces rebleeding rates.

TIPS performed for secondary prophylaxis is associated with one of the lowest rebleed rates. The drawback is a relatively high rate of hepatic encephalopathy associated with the procedure, which can become difficult to manage. More importantly, the reduced rate of rebleeding is not accompanied by a decrease in mortality. For this reason, the risks associated with it relegate TIPS to more of a rescue therapy. If a rebleed does occur despite prophylactic β-blockade and EVL, TIPS may be the only option (assuming one has not already been placed).

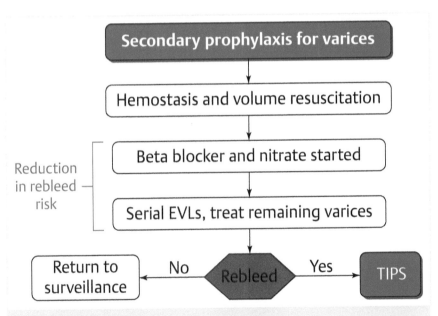

Fig. 6.12 Simplified algorithm for secondary prophylaxis after a variceal bleed. EVL, endoscopic variceal ligation; TIPS, transjugular intrahepatic portosystemic shunt.

6.6 Ascites

Ascites is the most common complication associated with cirrhosis. Portal hypertension–related splanchnic vasodilation activates the renin–angiotensin pathway, leading to sodium and water retention. As the hydrostatic pressure in the splanchnic vessels increases, fluid spills out into the peritoneal cavity.

In some cases, ascites is actually the first sign of decompensated cirrhosis. Patients present with a distended abdomen and often some associated discomfort. Diagnosis is made with a combination of labs and abdominal imaging (ultrasound or CT). Ascites can be graded as mild, moderate, or large. New-onset ascites should be worked up with a diagnostic paracentesis to establish the underlying cause; this is important to determine the treatment approach. In cirrhosis-related ascites, fluid studies typically show polymorphonuclear (PMN) cell count less than 250, a serum-ascites albumin gradient (SAAG) greater than or equal to 1.1, and total protein less than 2.5 g. In the real world, some clinicians just skip the diagnostic paracentesis if the patient has known cirrhosis.

Clinically apparent ascites is managed initially with medication. First-line treatment is with diuretics (especially spironolactone and furosemide). Patients need to limit sodium intake to 2 g/d. Additionally, in alcoholic cirrhosis, abstinence from alcohol can have a dramatic effect on reducing ascites.

If ascites is refractory despite administration of the maximum tolerable and safe dosing of diuretics, and compliance with lifestyle modification, it is usually an indication that liver disease has become advanced and completely irreversible. Even with large-volume paracentesis, the fluid will rapidly reaccumulate. At this point the options are limited to (1) serial paracentesis, (2) TIPS creation, or (3) liver transplant for those who qualify.

Serial paracentesis is often the initial approach and may be used as a temporary strategy for those who will ultimately get a TIPS or transplant. The frequency of paracentesis is typically about 2 weeks. Sometimes IR can assist by placing a tunneled peritoneal catheter for patients in instances where serial paracentesis is not feasible; however, this comes with the undesirable increased risk of infection.

TIPS can be effective for refractory ascites in patients without contraindications, usually only after the patient is found to have difficulty adhering to scheduled serial paracentesis.

6.7 Liver Transplantation and Complications

Patients with end-stage liver disease have a poor prognosis, and liver transplantation is often the best option for those who are candidates. The number of liver transplants performed for both chronic and acute liver failure has increased significantly over the last few decades. Unfortunately, complications are not uncommon after liver transplantation. Interventional radiologists play an important role in the multidisciplinary management of these patients.

Liver Transplant Candidacy

There are a finite number of livers available for transplant and an increasing number of patients awaiting one. A great deal of thought goes into prioritizing these patients, especially in regard to predicting immediate mortality risk. The goal is to allocate liver transplants to have the greatest benefit for the greatest number of people. Patients with fulminant liver failure are given the highest priority; death is imminent if they do not receive a new liver. Patients with chronic end-stage liver disease are prioritized using MELD scores. Unsurprisingly, cirrhosis is the most common indication for a liver transplant.

The MELD score was initially created and used to prognosticate a patient's 3-month mortality risk following TIPS. It was later validated as a tool for determining the 3-month mortality risk in *all* patients with chronic liver disease.

Patients with MELD scores greater than 15 are considered transplant candidates, and are placed on the national liver transplant waitlist. MELD scores are updated frequently. As the MELD score rises, patients move higher on the list.

In certain disease states, MELD exception points are given. The concept of exception points can be best illustrated in patients with cirrhosis and HCC. Small HCCs often do not disqualify patients outright from liver transplant candidacy; however, a patient with stage II HCC may not have liver dysfunction severe enough to give a high MELD score. Because of this, they may be low on the transplant list for a longer period of time, allowing the cancer to advance to a point of disqualifying from transplant candidacy. The solution to this problem is allocation of additional MELD points, termed exception points. Exception points essentially boost the chances of receiving a transplant. Several disease states afford the patient MELD exception points.

When transplantation is a realistic goal, patients undergo a complete work-up to assess fitness for undergoing a major surgery, rule out malignancies or infections elsewhere in the body, and ensure they have the means to comply with the intensive post-surgery regimen.

Contraindications for liver transplantation include poor cardiopulmonary reserve, incurable cancer elsewhere, including metastatic HCC and extrahepatic spread of cholangiocarcinoma. If the pretransplant psychosocial evaluation suggests that a patient may not comply with the post-transplantation expectations (taking daily immunosuppressives, coming to the regular follow-up appointments, abstaining from alcohol/drug use, etc.), the patient may not get a transplant, even if they are otherwise candidates.

Older age, renal insufficiency, hypertension, and diabetes are not prohibitive, but are known risk factors for poor short- and long-term outcomes in transplant recipients. Post-transplant surveillance is more intensive for these patients.

Liver Transplant Type, Technique, and Post–Liver Transplant Anatomy

There are several types of liver transplants. A full-size liver transplant is harvested from a deceased donor. A reduced-size liver transplant is also harvested from a deceased donor but is reduced in size prior to transplantation. With a living-related donor transplant, either the left or right hepatic lobe of a living donor is transplanted into the recipient. With a split liver transplant, the donor cadaveric liver is split into two grafts and each graft is distributed to a separate recipient.

The anatomy of a transplanted patient will differ based on the type of transplantation, the size of the donor liver, and pre-existing aberrant anatomy. It is important that you understand the transplant anatomy prior to any intervention.

A liver transplantation begins with resection of the recipient's diseased liver and all of the vascular/biliary connections. The donor liver is then introduced into the

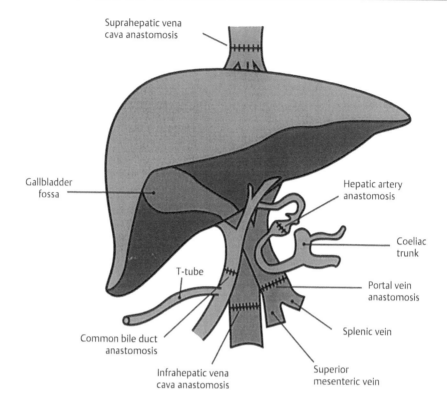

Suprahepatic vena
cava anastomosis

Gallbladder
fossa

Hepatic artery
anastomosis

Coeliac
trunk

T-tube

Portal vein
anastomosis

Common bile duct
anastomosis

Splenic vein

Infrahepatic vena
cava anastomosis

Superior
mesenteric vein

Fig. 6.13 Surgical anastomoses in a liver transplant. (Source: Standard Orthotopic Cadaveric Liver Transplantation. In: Sidhu P, Baxter G, eds. Ultrasound of Abdominal Transplantation. 1st Edition. Thieme; 2002.)

recipient's abdomen. The venocaval anastomosis is performed first, followed by the portal venous, arterial, and biliary anastomoses (▸ **Fig. 6.13**).

Anastomosis of the IVC can be performed end-to-end or by the "piggyback" technique. In the end-to-end anastomosis, a portion of the recipient's IVC is resected along with the diseased liver and replaced with that corresponding section of donor IVC. End-to-end anastomosis has gone out of style as it requires veno-venous bypass and occlusion of the IVC, which may not be feasible in certain patients. The piggyback technique involves leaving the recipient's retrohepatic IVC in place when performing the hepatectomy. Donor IVC is transplanted along with the liver and anastomosed to the stump of the recipient hepatic vein, or side to side with the recipient IVC.

The donor celiac axis is anastomosed to the recipient hepatic artery at the bifurcation of the left and right hepatic arteries, or at the takeoff of the gastroduodenal artery. Recipients with an inadequate hepatic artery may undergo a donor iliac artery interposition graft, anastomosed directly to the recipient aorta. This is called a Carrel patch.

Portal venous anastomosis occurs in an end-to-end fashion from the donor main portal vein to the recipient's main portal vein. In the setting of a split or partial graft, end-to-end anastomosis occurs from the donor's right or left portal vein to the recipient's main portal vein.

Biliary ductal anastomosis can be performed through duct-to-duct reconstruction (choledochocholedochostomy [CDC]), which is preferred, or otherwise a duct-to-bowel reconstruction (Roux-en-Y choledochojejunostomy [CDJ]). In certain cases (sclerosing cholangitis, biliary atresia, duct size mismatch) duct-to-bowel anastomosis is the only option. Some patients may have multiple sites of CDJ.

Post–Liver Transplant Complications

In the immediate post-LT period, elevation of LFTs is common, likely due to ischemia during surgery and reperfusion injury. Transaminases can rise up to four to five times the upper limit of normal shortly after surgery. In uncomplicated cases, LFTs begin normalizing within about a week. There are also expected abnormal post-transplant imaging findings including right-sided pleural effusion, minimal ascites, perihepatic hematoma, and periportal edema. These usually subside within a few weeks.

Patients with transplant complications may be initially asymptomatic since the allograft is not innervated. Post-LT complications should be suspected when there are *persistent* lab abnormalities, or when the LFTs normalize but then go back up. Complications at the anastomoses may also be detected in asymptomatic patients during the routine post-transplant graft evaluation by ultrasound. Cross-sectional imaging may be helpful in deciphering between the multitude of complications that can occur in liver transplant recipients.

The most common cause of graft failure is acute rejection, followed by vascular and biliary anastomotic complications. Acute rejection should be suspected in post-LT patients with fever and globally altered LFTs, although definitive diagnosis can only be made through liver biopsy. Rejection is typically managed with high-dose corticosteroids, but it may require the addition of second-line immunosuppressive therapies.

Complications at the hepatic arterial anastomosis are the most common type of anastomotic problem. Hepatic artery thrombosis is managed with thrombolysis, albeit cautiously given the increased risk of bleeding. Hepatic artery stenosis is managed with angioplasty. Stenting is avoided initially as it can make future revascularization attempts difficult (surgical or percutaneous). As such, stenting is considered *only* when a stenosis recurs, or if a flow-limiting dissection occurs during angioplasty. Hepatic arterial stenosis can also result in biliary ischemia, since the hepatic artery supplies the bile ducts. Less common complications include hepatic artery pseudoaneurysms and intrahepatic arterioportal fistulae secondary to liver biopsies. Pseudoaneurysms are treated with coil embolization, while fistulae may be observed in many patients, but may require endovascular therapy when they cause significant symptoms.

Biliary complications usually manifest in the early postoperative period (< 3 months). Biliary leak can occur at the cystic duct remnant, at the ductal anastomosis, or at the cut edge of the liver. If a surgical drain is present, bile leaks will manifest as an increase in bilious output. If a surgical drain is not present, bile will accumulate in the peritoneal cavity and result in abdominal pain, distension, and jaundice. Bile leaks require biliary diversion via an endoscopic stent or percutaneous drain placement for several weeks until the defect has healed. Large intraperitoneal biliary collections should also be drained directly.

Biliary strictures usually occur at the site of surgical anastomosis or secondary to hepatic artery ischemia, and present with jaundice/rising direct bilirubin. While other LFT abnormalities may also be present, an elevated and uptrending direct bilirubin is the most specific sign. Strictures are treated with plasty and stenting if they are causing significant biliary stasis. Note that percutaneously accessing the biliary tree in a transplanted liver is generally more difficult due to postsurgical anatomy, and in the setting of leak it can be extremely difficult due to decompression of the ducts.

Complications at the portal vein and the hepatic vein/IVC anastomosis are less common. When they occur, portal vein complications can cause worsening portal hypertension (ascites, varices, etc.), and hepatic vein anastomotic complications can cause allograft enlargement, hepatic dysfunction, and even lower extremity edema. Like hepatic artery stenoses, venous stenoses are also initially managed with angioplasty, with stenting reserved for refractory or recurrent cases.

Suggested Readings

[1] Ahmed O, Mathevosian S, Arslan B. Biliary interventions: tools and techniques of the trade, access, cholangiography, biopsy, cholangioscopy, cholangioplasty, stenting, stone extraction, and brachytherapy. Semin Intervent Radiol. 2016; 33(4):283–290

[2] Friedewald SM, Molmenti EP, DeJong MR, Hamper UM. Vascular and nonvascular complications of liver transplants: sonographic evaluation and correlation with other imaging modalities and findings at surgery and pathology. Ultrasound Q. 2003; 19(2):71–85, quiz 108–110

[3] Garcia-Tsao G, Sanyal AJ, Grace ND, Carey W; Practice Guidelines Committee of the American Association for the Study of Liver Diseases. Practice Parameters Committee of the American College of Gastroenterology. Prevention and management of gastroesophageal varices and variceal hemorrhage in cirrhosis. Hepatology. 2007; 46(3):922–938

[4] Gulaya K, Desai SS, Sato K. Percutaneous cholecystostomy: evidence-based current clinical practice. Semin Intervent Radiol. 2016; 33(4):291–296

[5] Keller FS, Farsad K, Rösch J. The transjugular intrahepatic portosystemic shunt: technique and instruments. Tech Vasc Interv Radiol. 2016; 19(1):2–9

[6] Patel A, Fischman AM, Saad WE. Balloon-occluded retrograde transvenous obliteration of gastric varices. AJR Am J Roentgenol. 2012; 199(4):721–729

[7] Pomerantz BJ. Biliary tract interventions. Tech Vasc Interv Radiol. 2009; 12(2):162–170

[8] Quiroga S, Carmen Sebastià M, Margarit C, Castells L, Boyé R, Alvarez-Castells A. Complications of orthotopic liver transplantation: spectrum of findings with helical CT. Radiographics. 2001; 21(5):1085–1102

[9] Runyon BA; Practice Guidelines Committee, American Association for the Study of Liver Diseases (AASLD). Management of adult patients with ascites due to cirrhosis. Hepatology. 2004; 39(3):841–856

[10] Saad WE. Transjugular intrahepatic portosystemic shunt before and after liver transplantation. Semin Intervent Radiol. 2014; 31(3):243–247

[11] Saad WE, Darcy MD. Transjugular intrahepatic portosystemic shunt (TIPS) versus balloon-occluded retrograde transvenous obliteration (BRTO) for the management of gastric varices. Semin Intervent Radiol. 2011; 28(3):339–349

7 Oncology

Shantanu Warhadpande, Alex Lionberg, Junjian Huang, Carl Schmidt, and Jonathan G. Martin

It has become abundantly clear that the care of cancer patients is best approached by a multidisciplinary team, including interventional radiologists and medical, surgical, and radiation oncologists. Tumor boards provide an opportunity for experts to collaboratively discuss individualized care for each patient. As the role of interventional oncology (IO) continues to expand, it is vitally important that every interventional radiologist has the relevant clinical knowledge to understand the complexities of cancer treatment, beyond just the technical aspects of the procedure. This chapter is an introduction to the clinical care of cancer patients who benefit from IO procedures, some of which have been firmly established and others which are newly emerging.

7.1 Hepatocellular Carcinoma

Approach to a New Liver Mass

Patients with liver lesions are usually referred to a specialist after a lesion has been detected on imaging. Before the patient even walks into the clinic, there is already a good sense of what you're dealing with based on imaging characteristics (▶ Table 7.1). In some cases, the imaging is suboptimal, and further studies are needed. Ultrasound, CT, and MRI all have a role in liver imaging, each with its advantages and disadvantages (▶ Table 7.2).

Liver lesions are often asymptomatic, and diagnosis may be solely based on imaging. A thorough history and examination is mandatory for all potential IO patients, regardless of the presumed diagnosis. Risk factors can help narrow the differential, especially if imaging characteristics are ambiguous. For example, a young female on birth control is more likely to develop an adenoma, while a patient with cirrhosis should make you think about hepatocellular carcinoma (HCC). The physical examination should look for

Table 7.1 Characteristic imaging appearance of liver lesions

Liver lesion differential	Imaging characteristics
Adenoma	Imaging varies significantly, most commonly arterial hyperenhancement with enhancement equal to normal liver in later phases
Focal nodular hyperplasia	Arterial hyperenhancement with enhancement equal to liver on later phases, nonenhancing central scar is the key diagnostic feature
Hemangioma	Discontinuous, progressive, peripheral nodular enhancement
HCC	Arterial hyperenhancement with washout (decreased contrast relative to normal liver) in later phases; often with a capsule
Cholangiocarcinoma	Delayed, progressive, persistent enhancement
Metastatic lesions	Highly variable, often demonstrates peripheral enhancement or arterial hyperenhancement. Usually multiple in number

Abbreviation: HCC, hepatocellular carcinoma.

cirrhotic stigmata (jaundice, scleral icterus, etc.), signs of extrahepatic malignancy, and an assessment of functional status. Baseline labs should include complete blood count (CBC), liver function tests (LFTs), coags, hepatitis panel, and tumor markers.

Working up a Suspected Liver Malignancy

The first step when working up a suspected liver neoplasm is determining if the patient has cirrhosis. For those with cirrhosis, the diagnosis will almost always be HCC (▶ Fig. 7.1). In these patients, the diagnosis can be made with imaging alone.

In a noncirrhotic liver, a malignant-appearing lesion is more likely to be metastatic disease. These patients should undergo a thorough work-up including age-appropriate screening, as well as dedicated CT imaging of the chest, abdomen, and pelvis. Further evaluation might include MRI (especially if the liver lesion is indeterminate on CT), or percutaneous biopsy (**Procedure Box 7.1**).

Tumor markers can be helpful, but not always. If they're elevated, it adds to your evidence, but negative markers do not rule out a malignancy. If HCC is the presumed diagnosis, a baseline alpha fetoprotein (AFP) should be measured. AFP, CA 19-9 and carcinoembryonic antigen (CEA) are mainly used to monitor treatment response to HCC, cholangiocarcinoma, and colorectal cancer, respectively.

Table 7.2 Differences in liver imaging modalities

Modality	Advantages	Disadvantages
CT	Comprehensive look at abdominal anatomy; fast	Radiation; requires contrast; poor evaluation of the biliary system
MRI	Better characterization of the biliary system; most sensitive for lesion detection and characterization	Motion limits evaluation of the bowel; takes longer to do; most expensive
Ultrasound (US)	Quick, portable, cheap; good for screening	Limited ability to detect lesions; poor lesion characterization

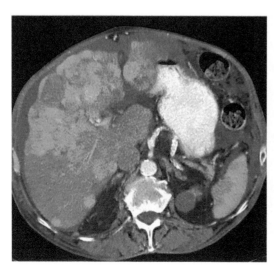

Fig. 7.1 Contrast-enhanced CT showing numerous liver masses with the characteristic appearance of hepatocellular carcinoma. (Source: Herzog C. Diffuse hepatocellular carcinoma (HCC). In: Burgener F, Zaunbauer W, Meyers S, et al., eds. Differential Diagnosis in Computed Tomography. 2nd edition. Stuttgart: Thieme; 2011.)

Once a liver lesion is diagnosed as HCC, the extent of liver disease needs to be determined. The overwhelming majority of patients who develop HCC have some degree of cirrhosis. One of the many ways liver dysfunction can be categorized is by the Child–Pugh and the model for end-stage liver disease (MELD) scores.

The Child–Pugh score was originally intended to predict operative mortality but is now a prognostic indicator for determining the severity of liver disease and the need for transplant in cirrhotics. The score is based on the patient's total bilirubin, serum albumin, prothrombin time (PT)/international normalized ratio (INR), degree of ascites, and hepatic encephalopathy (▶Table 7.3).

MELD takes into account serum bilirubin, serum creatinine, PT/INR, and serum sodium in some cases. Calculators for the MELD score are available online, with numerical scores corresponding to a 3-month mortality rate (▶Table 7.4).

Procedure Box 7.1: Percutaneous Biopsy　ⓘ

Biopsies can be performed with either ultrasound or CT guidance. There are several key steps to keep in mind when performing biopsies. First, ensure the target lesion is safely accessible before starting. If the lesion is too deep for the available needles or if there are vital structures between the skin and target, biopsy should not be performed. Next, keep in in mind where the lesion is and be prepared for the organ-specific complications that can arise postbiopsy. Biopsies may seem simple, but serious complications can and do occur.

Fine-needle biopsies use 20- to 25-gauge needles, which are relatively atraumatic and can even go through bowel without causing problems in most cases; however, they may not provide tissue samples large enough for accurate diagnosis. Core biopsy needles are typically 14 to 20 gauge, and can provide more substantial samples. Core biopsies are ideal when the patient has a lesion without a known primary malignancy, and a larger chunk of tissue is needed for diagnosis. These needles generally should not go through bowel.

For liver biopsies, it is important to determine whether the patient has ascites and/or advanced cirrhosis, which can make puncture of the liver capsule difficult and increase the risk of bleeding. Hepatic dome tumors may require a transpleural approach. Superficial lesions should not be approached directly, but instead using a path that allows the needle to traverse some parenchyma before hitting the target lesion. This way, if bleeding occurs, there is a greater likelihood the needle tract will thrombose and result in hemostasis.

Table 7.3 Child–Pugh scoring

	1 point	2 points	3 points
Total bilirubin	< 2	2–3	> 3
Serum albumin	> 3.5	2.8–3.5	< 2.8
Prothrombin time	< 4	4–6	> 6
Ascites	None	Mild/controlled	Moderate/severe/refractory
Hepatic encephalopathy	None	Grade I–II	Grade III–IV

Child–Pugh A: 5–6 points (2-year survival 85%)
Child–Pugh B: 7–9 points (2-year survival 57%)
Child–Pugh C: 10–15 points (2-year survival 35%)

The patient's functional status is also important when starting to think about treatment options. It can be determined using a tool such as the Eastern Cooperative Oncology Group (ECOG) performance scale. The Barcelona Clinic Liver Cancer (BCLC) and the Hong Kong Liver Cancer (HKLC) staging classification systems incorporate both the extent of the disease and performance status to help determine the treatment strategy. Albumin–Bilirubin (ALBI) score is one other grading system you might hear about. In current clinical practice, the BCLC, HKLC, and ALBI are used as rough guides rather than part of a rigid algorithm.

Management of HCC

HCC treatment options include resection, transplantation, chemoembolization, radio-embolization, ablation, stereotactic body radiation therapy (SBRT), and systemic chemotherapy (▶ Fig. 7.2).

Table 7.4 MELD score

MELD score	3-month mortality
> 40	71%
30–39	53%
20–29	20%
10–19	6%
< 9	2%

Abbreviation: MELD, model for end-stage liver disease.

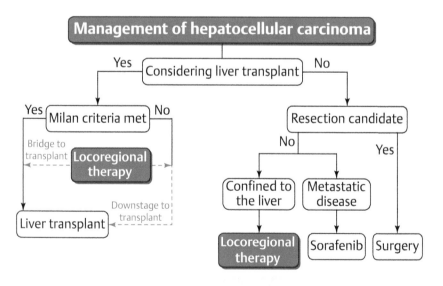

Fig. 7.2 Simplified algorithm for management of hepatocellular carcinoma. Locoregional therapy includes transarterial radioembolization/chemoembolization and percutaneous ablation.

Resection

For nontransplant candidates with HCC, surgical resection is the preferred option, since it has the highest potential to be curative. To determine the resectability of HCC, a number of anatomic and functional factors need to be considered.

Patients with Child–Pugh A cirrhosis may tolerate even a major liver resection so long as they do not have portal hypertension. Patients with Child–Pugh B cirrhosis and no portal hypertension may tolerate a moderate or minor hepatectomy (particularly laparoscopic operations). Major hepatectomy is usually contraindicated. Patients with Child–Pugh C cirrhosis and any patient with portal hypertension are generally not candidates for *any* liver resection.

In a noncirrhotic with HCC, up to 80% of the liver can be removed without compromising long-term liver function. In cirrhotic patients with HCC, no more than 50 to 60% of the liver volume can be resected. Interventional radiologists can help these patients by performing a preoperative **portal vein embolization** (**Procedure Box 7.2**). Embolization of the portal vein supplying the liver segments to be resected is performed weeks to months in advance of the surgery. The liver responds by hypertrophy of the nonembolized liver segments. As a result, the liver remnant may become large enough to allow for safe resection of the cancer-containing segments (▶ **Fig. 7.3**).

Procedure Box 7.2: Portal Vein Embolization ⓘ

Portal vein embolization is performed to cause hypertrophy of the future liver remnant prior to partial hepatectomy. A needle is used to percutaneously access the portal system (▶ **Fig. 7.4**). Most commonly, the procedure targets the right hepatic lobe; if the left lobe is diseased and planned for resection, the right lobe is usually already large enough to maintain adequate function. Whereas, if the right lobe is diseased, the smaller left lobe may need to hypertrophy beforehand.

Once the portal vein is accessed percutaneously, a catheter is used to select the branch of the portal vein feeding the lobe to be resected, and embolization can proceed. A variety of embolic materials have been used for preoperative portal vein embolization including coils, gelatin sponge, n-butyl cyanoacrylate (NBCA), polyvinyl alcohol (PVA), tris-acryl microspheres and ethanol. Nonabsorbable materials are preferred because surgery is usually performed weeks to months after PVE.

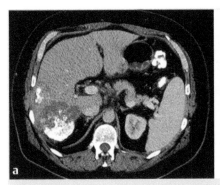 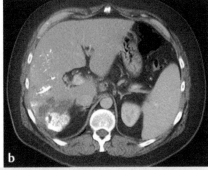

Fig. 7.3 This patient underwent a right portal vein embolization (PVE) in preparation for a right hepatectomy. Note the difference in size of the left hepatic lobe **(a)** before and **(b)** after PVE.

Generally, as long as a liver mass does not disturb the hepatic inflow (via the hepatic artery and portal vein) and hepatic outflow (via at least one hepatic vein), it can be resected in most patients. Central lesions cannot be resected for this reason. Finally, as with any surgical patient, respiratory and cardiac comorbidities factor into overall procedural risk.

Transplantation

A cirrhotic liver will continue to be a breeding ground for new areas of HCC. A liver transplantation offers the patients not only a cure of their current malignancy, but also addresses the underlying liver dysfunction and predisposition for developing more cancer. Transplantation is a definitive treatment option reserved for early-stage HCC patients with cirrhosis, though they have to be transplant candidates. In most institutions, the Milan criteria is used to identify transplant candidacy. This takes into consideration the tumor size, number, and location (▶ Table 7.5). In 1996, a paper published by Mazzaferro et al showed that outcomes for transplanted HCC patients that met this criteria were similar to cancer-free transplanted patients. The study is criticized for its limitations, and data published since then suggests that more inclusive criteria, allowing for somewhat larger tumors, do not adversely impact 5-year survival. The University of California San Francisco (UCSF) criteria is an alternative that takes this into account. For cancer and cancer-free patients alike, liver transplantation requires a great deal of planning and close follow-up. Transplantation is discussed in greater detail in Chapter 6.

Locoregional Therapy

The options for locoregional therapy include transarterial bland, chemo- or radio-embolization, and ablation. In general, locoregional therapy is an option when a patient

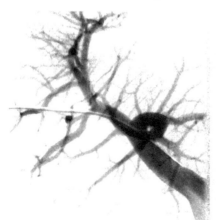

Fig. 7.4 Venogram demonstrating an opacified portal venous system following percutaneous access.

Table 7.5 The Milan criteria

Single HCC < 5 cm, or up to three nodules < 3 cm each

No evidence of gross vascular invasion

No regional nodal or distant metastases

Abbreviation: HCC, hepatocellular carcinoma.

with HCC is not a transplant or resection candidate. In some patients who meet or are close to meeting transplant candidacy, these procedures can be used as adjunctive therapy until they are definitively treated with a new liver. In select cases, locoregional therapy itself can be potentially curative.

For patients within the Milan criteria, the primary goal is to prevent the patient's current lesions from growing to the point of nullifying transplant eligibility. The interventional radiologist plays a role in **"bridging to transplant"** when locoregional therapy is performed to halt tumor progression and maintain the patient's transplant candidacy. The use of bridging therapy can prevent qualified transplant recipients from dropping off the list due to disease progression. Transplant guidelines now make all patients wait 6 months before MELD exception points are given. This waiting period allows tumors with aggressive biology to declare themselves. Less aggressive tumor biology portends better outcomes for transplantation, though the longer wait for exception points can still be detrimental to these patients. Bridging therapies will be even more important to address this going forward.

For patients who are just outside the Milan criteria for transplantation, the question then becomes whether the patient's tumors can be sufficiently reduced in size and number to make them eligible for transplantation. If yes, therapy should be directed toward this goal. An example is a patient who has one 2-cm mass and one 4-cm mass, which puts him outside of the Milan criteria. If locoregional therapy is performed and the 4-cm mass decreases in size to 2.5 cm, the patient is now eligible for liver transplant. This is called **"downstaging to transplant."**

If downstaging is not feasible, attention is turned toward prolonging life before the patient succumbs to the disease. Ablation and embolization can both be performed and repeated if necessary, with the aim of reducing or slowing disease progression, adding months or even years of survival.

Thermal **ablation** by radiofrequency (RFA) or microwave (MWA) is a good option for small (< 3–5 cm) HCC lesions. RFA and MWA involve percutaneous (occasionally laparoscopic or open surgical) insertion of a probe into the tumor and heating it to the point of necrosis (**Procedure Box 7.3**). Lesions larger than 3 cm can be ablated, but recurrence rates are higher. Generally speaking, ablation is avoided for central lesions very close to the confluence of bile ducts or in close proximity to blood vessels. Proximity to blood flow tends to limit ablation efficacy as the vessels cause a heat sink effect, keeping temperatures from reaching the desired therapeutic level. In select cases (an isolated, small HCC lesion), ablation *can* be curative.

Transarterial chemoembolization (TACE) involves injecting chemotherapy into a branch of the hepatic artery feeding the tumor. The reason this works is because of the dual blood supply of the liver. Liver malignancies are supplied predominantly from the hepatic artery branches (> 80%), while normal liver parenchyma is supplied mostly by the portal vein. By selectively treating the arterial system, TACE can be used to target the cancer without causing major damage to the liver parenchyma (**Procedure Box 7.4**).

There are several different types of transarterial embolization, which differ based on materials used. In conventional TACE, the cocktail injected includes a chemotherapeutic drug, lipiodol, and an embolic substance.

The chemotherapeutic drug used for TACE varies, and no studies have concluded that one is definitely better than another. Options include some combination of emulsified doxorubicin, cisplatin, and mitomycin. Alternatively, an embolic agent can be used without any chemotherapy, which is called bland embolization. Yet another option is the use of drug-eluting beads (DEB-TACE), which slowly elutes a chemotherapy agent, often doxorubicin.

Ablation techniques offer the ability to kill tumors percutaneously, without the need for open surgical resection or potentially toxic chemotherapy. The most common forms of ablation involve the application of heat (RFA or MWA) or cold (cryoablation). One advantage of cryoablation over RFA/MWA is that the resultant ice ball can be directly visualized on CT scans. Visualization of the ice ball is especially important when there are vital structures near the target lesion, such as when the colon lies within close proximity to an RCC. Patients usually experience minimal pain with cryoablation, while heat can cause significant pain. With RFA and MWA, heat sink effect needs to be taken into account. When ablating a lesion close to a blood vessel, the flow of blood tends to carry the heat away, decreasing the maximum temperature reached within the tissue. This results in a suboptimal burn and may lead to an incomplete treatment.

The initial approach to an ablation is similar to the approach to a percutaneous biopsy. The lesion is identified under CT or ultrasound, and a safe access is planned. Special attention is paid to adjacent organs, and adjunctive techniques like hydrodissection may be used to move sensitive tissues away from the ablation zone. Ablation equipment (size and number of probes/needles) is selected so as to sufficiently cover the entire lesion, including a margin of normal tissue to ensure complete and effective therapy.

Under CT or ultrasound guidance, the probes are placed through the lesion, and heat or cold then applied. Ablation devices vary, but thermal effects are typically applied for approximately 10 to 20 minutes. Ultrasound and CT can be used to evaluate treatment effect during ablation, and the probes can be repositioned as needed.

When a satisfactory result is obtained, the needles are removed and a postablation scan is performed to ev for bleeding or other complications, such as unintended damage to adjacent tissues. Repeat contrast-enhanced scans are performed in the coming months to identify resolution or areas that may require additional treatment.

Lipiodol is poppy seed oil that is injected along with the chemotherapy. It is taken up by the tumor and provides a radiopaque appearance on follow-up imaging. Retained lipiodol on follow-up imaging is an indicator of appropriately-targeted therapy, and correlates with treatment response in many patients. The embolic agent (Gelfoam, PVA, microspheres) is injected after the chemotherapy–lipiodol mixture.

Lobar embolization involves infusion of the materials from a more proximal point in the hepatic artery and is preferred when there are multiple tumors (or one large tumor) supplied by that hepatic artery branch (▶ Fig. 7.5). *Segmental* embolization is preferable when there is a single smaller tumor, and is performed by positioning the catheter more distal, in a second- or third-order artery.

Contraindications to chemoembolization are less stringent than for surgery, though patients still need to be selected appropriately (▶ Table 7.6).

Transarterial chemoembolization should not be performed when the patient's functional liver reserve is too low. Patients undergoing embolization for HCC invariably have background hepatic dysfunction secondary to cirrhosis. When the embolization is performed, although the malignant lesions are targeted, at least some liver parenchyma will also be affected by the treatment. If the patient's liver function is poor, this may tip them over into fulminant hepatic failure and death. Most of the TACE contraindications are defined as such so that patients at greatest risk for these complications will be excluded from eligibility.

Procedure Box 7.4: Transarterial Chemoembolization and Radioembolization ⓘ

TACE and Y-90 therapies offer an alternative locoregional treatment for malignancies in the liver, allowing high doses of chemotherapy-eluting or beta-radiation–emitting embolic material directly to the tumors, while minimizing systemic side effects. The procedure is essentially the same for both TACE and Y-90.

After obtaining femoral access, a superior mesenteric artery (SMA) arteriogram with delayed imaging is performed to confirm portal vein patency and exclude common variants such as an anomalous origin of the right hepatic artery; a recent contrast-enhanced CT or MR may obviate the need for this step. The celiac artery is then accessed and an arteriogram performed to map out the arterial anatomy. A catheter is advanced into the common hepatic artery if possible, which is left in place for the duration of the procedure. Through this catheter, a microcatheter/guidewire system is used to select the branch of interest.

During a TACE, infusion materials may be delivered from a proximal point in the hepatic arterial system (right hepatic or left hepatic artery), which is known as lobar embolization. Lobar embolization is usually preferred when there are multiple lesions in the liver, which cannot be treated separately. If treating a small tumor, individual segmental arterial branches can be selected, and superselective embolization performed. If the lesion is large, the microcatheter may need to be positioned more proximally in the artery. Embolic material is slowly injected under direct fluoroscopic visualization, taking care not to inject too hard or beyond the endpoint of sluggish forward flow, which could cause reflux of embolic material into non-target territories.

With TARE, reflux is a much more catastrophic event than in TACE, and additional steps are taken to minimize potential reflux. This includes using the initial MAA planning study to ensure there is no extrahepatic shunting and to identify any problematic vessels that might provide a route for reflux. During the TARE procedure, these problematic vessels may need coil embolized to seal them off.

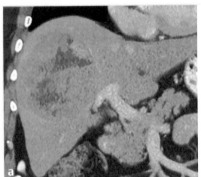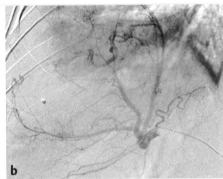

Fig. 7.5 (a) This patient was evaluated for a possible extended right hepatectomy for a large hepatocellular carcinoma but was deemed a nonsurgical candidate given the tumor size, location (abutting the hepatic inflow vessels), and the patient's comorbidities. Locoregional therapy with transarterial chemoembolization was pursued. (b) Hepatic artery digital subtraction angiography image shows significant mass effect on the vessels as they course around the large tumor.

Table 7.6 Contraindications to TACE

Very large bilobar tumor burden (> 50%)

Impaired portal vein blood flow (portal vein thrombosis, hepatofugal blood flow)

Decompensated cirrhosis (tense ascites, clinical encephalopathy, hepatorenal syndrome)

Renal insufficiency

High bilirubin

Abbreviation: TACE, transarterial chemoembolization.

As previously described, chemoembolization involves disruption of the preferential arterial supply to the malignancy and preserving the portal venous supply. If the portal vein is occluded to begin with, the parenchyma is reliant on arterial blood supply. Portal vein thrombosis is not uncommon in the setting of cirrhosis, and therefore the patency of the portal vein must be confirmed prior to treatment. This can be done by ultrasound, CT, MRI, or delayed portal venous phase angiography.

Similarly, if there are other signs of background liver dysfunction, including elevated total serum bilirubin (usually > 2 mg/dL), or decompensated cirrhosis (tense ascites, clinical encephalopathy, hepatorenal syndrome), embolization is generally not considered safe. If the liver is completely tumor filled, the level of intervention required for effective therapy is more likely to result in harm (fulminant liver failure) than any significant benefit.

Complications of chemoembolization are related to ischemic damage to the liver or from nontarget embolization. Biliary tree injuries and hepatic abscesses are examples of complications that result from parenchymal damage. Biliary injuries are more common because the biliary system, unlike hepatocytes, is primarily supplied by the hepatic arteries. Reflux of embolic material can result in gastroduodenal embolization, resulting in gastric/duodenal ulceration.

Approximately 90% of patients will have **postembolization syndrome** following transarterial embolization, characterized by a constellation of symptoms including low-grade fever, nausea, vomiting, right upper quadrant pain, and transaminitis. CT imaging during this period may show findings that mimic an abscess, so it is important to recognize this as normal. It should evolve/involute over time, whereas an abscess will persist or increase. If postembolization syndrome is suspected, imaging may only lead to confusion, and should therefore be avoided. Postembolization syndrome is usually transient and resolves within a week.

Yttrium-90 **radioembolization,** also called transarterial radioembolization (TARE) or selective internal radiation therapy (SIRT), is similar to TACE, but with a few important differences (**Procedure Box 7.4**). Instead of chemoembolic material, radioactive Y-90–labeled microspheres (resin or glass) are delivered into the hepatic artery branch supplying the tumor. Whereas TACE/bland embolization causes hepatocyte necrosis, TARE with Y-90 leads to tumor shrinkage mostly by apoptosis, and does not cause a postembolization syndrome. One other advantage of TARE over TACE is that it can be performed in the setting of portal vein thrombosis. Because the arterial inflow is less disrupted by the relatively smaller embolic character of these particles, the normal liver parenchyma will continue to receive adequate perfusion for normal hepatic function. Y-90 contraindications are similar to those for TACE with a few notable additions (▶**Table 7.7**).

Radioembolization requires an arterial mapping procedure prior to the embolization. This is to avoid nontarget embolization, to ensure the procedure will besafe to perform, and to calculate the dose that should be delivered to achieve the desired effect.

A major concern with TARE is the potential delivery of the radioactive material into nontarget organs, such as the lung or GI tract. Before the radioembolization, an angiogram is performed in the IR suite to visualize the hepatic vasculature. If vessels are identified which cannot be avoided by catheter positioning alone, including branches to the skin, stomach, duodenum, or feeding distant organs, IR may embolize them prior to radioembolization.

After any accessory vessels have been embolized, the next step is a catheter infusion of Tc-99m microaggregated albumin (MAA) to the hepatic artery. The MAA mimics the beads used with radioembolization, and the radiolabel allows the use of scintigraphy to demonstrate the distribution of infused materials (▶ Fig. 7.6). A nuclear medicine scan is performed after the infusion to determine the fraction of drug being shunted to the lungs or other extrahepatic locations. A small amount of shunting of blood from liver to the lungs is a normal process, but can occur at levels which make radioembolization unsafe. If the dose of radiation delivered to the lungs is greater than 30 Gy in a single treatment or greater than a cumulative dose of 50 Gy across multiple treatments, radioembolization should not be performed. The MAA study calculates a shunt fraction to the lungs that is used along with the tumor volume and other factors to calculate the treatment dose. There should *never* be shunting to the GI tract; even the smallest shunt fraction to the GI tract is unacceptable.

In TACE, a small amount of nontarget embolization to the GI system is likely to have a transient effect. With TARE, however, even a very small number of radioembolization particles are likely to cause significant enteritis or ulceration. Similarly, a dose to the gallbladder may result in acute cholecystitis, a sufficiently high dose to the lung may cause radiation pneumonitis, and nontargeted dose (by way of the falciform artery) to the periumbilical skin may cause radiation necrosis. Although potentially severe, these complications are quite rare at high-volume centers.

Table 7.7 TARE contraindications

TARE absolute contraindications	TARE relative contraindications
Pregnancy	Prior liver radiotherapy
Uncorrectable hepatopulmonary shunting	Malignant infiltration of portal vein
Uncorrectable GI vascular reflux	Elevated bilirubin
Breastfeeding	

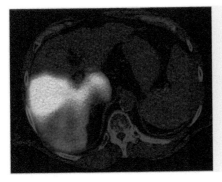

Fig. 7.6 A microaggregated albumin (MAA) planning study is performed before a Y-90 radioembolization treatment. This nuclear medicine scan was obtained after intra-arterial injection of a radiotracer into the hepatic artery. MAA mapping ensures that radiotracer activity is confined to the targeted liver lesion and not unexpectedly shunted to the GI tract or the lungs.

Stereotactic Body Radiation Therapy

SBRT is short course radiation delivered by radiation oncologists. Radiation can be delivered to the tumor, but unavoidably affects portions of normal liver and other adjacent organs within the beam, limiting the total dose that can be used. In contrast, Y90 radioembolization allows a much higher dose to be delivered selectively to the tumor, and the short distance of travel of beta-radiation in soft tissue prevents significant exposure to tissues beyond the treatment zone.

Systemic Chemotherapy

When patients have very advanced disease, systemic chemotherapy is the last option. Systemic chemotherapy for HCC is limited to the biologic drug **sorafenib.** The survival benefit of sorafenib is marginal, typically measured in weeks to months. It is also associated with treatment-limiting side effects in many patients with cirrhosis. Sorafenib can be used for patients who are terminal but want a few more weeks of life.

7.2 Liver Metastases

In Western countries, metastatic disease is by far the most common cause of solid liver neoplasms, with GI tract, breast and lung being the most common primaries. Patients may present with signs and symptoms of hepatic disease as the first indication of cancer elsewhere in the body. Many types of metastatic disease to the liver can be treated by IR; the most common are metastatic colorectal cancer and metastatic neuroendocrine tumors. We think about metastatic disease in the liver a little differently than HCC, though many of the treatment considerations are the same.

Management of Colorectal Cancer Metastasis to Liver

For patients with colorectal cancer and liver metastasis (mCRC), it is important to know if there are tumors in the liver at the initial discovery of the primary lesion (synchronous disease) versus discovery of liver tumors *after* the initial diagnosis/treatment of the primary lesion (metachronous disease).

In the patients with synchronous disease, surgeons want to determine if it's possible to resect all the lesions, primary and metastatic. As with HCC, liver resection of CRC metastasis is potentially curative if there is no other metastatic disease. Resection should always be the first consideration if it is feasible (▶**Fig. 7.7**). Timing of the

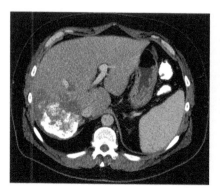

Fig. 7.7 This patient with colorectal cancer was found to have a liver metastasis at the time of diagnosis (synchronous disease). Following a hemicolectomy he underwent portal vein embolization to hypertrophy his left hepatic lobe, and soon after underwent a successful right hepatectomy.

resection may be affected by other factors such as the need for an urgent operation to deal with a symptomatic primary or the need to undergo neoadjuvant chemotherapy.

In liver-predominant metachronous disease (liver metastasis found after the primary has already been treated), patients undergo partial hepatectomy if possible. If they are not resection candidates, chemotherapy is the next viable option. Systemic chemotherapy such as 5-fluororuracil (5-FU) + oxaliplatin (FOLFOX), 5-FU + irinotecan (FOLFIRI), and bevacizumab are available to be used in selected colorectal cancer patients. It is possible that induction chemotherapy can result in an unresectable tumor shrinking and becoming resectable. The problem here is that the response rates to chemotherapy in mCRC patients is substantially diminished once they have already undergone a course of the first-line chemotherapy agents and their disease has progressed.

Currently, locoregional therapy performed by interventional radiologists is used for patients with mCRC who have exhausted options for chemotherapy. Ablation, TACE, and Y-90 are all options for liver-predominant mCRC. As with HCC, ablation is suited for patients with small but unresectable lesions (< 5 cm).

Management of Neuroendocrine Tumors in the Liver

Liver-predominant metastatic neuroendocrine tumors (mNET) arise commonly from a pancreatic or GI origin. Classically, these become symptomatic *after* they are metastatic to the liver, as the "first-pass" effect of the liver is bypassed. Presenting symptoms include flushing, diarrhea, wheezing, and palpitations. Diagnosis is made by measurement of serum 5-hydroxyindole acetic acid (5-HIAA) or other vasoactive peptides. Contrast-enhanced CT of the chest, abdomen, and pelvis may be effective at detecting larger tumors, but a primary lesion in the bowel can often be hard to detect on CT. Nuclear medicine imaging with radiolabeled octreotide (Octreoscan) or metaiodobenzylguanidine (MIBG) are more sensitive for primary lesion localization. About 5 to 10% of primaries will never be found.

Metastasis to the liver will usually be evident on CT imaging, but a PET-CT is often helpful. The liver metastasis typically does not lead to significant functional liver disease, and most patients will have an indolent course. The main reason for treating the metastatic neuroendocrine lesions in the liver is hormonal and bulk symptom control.

Options for treatment of mNET include therapy with somatostatin analogues, cytotoxic chemotherapy, resection, chemoembolization, and radioembolization.

Somatostatin analogues, such as octreotide, are effective at suppressing the release of tumor-related hormones and alleviating symptoms. This is often the preferred approach for low-grade tumors in order to avoid more invasive treatment. Some studies suggest that somatostatin analogues have the ability to stabilize or even shrink the tumor burden. Systemic chemotherapy for the most part has low response rates and a high toxicity profile. Because of this, chemotherapy is usually reserved for clinical trials only.

For isolated primaries, surgical resection can be curative and is the standard of care. Liver resection in the setting of metastatic disease is more controversial, as the benefits are questionable in light of the often slow growth of the tumors. That said, select patients do undergo hepatic resection, with both curative and palliative intent. Data suggest there is a benefit in terms of symptomatic relief and progression-free survival to support this.

Therapy with chemoembolization or radioembolization is a good option for symptomatic control of mNET that is unresectable or refractory to medical management (▶ Fig. 7.8). Prior to the procedure, patients are given a prophylactic dose of octreotide to account for the release of large amounts of vasoactive hormones from treated tumor, which could otherwise lead to hypertensive crises.

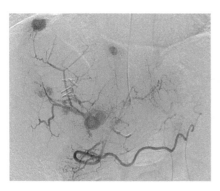

Fig. 7.8 A patient treated with transarterial chemoembolization for symptomatic, metastatic neuroendocrine tumors in the liver (primary NET was in the small bowel). Digital subtraction angiography image shows multiple hypervascular lesions in the liver. (This image is provided courtesy of Joshua Pinter, MD, University of Pittsburgh Medical Center.)

In 2018, a new peptide receptor radionuclide therapy for mNET (of gastropancreatic origin) was approved. Lutetium-177-Dotatate involves loading a radionuclide onto a somatostatin-receptor antagonist. The somastatin-receptor antagonist will target and bind the NET cells while the radionuclide Lu-177 delivers targeted radioactivity to kill the cells. While still quite new, you may see this therapy used more and more in patients with mNET refractory to other therapies.

7.3 Ablation Therapy for Malignancies

Radiofrequency ablation, microwave ablation, and cryoablation have been used for many years in the treatment of solid tumors outside the liver, particularly for the kidney. For other solid organ malignancies, ablation has not made it into the treatment algorithms. Despite this, you should have a basic understanding of how ablative therapies are being used.

Non-small Cell Lung Cancer and Secondary Lung Lesions

Many lung lesions will be found either incidentally on chest imaging or on low-dose screening CT scans in smokers. Lesions that are radiographically concerning for malignancy will be biopsied either with CT guidance by an interventional radiologist, bronchoscopy by a pulmonologist, or through a video-assisted thoracoscopic surgery (VATS) by a surgeon.

When reviewing a case for a possible CT-guided lung biopsy, you should be able to determine if there is a safe window for reaching the nodule or mass. The ideal lesion is peripherally located and at least a centimeter in diameter. Also consider the trajectory; the needle should be oriented as close to perpendicular to the pleura as possible, which may be challenging if there are ribs or a scapula in the way. More central lesions increase the risk of vascular injury and associated hemorrhage. These tend to be closer to an accessible bronchus and are better approached by bronchoscopy if that is an option. Anything near the diaphragm is another tricky location since breathing will tend to make the nodule a moving target and increase the number of passes needed for a diagnostic sampling. Locations that are not amenable to bronchoscopy or CT-guided techniques may be better approached with VATS.

A small amount of hemoptysis is normal with lung biopsies. Larger-volume hemoptysis is infrequent but may be potentially life threatening if it occurs as a result of injury to a major artery. Pneumothorax is a relatively common complication with CT-guided lung biopsies, occurring somewhere in the range of 20% of all cases. All patients that undergo a biopsy should have a chest X-ray 2 hours after the procedure to rule it out, however, a pneumothorax is usually identified well before that. The patient may become short of breath during the procedure, but more commonly it is detected on the completion CT scan. Small pneumothoraces are typically asymptomatic and will resolve on their own, and less than half of all postbiopsy pneumothoraces require a chest tube. There is no definite size cutoff for deciding when a chest tube needs to be placed, so it is more of a clinical judgement based on the presence of symptoms and the patient's baseline respiratory status, in addition to the size of the pneumothorax. If it is detected with the biopsy needle still in place, a chest tube is easily placed using the existing tract, thereby avoiding another puncture.

For patients diagnosed with **non–small cell lung cancer (NSCLC)**, treatment options include surgical resection, systemic chemotherapy with a cisplatin agent, radiation therapy, and ablation.

Surgical treatment with lobectomy or segmentectomy is the standard treatment for stage I and II disease. Stage I NSCLC patients do not receive adjuvant chemotherapy unless the tumor size is larger than 4 cm. Most stage II patients receive adjuvant chemotherapy after resection.

Radiation therapy (SBRT) is used in two different ways. When patients with stage I or stage II NSCLC undergo resection and are found to have positive margins, this is followed with radiation therapy. Radiation is also the standard-of-care treatment for patients who are not healthy enough to undergo surgery.

Ablative therapy in the lung is occasionally used in stage I and II NSCLC. Like radiation, its use is limited to patients who are poor surgical candidates. However, ablation is typically only used when SBRT is not possible for one reason or another. The reason for this is likely due to the abundance of research showing the benefit of radiation, and a relative paucity of research related to ablation. Despite this, research so far is promising, and lung ablations may have a growing role in the future. When ablating lung tumors, consideration should be given to risk of pneumothorax, abscess formation, pneumonia, and proximity of the lesion to vital structures.

Metastases to the lung can also be ablated but the role is even less defined. These should be approached on a case-by-case basis.

Renal Cell Carcinoma

Renal lesions are a common finding on cross-sectional imaging. The key step in evaluating a renal lesion is determining if it is cystic or solid. Cystic lesions are further described by the Bosniak classification. Simple cysts are classified as Bosniak I and require no follow-up. Bosniak II cysts are considered complex, as evidenced by the presence of thin septa or subtle enhancement, and in some cases require follow-up. Bosniak III and IV lesions are characterized by thick septations and calcifications, and may be partially solid. These are more concerning findings. Bosniak III/IV lesions and all solid renal masses need further evaluation with ultrasound/MRI. Note that biopsy of renal masses is highly controversial and many suspicious-appearing lesions are not definitively diagnosed until they are resected.

Primary renal malignancies are far more common than metastases. **Renal cell carcinoma** (RCC) is the most common primary tumor of the kidney. RCCs are generally silent, and are most often found incidentally on cross-sectional imaging or following metastatic spread.

The management of RCC is dependent on the tumor size, the extent of disease outside the kidney, and the patient's functional status. Treatment options include nephrectomy, active surveillance, or tumor ablation.

Nephrectomy, total or partial, is the gold standard for management of primary RCC. For tumors that are large (> 7 cm), invade surrounding structures, or are centrally located in the kidney, a radical nephrectomy is preferred. For smaller tumors without spread to surrounding structures, a partial nephrectomy can be performed. A partial nephrectomy is termed *nephron-sparing*. Nephron-sparing interventions are especially important in patients who have bilateral lesions, those who have a solitary kidney, and for patients with chronic kidney disease.

While nephrectomy can be curative, unfortunately not all patients are surgical candidates. Poor surgical candidates have two options: active surveillance or ablation.

Active surveillance is an option for patients who have a small tumor. It is worth considering for older patients with other medical problems and a limited expected lifespan. Small lesions tend to grow slowly, so these patients will most likely die with RCC rather than because of it. Routine cross-sectional studies are used periodically to monitor the lesion's growth. If significant growth is seen, a discussion about interventions can be revisited.

Another nephron-sparing intervention is percutaneous ablation (▶**Fig. 7.9**). The procedure is ideal for small (< 4 cm) and peripherally located tumors (especially exophytic lesions surrounded by perinephric fat). While ablation is most often used for nonsurgical candidates, a 2015 study by Thompson et al showed that renal ablation techniques are as effective as surgery for stage T1 lesions, in terms of local control and tumor-free survival. Despite this, ablation is not yet a part of the consensus treatment algorithms for this group of patients.

Cryoablation, RFA, and MWA can all be effectively utilized in the kidney, similar to liver malignancies. Cryo- and RF ablation have been used for many years. Though newer, microwave ablation is becoming more and more popular. When treating RCC with these techniques, the ablation zone should include tissue 0.5 to 1 cm beyond the tumor to maximize the chances of complete lesion destruction. The major risks with cryoablation are bleeding and hematuria, whereas with RFA the risks are nerve and/or urinary tract injury.

Patients with advanced disease not responsive to the above are typically treated systemically with immunotherapy and/or antivascular endothelial growth factor (anti-VEGF) drugs.

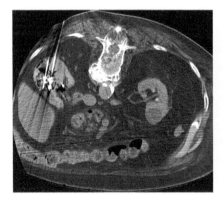

Fig. 7.9 This patient with a 5.6-cm renal cell carcinoma in the right kidney was a poor surgical candidate. He was offered a microwave ablation by IR. Intraprocedural CT image shows two microwave probes within the lesion. (This image is provided courtesy of Joshua Pinter, MD, University of Pittsburgh Medical Center.)

Bone Metastases

Many solid tumors can metastasize to bones, which are prone to pathological fractures and cause significant pain. Pain palliation is an important consideration in patients with symptomatic bone metastases, and a multidisciplinary approach is often used in management.

Medical therapy with analgesics, steroids, and bisphosphonates can all be helpful in relieving pain. Radiation therapy is frequently used as well. The majority of patients see a decrease in their pain following several radiation treatments. Adjuvant radiation is used postsurgery to reduce local recurrence and promote bone healing.

Surgical management has a limited role as a palliative measure. Long bone lesions that have caused (or are in danger of causing) a fracture may be treated surgically. Neurologic impairment secondary to lesions of the spine are also treated in select cases. Surgical management is obviated if the expected recovery time is greater than the patient's life expectancy.

Many of these treatment approaches fail to completely relieve pain from bony lesions, with recurrence of pain not uncommon. If radiation has failed or is deemed unlikely to provide benefit, ablation may be an option. Ablative therapies have been shown to be effective in alleviation of pain secondary to these bony metastases. Cryoablation of these lesions has also been shown to incur good local tumor control. Currently these are only being done at a small number of institutions.

Suggested Readings

[1] Atwell TD, Callstrom MR, Farrell MA, et al. Percutaneous renal cryoablation: local control at mean 26 months of followup. J Urol. 2010; 184(4):1291–1295

[2] Boas FE, Bodei L, Sofocleous CT. Radioembolization of colorectal liver metastases: indications, technique, and outcomes. J Nucl Med. 2017; 58(Suppl 2):104S–111S

[3] Hickey R, Vouche M, Sze DY, et al. Cancer concepts and principles: primer for the interventional oncologist-part I. J Vasc Interv Radiol. 2013; 24(8):1157–1164

[4] Hickey R, Vouche M, Sze DY, et al. Cancer concepts and principles: primer for the interventional oncologist-part II. J Vasc Interv Radiol. 2013; 24(8):1167–1188

[5] Lencioni R, Crocetti L, Cioni R, et al. Response to radiofrequency ablation of pulmonary tumours: a prospective, intention-to-treat, multicentre clinical trial (the RAPTURE study). Lancet Oncol. 2008; 9(7):621–628

[6] McMenomy BP, Kurup AN, Johnson GB, et al. Percutaneous cryoablation of musculoskeletal oligometastatic disease for complete remission. J Vasc Interv Radiol. 2013; 24(2):207–213

[7] Salem R, Gordon AC, Mouli S, et al. Y90 radioembolization significantly prolongs time to progression compared with chemoembolization in patients with hepatocellular carcinoma. Gastroenterology. 2016; 151(6):1155–1163.e2

[8] Thompson RH, Atwell T, Schmit G, et al. Comparison of partial nephrectomy and percutaneous ablation for cT1 renal masses. Eur Urol. 2015; 67(2):252–259

8 Arterial Disease

Shantanu Warhadpande, Alexander Maad El-Ali, Andrew Niekamp, Kurt Stahlfeld, Geogy Vatakencherry, and Kyle J. Cooper

8.1 Peripheral Artery Disease

Peripheral artery disease (PAD) refers to progressive narrowing of the aorta and the major arteries of the extremities and organs, essentially the body's entire circulation except the brain and heart. PAD is almost always due to atherosclerosis, which is cholesterol and inflammatory cell buildup in the vessel wall. While less common, other causes of PAD include emboli, extrinsic compression, trauma, adventitial cystic disease, peripheral aneurysms, and vasculitis.

As atherosclerosis is a systemic condition, patients with PAD also commonly have coronary artery and cerebrovascular disease. The long-term cardiovascular morbidity and mortality in these patients is high, and much of the medical management strategy is centered around reducing overall cardiovascular risk.

The most commonly affected vessels in PAD are those of the lower extremity, with nearly half of all PAD patients experiencing symptoms from the disease. Management of the symptomatic PAD patient differs from that of the asymptomatic patient.

Approach to the Asymptomatic Patient with Suspected PAD

Asymptomatic PAD may be diagnosed in the outpatient setting, often by a primary care physician or cardiologist. Given the number of comorbid conditions associated with PAD, it should be highly suspected in smokers, diabetics, patients older than 50 (especially males), and those with hypertension, hyperlipidemia, coronary artery disease, or prior stroke. Making the diagnosis is important, even in asymptomatic patients. Having PAD is an indicator of high risk for vascular disease throughout the body, and initiation of appropriate medical therapy in an asymptomatic patient could prevent a heart attack or stroke.

Patients with risk factors should be initially screened for PAD with a thorough history. It's important to ask about leg pain with exercise, leg pain at rest, and the presence of nonhealing wounds. On physical exam, you want to check for pulse strength and bruits throughout the body. A detailed visual inspection of the legs and feet is important. Any nonhealing ulceration, skin discoloration, or gangrene may signify advanced disease. Keep in mind, a patient may have a normal exam in the legs, but evidence of vascular disease elsewhere. You need to listen for carotid bruits, measure blood pressure in both arms (a difference between the two may be a clue to subclavian stenosis), and palpate the abdominal aorta.

Patients with suspected PAD can be further evaluated with a resting ankle-brachial index (ABI) (▶ Table 8.1). The test is basically a calculation of the ratio of the ankle blood pressures in each leg to the brachial pressures in each arm. An ABI less than 0.9 is consistent with PAD, but a normal value doesn't rule it out.

If suspicion remains high in patients with a normal or borderline ABI, they are further evaluated with an exercise ABI. This is especially useful to differentiate PAD from the other types of exertional extremity pain (osteoarthritis, spinal stenosis, venous hypertension). An exercise ABI with 15% or greater decrease compared to the pre-exercise value is abnormal and consistent with PAD.

Table 8.1 Ankle–brachial index

ABI	Interpretation
> 1.3	Falsely high value
0.9–1.3	Normal
0.7–0.9	Mild PAD
0.4–0.7	Moderate PAD
< 0.4	Severe PAD

Abbreviation: PAD, peripheral artery disease.

Falsely elevated ABIs (> 1.3) are common in patients with chronic kidney disease and diabetes, related to calcification causing noncompressibility of the artery. If this is seen, the ABI should be supplemented with a toe-brachial index (TBI). The vessels of the great toe are often spared, even in the setting of severe calcification more proximally. A TBI of less than 0.7 is diagnostic of PAD.

Approach to the Symptomatic Patient with Suspected PAD

When a patient presents with lower extremity pain, keep in mind the nonvascular etiologies of leg pain (▶ **Table 8.2**). Symptoms of PAD range from mild to debilitating, often described as cramping or aching. Pain is caused by nerve and muscle ischemia, affecting muscle groups distal to the level of flow restriction (calf pain due to femoral–popliteal occlusions; buttock and thigh pain from aortoiliac occlusions, etc.). Symptomatic PAD presents in one of three ways: intermittent claudication, atypical leg pain, or critical limb ischemia. Vascular specialists commonly use the Rutherford scale to stratify symptomatic patients (▶ **Table 8.3**).

Intermittent claudication (IC) is the mildest form of symptomatic PAD, comprising stages 1 to 3 on the Rutherford scale. It is characterized by extremity pain that occurs after walking a certain distance and is relieved with rest. The distance to symptom onset is consistent and reproducible but can be shortened when walking uphill or going up stairs.

Atypical leg pain is related to IC but occurs when patients do not have the classic intermittent claudication symptoms. Rather, they may have pain after walking that isn't debilitating enough to stop walking, or other nonspecific lower extremity symptoms. This is the catch-all category of lower extremity symptoms that don't neatly fit the bill of claudication. Thus, even if the patient doesn't have a classic story for claudication, be aware that PAD can present with atypical leg symptoms.

Critical limb ischemia (CLI), comprising stages 4 to 6 on the Rutherford scale, is characterized by pain at rest, ulceration of the skin, nonhealing wounds, and/or gangrene. While intermittent claudication and critical limb ischemia are both variants of PAD, only the latter is limb-threatening.

Symptomatic patients with suspected peripheral vascular disease will get an ABI. When critical limb ischemia is suspected, a number of studies are done together to confirm the diagnosis and localize the atherosclerotic burden for treatment planning. Ultrasound is often used to locate and gauge severity of the disease. Normal triphasic Doppler waveforms will change to damped monophasic waveforms beyond the level of a significant stenosis or occlusion. Additional tests include segmental pressure measurements, pulse volume recordings (PVRs), transcutaneous oxygen pressure measurements

Table 8.2 Differential diagnosis for lower extremity pain and differentiating features

Etiologies of lower extremity pain	Differentiating features
Neurogenic pain	Sharp pain that radiates down the leg; pain can be reproduced/alleviated with maneuvers that change back position
Musculoskeletal pain	Pain over muscles and joints, usually accompanied with tenderness to palpation; pain occurs with activity
Pain due to venous disease	Pain, "heaviness," "tightness" in entire leg after walking; pain relieved with elevation of the leg
Claudication	Leg muscle pain that is reproducible with walking certain distances; pain relieved quickly with rest

Table 8.3 Rutherford's classification for chronic limb ischemia

Stage 0	Asymptomatic
Stage 1	Mild claudication
Stage 2	Moderate claudication
Stage 3	Severe claudication
Stage 4	Pain at rest
Stage 5	Tissue loss/ulceration
Stage 6	Extensive tissue loss/ulceration/gangrene

($TcPO_2$) and skin perfusion pressure (SPP). Each of these tests is designed to help delineate the level of disease or distinguish between ischemic and nonischemic ulceration. They can also help predict the likelihood of wound healing after intervention. A full discussion of these tests is beyond the scope of this book.

Some clinicians rely on CT angiography as it tends to be a quick test to stratify location and burden of disease in the various segments of the peripheral arterial bed, including aortoiliac, femoral–popliteal, and tibial–pedal disease.

Management of PAD

Medical management is extremely important for all patients with PAD, regardless of the Rutherford class. Patients are put on an antiplatelet agent, either aspirin or clopidogrel, and a moderate- or high-intensity statin. Hypertension and diabetes should be controlled according to established guidelines, and smoking cessation strongly encouraged. Optimized medical therapy and lifestyle modification can slow the progression of atherosclerotic disease and help to prevent future cardiovascular events.

The diagnosis of PAD in an asymptomatic patient is a warning sign, alerting us to atherosclerotic disease likely present throughout the patient's body. If peripheral arteries are affected, coronary, carotid, renal, and mesenteric arteries may be affected as well. All PAD patients should undergo screening for subclavian stenosis, carotid stenosis, and abdominal aortic aneurysm (AAA), regardless of age, gender, or smoking status.

In symptomatic patients with *intermittent claudication only*, the management goals include symptom control, improvement in ambulatory status, and cardiovascular risk reduction. Because intermittent claudication is not limb-threatening, patients can be managed on an outpatient basis. After initiating optimal medical therapy, most patients will benefit from **supervised exercise therapy.** This involves participation in 30 minutes of walking, typically at least three times a week. During the exercise, patients walk to the point of maximum claudication (and just beyond, if possible), rest until the pain abates, and then repeat. Only walking time is counted toward the 30-minute goal. The CLEVER trial showed that participation in supervised exercise therapy improved pain-free walking distances comparable to treatment with endovascular therapy.

Exercise programs have excellent long-term durability and the added benefit of improving overall cardiovascular health. The initial trial of exercise should last around 3 months before symptoms are reassessed. While many patients were previously forced to perform this program at home due to lack of coverage by insurance companies, supervised exercise therapy is now being covered by Medicare and most insurance providers.

If symptoms persist despite exercise therapy, the patient may be started on **cilostazol,** a phosphodiesterase inhibitor. Cilostazol has both antiplatelet and vasodilatory effects. It has been shown to increase pain-free walking distances, but does not affect progression of the disease. Many patients are intolerant due to side effects (headache, diarrhea, dizziness, palpitations), and it is contraindicated in those with heart failure.

Most patients with claudication see considerable improvement with conservative therapy. The minority who continue to have lifestyle-limiting claudication despite an adequate trial of conservative therapy may be candidates for an invasive intervention. Diabetic patients tend not to improve as quickly or as completely as their nondiabetic counterparts, and more frequently require an intervention to achieve an acceptable level of symptomatic improvement.

For patients with *critical limb ischemia* (rest pain, ulcerative skin changes, nonhealing wounds, gangrene), the disease has progressed to the point of becoming limb-threatening. The goal of therapy for these patients is, first and foremost, limb salvage. Early intervention and revascularization can reduce tissue loss, relieve rest pain, and allow for existing wounds to heal. If limb salvage is not possible or fails, amputation may be necessary.

When there is an indication to revascularize an extremity, vascular specialists have two options: surgery or endovascular procedures (▶ **Fig. 8.1**). Deciding which treatment method is most appropriate can be a complicated decision, and is often influenced by the experience of the operator.

Surgical options for treating PAD include endarterectomy and bypass. **Endarterectomy** involves surgical exposure of the diseased arterial segment and physical removal of the thrombosed plaque through an arteriotomy. This is often combined with **patch angioplasty,** which includes sewing a bioprosthetic or artificial patch onto the arteriotomy site during closure to widen the lumen and accommodate for postsurgical scarring. **Bypass** involves surgically suturing the proximal portion of a conduit (either a vein or a synthetic graft) upstream to the diseased segment of the artery, and suturing the distal portion of the conduit downstream of the diseased segment, effectively rerouting blood past the diseased arterial segment. Common bypasses you will see include aortofemoral/aortobifemoral, axillofemoral, femoral–femoral, femoral–popliteal, and femoral–tibioperoneal.

To maximize graft patency, the proximal and distal anastomosis sites should be disease-free segments, allowing for adequate inflow and outflow from the graft. Autologous veins, often harvested greater saphenous veins, tend to have much higher patency rates than synthetic grafts (polytetrafluoroethylene [PTFE]). Whenever

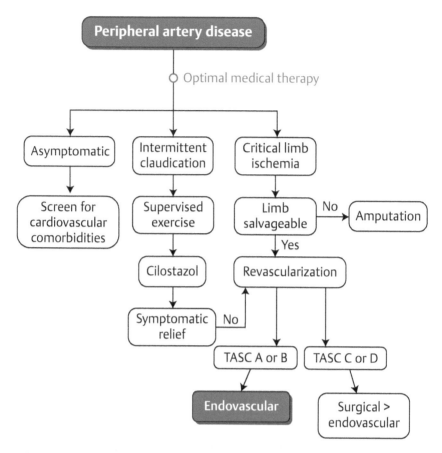

Fig. 8.1 Simplified algorithm for management of peripheral arterial disea. Note that many TASC C and D lesions are now being treated endovascularly. The decision to proceed with surgical revascularization over endovascular revascularization takes into account the patient's comorbidities, surgical risk, and the lesion characteristics.

possible, prebypass vein mapping should be performed to determine the quality of veins available for harvest.

Endovascular treatment for PAD has been used since the 1960s as a means of opening up arteries and increasing downstream flow. This typically involves some combination of angioplasty, stenting, and/or atherectomy. As a general rule, endovascular treatments are most successful in larger arteries with focal stenoses. In the setting of multilevel disease *in claudicants,* treating aortoiliac disease alone is often sufficient for symptomatic improvement. The procedure employed depends on the location, length of diseased segment, and the presence or absence of calcification.

Specialty wires, new device technology, and novel techniques have allowed interventional radiologists to treat arterial occlusions that previously would not have been amenable to endovascular therapy. Previously "uncrossable" occlusions have become treatable due to increased comfort and expertise with tibial and pedal retrograde access. An advanced technique aided by new technology involves crossing arterial lesions by guiding a wire in the subintimal space just proximal to the lesion and dissecting alongside the lesion. Once past the occluded segment, reentry devices can be used to regain access from the subintimal space back into the native arterial lumen, at which point a stent is typically deployed across the entire diseased segment. In addition, drug-eluting technology on balloons and stents have improved the patency of endovascular interventions.

Endovascular Interventions versus Surgery for PAD

The **Transatlantic Inter-Society Consensus (TASC II) guidelines** classify patients according to lesion location and burden. TASC breaks down lower extremity PAD into three subsets: aortoiliac (inflow), femoral–popliteal (outflow), or tibioperoneal (runoff) disease. Disease severity and complexity is then graded for each subset on a four-point scale, from A to D. Here's a simplified way of thinking about TASC lesions. TASC A and B disease includes short-segment stenoses or occlusions, unilateral or bilateral (▶Fig. 8.2). TASC C lesions tend to be a little longer. TASC D disease covers diffuse, multifocal, or large-vessel stenoses/occlusions (▶Fig. 8.3).

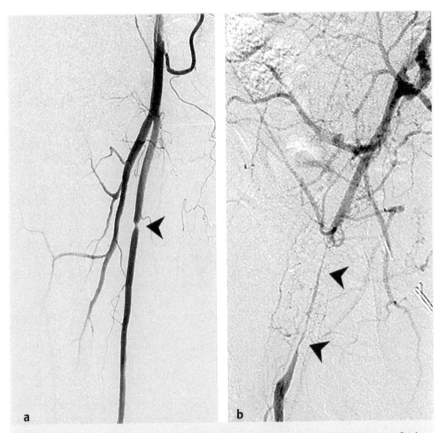

Fig. 8.2 **(a)** Angiographic images demonstrating a short TASC A stenosis involving the superficial femoral artery and **(b)** a longer TASC B stenosis involving the common femoral artery.
(These images are provided courtesy of Matthew Czar Taon, MD, Kaiser Permanente Los Angeles.)

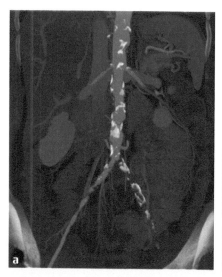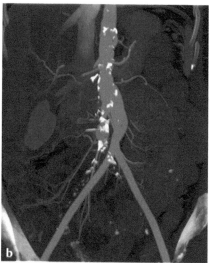

Fig. 8.3 **(a)** CT of the abdomen and pelvis showing extensive aortoiliac atherosclerotic disease consistent with a TASC D lesion. **(b)** This lesion was treated with an aortobifemoral bypass. (These images are provided courtesy of Matthew Czar Taon, MD, Kaiser Permanente Los Angeles.)

TASC II classification is a guide to the complexity of a lesion based on lesion length, location, and involved vasculature, which can be an aid in determining the technical difficulty of endovascular revascularization.

For all subsets (aortoiliac, femoral–popliteal, or tibioperoneal disease), endovascular therapy is considered first line for TASC A and B disease. Surgery is often favored in patients with TASC C and D disease (▶ **Fig. 8.3**). It is important to note that as technology and experience with endovascular therapy has improved, the trend has been toward increasing use of endovascular techniques for TASC C and even TASC D lesions, particularly in patients with poor surgical candidacy. In the hands of a skilled interventionalist, endovascular treatment is *technically* feasible in all but the most recalcitrant lesions.

Given these advances, many endovascular specialists have embraced an endovascular-first approach to PAD cases. Many vascular patients tend to have multiple medical comorbidities which make them poor surgical candidates; in these patients, a less invasive approach is preferred. If surgery is being considered, the adequacy of the autologous vein conduit should be evaluated.

In addition to disease burden, the artery involved may determine if surgery is favored over endovascular therapy. For example, many vascular specialists prefer treating common femoral artery disease surgically, given the relatively straightforward surgical approach to this area, and the risks associated with endovascular treatment, including stent fracture or dissection. Similarly, popliteal artery disease is also more commonly treated with surgical bypass given its location and the risk of stent malfunction when deployed across a joint.

Another important consideration is the patient's overall prognosis and expected lifespan. Findings from the BASIL trial (2005) suggested that for patients with longer expected life-spans, surgical bypass should be preferred. Despite the increased morbidity associated with bypass surgery, patients expected to live longer may benefit most from the higher patency rate of a bypass. For those with shorter expected lifespans, endovascular stenting is preferred.

While considered a landmark paper, the BASIL trial data is over a decade old. More recently published studies have validated the endovascular-first approach as safe and efficacious, even for younger patients. As technology and techniques continue to improve, the endovascular and surgical treatment algorithms will need to be redefined.

8.2 Acute Limb Ischemia

The natural history of peripheral artery atherosclerotic disease is a gradual narrowing of the arteries, with progressive symptom severity corresponding to the degree of luminal stenosis. Ischemia can, however, develop rapidly when an artery becomes acutely occluded. This is referred to as **acute limb ischemia (ALI)**. There is often a very high risk of limb loss with ALI if not treated immediately, as many patients lack the collateral blood supply seen in those with chronic arterial occlusions.

Work-up of a Patient with Acute Limb Ischemia

ALI must be included in the differential for all patients presenting with acute limb pain. The classic signs of ALI include the 6 P's: pain, pallor, pulselessness, paresthesias, poikilothermia (cool to touch), and paralysis. Pain is typically the earliest and most consistent sign, while the others may be more variable.

There are two major causes of ALI: in situ thrombosis and occlusion due to emboli. Management is different for each.

Patients with known peripheral vascular disease presenting with acute limb ischemia most likely have **in situ thrombosis.** This type of occlusion is caused by rupture of an unstable atherosclerotic plaque, with rapid accumulation of clot leading to vessel obstruction (analogous to how coronary artery disease leads to myocardial infarction [MI]).

Those presenting with ALI and no history of PAD should be strongly suspected to have an **embolic occlusion,** especially when they have no PAD risk factors and good pulses in the contralateral limb. A cardiac source (from atrial fibrillation) is most typical, but embolus can also originate from aortic or peripheral artery aneurysms. An embolus travels downstream in the artery and lodges itself, usually at a branch point.

ALI is a clinical diagnosis. Treatment should be initiated based on history and physical exam alone, though an ABI can confirm the diagnosis if necessary. The blood pressure reading below the level of the occlusion is usually zero. Many clinicians use arterial Doppler to identify the location of the occlusion and determine the urgency of intervention. CTA, if time permits, can also confirm the location and be used to guide therapy.

Management of a Patient with Acute Limb Ischemia

All patients with acute limb ischemia should be immediately started on a heparin drip. Anticoagulation decreases propagation of clot and worsening of limb ischemia. The urgency of additional treatment is based on the extent of damage to the limb. The vascular and peripheral neurologic exam is crucial in determining whether the limb is viable, threatened, or nonviable. Determining this is the most important initial step once ALI is suspected. This is categorized by the Rutherford classification for acute limb ischemia (▶ Table 8.4), which is distinct from the Rutherford classification for chronic disease.

Nerves are more sensitive to ischemia (irreversible damage within 6–8 hours), while muscle can tolerate hypoxia for longer periods. For this reason, sensory loss will always precede motor deficits. Venous Doppler signals are usually detectable, even in the absence of arterial signal, up until the point of profound ischemic damage.

Table 8.4 Rutherford's classification for acute limb ischemia

Category	Clinical findings	Limb viability	Treatment
Category I	1. Dopplerable arterial pulses 2. Venous signal present 3. Sensory intact 4. Motor intact 5. Acute onset of pain; may or may not have rest pain in extremity	Viable	Tx: embolectomy (< 48 h)
Category IIa	1. No dopplerable arterial pulses 2. Venous signal present 3. Decreased sensation 4. Motor intact 5. Rest pain in extremity	Marginally threatened	Urgent embolectomy (< 24 h)
Category IIb	1. No dopplerable arterial pulses 2. Venous signal present 3. Decreased sensation 4. Decreased motor strength 5. Rest pain in extremity	Immediately threatened	Immediate embolectomy; time is of the essence and the limb is still salvageable (< 4 h)
Category III	1. No dopplerable arterial pulses 2. No venous signal (thrombosis in venous system secondary to stagnant flow) 3. No sensation in limb 4. No motor strength in limb	Nonviable	Amputation; nonsalvageable limb. *Do not* attempt revascularization as ischemic tissue could release toxins leading to cardiac arrest

The presence of both sensory and motor deficits, as well as the loss of both arterial and venous Doppler signals indicates irreversible damage.

Determining the viability of the limb (viable, threatened, or nonviable) dictates the urgency of the intervention and type of intervention. According to the Rutherford classification, viable limbs (categories I and IIa) require invasive intervention, but not emergently. This can be managed by both surgical and endovascular treatments. With category IIb, the limb is imminently threatened and requires *immediate* surgical revascularization. Category III limbs are considered nonviable; revascularization could actually lead to the release of toxins from the dead tissue into the blood and increases the risk of cardiac arrest. Amputation is often the only solution.

Surgical options include embolectomy for embolic occlusions, and endarterectomy or bypass for in situ thrombosis. Surgical **embolectomy** involves a cutdown to the artery proximal to the occlusion, insertion of a catheter through a small hole in the artery and advancing it across the clot. Once across, a balloon at the tip is inflated and then the catheter is retraced, pulling the clot out with it. In contrast, endarterectomy involves exposure of the thrombosed artery and physical removal of the thrombosed plaque through a larger incision. If the plaque burden is too great, a bypass may be the only option. In reality, these techniques are often used in combination for many patients.

Endovascular treatments include catheter-directed thrombolysis and mechanical thrombectomy (**Procedure Box 8.1, Procedure Box 8.2**). **Catheter-directed thrombolysis** involves guiding a catheter into the clot and infusing thrombolytics, usually tissue plasminogen activator (tPA). It is best suited for fresh thrombus rather than chronic, organized clots (including chronic embolized material) (▶**Fig. 8.4**).

The TOPAS trial (Thrombolysis or Peripheral Artery Surgery) and the STILE trial (Thrombolysis for Ischemia of the Lower Extremity) both showed that for viable limbs (category I and IIa acute limb ischemia), lytic therapy is safe and effective. Thrombolysis has the advantage of lysing smaller, more distal thrombi in addition to the occlusive thrombus. As is the case anytime a thrombolytic is used, the major contraindications include active bleeding, and recent history of stroke or surgery.

Mechanical thrombectomy involves endovascular disruption and removal of the clot. Given the risk of downstream embolization, this has historically been done less frequently than catheter-directed thrombolysis, however, newer tools and embolic protection devices have increased interest in mechanical thrombectomy as a viable treatment option for ALI.

The main advantages of endovascular treatments over surgical treatments are shorter recovery time and the avoidance of general anesthesia (important since most of these patients have significant cardiopulmonary comorbidities).

Procedure Box 8.1: Catheter-Directed Thrombolysis for Acute Limb Ischemia   ℹ

After gaining arterial access (typically using a retrograde approach from the contralateral femoral artery), the occlusion is crossed using a guidewire. With the thrombus crossed, a special infusion catheter with multiple side holes is positioned such that it's tip within the thrombus itself. Contrast is injected to verify the catheter remains intraluminal. Thrombolytic agents are then administered slowly through the catheter, exiting the side holes and causing lysis of the thrombus. The patients are typically brought back between 4 and 24 hours after catheter placement for thrombolysis check, and to treat any underlying or persistent lesions.

Thrombolytic agents used include urokinase and tPA, with the latter being more common. The "pulse-spray" technique is commonly employed to deliver the lytic agents; this is where an initial bolus is delivered, followed by a continuous infusion overnight. Heparin should also be infused at slightly less than therapeutic doses through the sheath to prevent thrombus formation on the catheter or sheath. This should not be administered through the thrombolysis catheter simultaneously with the lytic agent, as precipitation can occur. Simultaneous full-dose anticoagulation is also not recommended due to the increased risk of bleeding complications.

Postprocedurally, patients should be admitted to the ICU for close monitoring and frequent lab draws. Patients should be monitored for complications secondary to thrombolytic therapy, including access site or remote bleeding, distal embolization, or compartment syndrome. Platelet counts, hemoglobin, and fibrinogen levels should all be closely monitored for the duration of the lytic infusion, to help identify those patients at high risk for catastrophic bleeding.

Mechanical thrombectomy involves the physical disruption and removal of thrombus and may be combined with thrombolytic agents administered during the procedure (pharmacomechanical thrombectomy). After gaining vascular access and identifying and crossing the occlusion, thrombus can be disrupted/removed in several ways.

(1) Suction thrombectomy: The vacuum created by simple aspiration of the catheter can be used to grab onto clots and suck them through the catheter lumen, or lodge them at the catheter tip, facilitating their extraction by removing the catheter from the sheath. Dedicated vacuum-assisted thrombectomy catheters exist which utilize larger catheter lumens with reinforced material resistant to collapse under negative pressure, although care must be used to not aspirate too much blood from areas of nonthrombosed flowing blood.

(2) Rheolytic thrombectomy: It utilizes a catheter which continuously instills and aspirates fluid through separate holes at the tip, which both disrupts the thrombus and creates a continuous vortex of negative pressure to remove fragmented thrombotic material. Unlike suction thrombectomy, this can be performed over a wire, maintaining distal access. Because of the fragmentation of thrombus and rapidly flowing fluid at the catheter tip, erythrocyte lysis will occur, which carries the risk of bradycardia (due to adenosine release) and renal injury. The number of pulses is determined by the catheter diameter and whether it is used in completely thrombosed or partially flowing segments of the vasculature. Patients should be counseled that red- or brownish-colored urine after the procedure is a normal side effect, and will decrease over time.

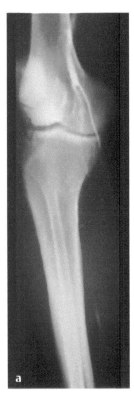 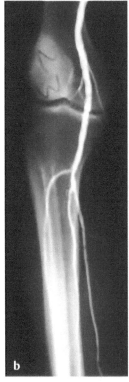

Fig. 8.4 (a) The popliteal artery abruptly cuts off just above the knee secondary to an acute embolus. Note that there is no collateral flow, which is typical for acute limb ischemia. **(b)** This lesion was successfully treated with thrombolysis, with follow-up imaging showing dissolution of the clot and restoration of normal arterial flow down the popliteal artery. (Source: Acute Ischemia of the Lower Extremities. In: Bakal C, Silberzweig J, Cynamon J, et al., ed. Vascular and Interventional Radiology. Principles and Practice. 1st Edition. Thieme; 2000.)

Regardless of the treatment chosen, after the acute clot has been addressed, reperfusion injury and resultant compartment syndrome can occur. Compartment syndrome presents with severe pain and swelling in the affected extremity. These patients will have severe pain even with gentle passive dorsiflexion/plantarflexion of their feet. If intracompartmental pressure is high enough, it can cause pressure necrosis of the nerves and resultant neurological deficits in the limb. In severe cases, venous obstruction and limb loss can occur.

Compartment syndrome requires an emergent fasciotomy, indicated by clinical diagnosis alone. Confirmative testing will only prolong time to treatment and increase the risk of permanent damage. Some clinicians will even perform a prophylactic fasciotomy after treating an ischemic limb to prevent compartment syndrome.

In all ALI patients, the inciting event also needs to be addressed. This includes optimal medical therapy in cases of PAD, and treating embolic disease if identified. Patients should get a baseline postprocedure ABI with segmental pressure measurements and Doppler tracings to be used for future comparison. Those that had a surgical bypass get a duplex ultrasound of the graft at every follow-up visit. Increased focal velocities within the graft, a graft velocity less than 40 cm/s, or an ABI drop of greater than 0.15 across the graft are clues to impending restenosis or occlusion. This requires further evaluation with either cross-sectional imaging or angiography.

8.3 Renal Artery Stenosis

Patients with essential hypertension are usually started on antihypertensives when lifestyle modification fails to adequately control the blood pressure. For those with persistently high blood pressure despite multiple antihypertensive agents, secondary hypertension should be considered. This includes hypertension due to renal artery stenosis, chronic renal failure, endocrine disorders, obstructive sleep apnea, and many others. As it is relevant to this chapter, renal artery stenosis will be discussed here.

Renal artery stenosis is usually the result of atherosclerosis (▶ Fig. 8.5). It classically affects the proximal third of the renal artery, often with associated vascular calcification. Stenosis results in decreased blood flow into the kidneys and upregulation of the renin–angiotensin system. The downstream effect is systemic vasoconstriction and hypertension. Because of the fixed stenosis in the renal artery, the upregulation of the renin–angiotensin system does not proportionally increase renal artery perfusion, and a constant pathological level of renin results. Another consequence of decreased renal blood flow is atrophy. When atrophy is unilateral, there's usually a compensatory hypertrophy of the contralateral kidney. If bilateral, both kidneys can become atrophied and lead to renal failure.

Renal artery stenosis should be suspected in patients with severe hypertension who have a sudden increase in serum creatinine after starting an ACE inhibitor, those with known severe atherosclerosis, or when imaging reveals asymmetry of the kidneys. Sometimes they can present acutely with flash pulmonary edema. This happens as a result of an upregulated renin–angiotensin system, with increasing fluid retention. An exam finding of an abdominal bruit can also be a clue, but this is not often detectable.

Management of Renal Artery Stenosis

First-line medical therapy for renovascular hypertension includes ACE inhibitors and angiotensin receptor blockers (ARBs). By inhibiting the renin–angiotensin pathway, the mechanism driving hypertension is blocked. This may seem counterintuitive as ACE inhibitors decrease glomerular filtration rate (GFR), and have a tendency to increase serum

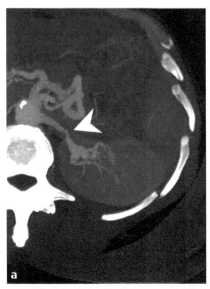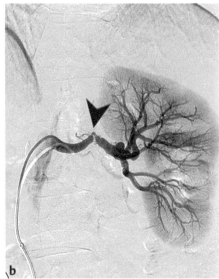

Fig. 8.5 **(a)** CT and **(b)** angiographic images of a left renal artery stenosis. (These images are provided courtesy of Matthew Czar Taon, MD, Kaiser Permanente Los Angeles.)

creatinine. However, the contralateral kidney usually compensates, and the creatinine bump is often insignificant. Nevertheless, creatinine does need to be monitored for signs of worsening renal function when RAS patients are treated with an ACE inhibitor or ARB. These drugs should be used cautiously in patients with known bilateral RAS. Many clinicians avoid them entirely, though it is not an absolute contraindication in bilateral disease. If an ACE/ARB causes kidney injury, it's usually reversible when the drug is stopped.

Multiple antihypertensive agents are commonly required for these patients. Other drug classes including thiazides, calcium channel blockers, or β-blockers can be added as needed. Maximum medical therapy for RAS also includes treatment of hyperlipidemia with a statin and lifestyle modifications (smoking cessation, weight loss, and glycemic control).

In the past, angioplasty and balloon-expandable stent placement was commonly used to treat renal artery stenosis. More recent data from the CORAL trial by Cooper et al in 2014 has shown that in most patients, endovascular therapy provides no long-term benefit compared to optimal medical therapy in terms of blood pressure control or long-term renal function. In fact, stenting actually has the potential to worsen the condition in some patients. Based on this evidence, the current management of choice for patients with RAS is pharmacologic and lifestyle modification.

When maximal medical management fails or is not tolerated, percutaneous revascularization can be considered. Intervention may also be appropriate in patients who suffer a clinically significant GFR drop on medical therapy, or those with recurrent pulmonary edema.

Endovascular angioplasty and stenting is the procedure of choice when intervention is required. Renal artery stenting is beneficial in the short term, but restenosis is common, and in some cases may even worsen the stenosis. It's important to have a discussion about expectations with the patients beforehand, so that they understand the likelihood of success with the procedure.

Generally speaking, ostial lesions require balloon-expandable stent placement while more distal lesions in the artery may be treated with angioplasty only. Stented patients are put on dual antiplatelet therapy for at least 3 months. Surveillance duplex ultrasound is done every 6 to 12 months to monitor for restenosis. When there is significant restenosis, repeat angioplasty or stent-relining may be necessary; surgical intervention may be required in refractory cases.

Surgical treatment with endarterectomy or bypass provides higher long-term patency and has a more lasting benefit, but is not commonly done. Renal artery stenosis patients tend to have many comorbidities, making the surgical risk prohibitively high. Surgery is only considered in patients who have failed both medical and endovascular treatment.

Although much less common, **fibromuscular dysplasia (FMD)** is another cause of renal artery stenosis that you should be aware of. Patients are classically young females who present with early-onset, treatment-refractory hypertension. They often lack the traditional risk factors for atherosclerosis. In such patients, suspicion for FMD should be high, and a CTA or renal ultrasound can be performed to confirm the diagnosis. The stenosis tends to be mid or distal along the renal artery, and has a characteristic string of beads appearance, although isolated stenoses or single or multiple aneurysms can also be seen.

Renal artery stenosis due to FMD is often treated endovascularly with balloon angioplasty alone; stents are rarely required. Patients with FMD frequently also develop involvement of the carotid arteries, which can lead to central nervous system symptoms. They usually get head-to-pelvis CTA to rule out any other concomitant arterial disease.

8.4 Mesenteric Ischemia

Bowel ischemia can present as a life-threatening acute problem or as an insidious chronic condition. Management differs depending on the acuity and etiology.

Acute Mesenteric Ischemia

Patients with **acute mesenteric ischemia** present with sudden onset, severe abdominal pain out of proportion to the abdominal exam. There are four major causes: embolic occlusion, in situ thrombosis, nonocclusive mesenteric ischemia (NOMI), and mesenteric venous thrombosis (▶ Table 8.5).

Embolic mesenteric occlusion occurs when an embolus, typically from the heart, occludes a visceral artery, with the superior mesenteric artery (SMA) most commonly affected. In *mesenteric artery thrombosis*, patients usually already have underlying chronic mesenteric atherosclerosis and postprandial abdominal pain (abdominal

Table 8.5 Causes of acute mesenteric ischemia and treatment

Causes of acute mesenteric ischemia	Treatment
Embolus	Surgical embolectomy
Mesenteric arterial thrombosis	Mesenteric vessel bypass with autogenous vein
Nonocclusive mesenteric ischemia	Catheter-directed vasodilators into culprit spasmed vessel
Mesenteric venous thrombosis	Correction of hypercoagulable state, possibly thrombectomy or TIPS

angina). *NOMI* results from a low-flow state related to vasopressor therapy or hypotension, common in the intensive care setting. *Mesenteric venous thrombosis* occurs in hypercoagulable patients, and results in ischemia due to venous outflow obstruction, bowel edema, and decreased bowel perfusion.

The typical patient presents with acute-onset, severe abdominal pain, but with a relatively benign exam. Labs tests may show a mild leukocytosis and a slight increase in lactic acid, but sometimes not even that. A high level of suspicion is required to identify and treat these patients in a timely fashion. Acute mesenteric ischemia should therefore be included on the differential for all cases of acute-onset abdominal pain.

Patients with acute mesenteric ischemia, regardless of underlying etiology, should be started on broad-spectrum antibiotics and anticoagulation (unless the patient is actively bleeding or has suffered ischemic colitis from hypoperfusion). The imaging modality of choice for suspected cases is CTA. It can be performed quickly and is widely available. Mesenteric duplex ultrasound is an alternative, though evaluation is often limited by body habitus and bowel gas obscuring views of the vessels.

The patient's abdominal exam dictates the urgency of the next step. As ischemia progresses, the lactic acid level and white count will rise. The development of peritoneal signs requires an emergent trip to the OR for ex lap and evaluation of bowel viability.

In acute mesenteric ischemia secondary to embolism, ex lap and open embolectomy are preferred. If the problem is due to acute-on-chronic thrombosis, and the patient is stable without peritoneal signs, catheter-directed thrombolysis of the occluded mesenteric vessel is an option. This is controversial though, as bowel viability cannot be determined by an endovascular approach. In many institutions, these patients still go to the OR for a bypass.

In the acute setting, the role of IR is most established for NOMI, in which catheter-directed infusion of vasodilators (papaverine, etc.) can be used to increase mesenteric perfusion.

Chronic Mesenteric Ischemia

Chronic mesenteric ischemia (CMI) is almost always due to visceral arterial atherosclerosis. For patients with CMI, symptoms typically do not develop until two of the three mesenteric arteries (celiac, SMA, and inferior mesenteric artery [IMA]) are stenotic or occluded. This is because the extensive network of collateral pathways can usually provide enough flow to maintain adequate perfusion if only one artery is affected. Once two arteries are affected, this collateral flow compensation is inadequate, and symptoms develop. The caveat to this is SMA disease, which can potentially cause chronic mesenteric ischemia in isolation.

Patients with CMI typically present with severe postprandial abdominal pain shortly after a meal, lasting 30 to 60 minutes. They tend to develop "food fear," avoiding oral intake and often losing a significant amount of weight. As with acute mesenteric ischemia, CTA is the initial study of choice, with abdominal US being the other option.

Treatment is pursued when the disease interferes with quality of life and has resulted in weight loss. Endovascular revascularization with angioplasty and stenting is the treatment of choice for CMI in most centers, through a surgical approach is sometimes performed. A 2015 meta-analysis by Cai et al found that despite lower periprocedural morbidity/mortality associated with endovascular revascularization, there was a higher 3-year recurrence rate in patients treated this way compared to those managed with surgery.

Surgical arterial bypass is considered in younger patients and good surgical candidates, given the durability of this treatment. That said, mesenteric bypass is a complicated, high-risk procedure. Most vascular specialists opt for an endovascular-first approach when possible.

Post-revascularization, stented patients should be placed on antiplatelet therapy and a statin, if not already started, with surveillance duplex ultrasound performed every 6 to 12 months to monitor for restenosis.

Median Arcuate Ligament Syndrome

Median arcuate ligament syndrome (MALS) is a rare cause of CMI, and occurs when the celiac axis is compressed by the median arcuate ligament. The median arcuate ligament is the curved, ligamentous connection between the two diaphragmatic crura. Significant arterial compression by this structure likely occurs more often than we realize, but is clinically silent in most patients.

The clinical presentation of MALS is postprandial pain and weight loss. An abdominal bruit may be heard. Most patients initially undergo a battery of examinations and endoscopies, all of which tend to be negative in a typical MALS patient. CTA is obtained when there is suspicion for underlying vascular disease, or when numerous other tests have failed to lead to a diagnosis. MALS is often a subtle imaging finding that can be missed unless it is specifically looked for. On CTA there will be an absence of atherosclerotic disease, and sometimes a focal stenosis with an indentation along the superior aspect of the celiac trunk, most easily seen on the sagittal reconstructions (▶Fig. 8.6).

Abdominal ultrasound with measurement of peak vessel velocities can be performed to confirm the MALS diagnosis. Respiratory maneuvers while performing the ultrasound are essential. Inspiration (diaphragm flattening and decreased tension on median arcuate ligament) results in improvement of the celiac compression, while expiration (diaphragm up and increased tension on median arcuate ligament) results in

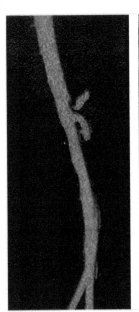
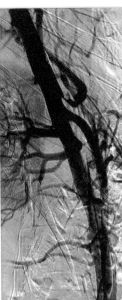

Fig. 8.6 Median arcuate ligament syndrome is most easily seen on sagittal images, which will show a hook-like configuration with a superior indentation of the celiac axis at its takeoff.

worsening of the compression. Inspiration/expiration would not be expected to affect peak vessel velocities in atherosclerotic disease.

Asymptomatic patients or patients with incidentally discovered MALS do not require treatment. For symptomatic patients, the first-line treatment for MALS is surgical decompression by dividing the arcuate ligament. If surgery fails to alleviate symptoms, endovascular stenting may be considered.

8.5 Aneurysmal Disease

Arteries are considered aneurysmal when the diameter is 1.5 times that of adjacent normal segments or age-matched controls. Formation of an aneurysm involves three pathological processes: proteolysis, inflammation, and smooth muscle cell apoptosis. The alterations in vascular wall composition result in a loss of wall strength and dilation of all three layers of the arterial wall—a true aneurysm. In contrast, a pseudoaneurysm usually involves vessel wall trauma with blood contained by only 1-2 layers of the vessel wall, often just the adventitia.

Depending on size, aneurysms present a risk of rupture due to the inherent weakness of the wall. Larger aneurysms can compress adjacent structures and result in pain, neurological deficits, or present as pulsatile, palpable masses.

Abdominal Aortic Aneurysms

As our population ages, the incidence of aortic aneurysmal disease has been increasing. Fortunately, treatment has improved significantly since the invasive aortic ligation techniques pioneered in the 1920s. It wasn't until 1991 that the first minimally invasive endovascular aneurysm repair (EVAR) procedures were introduced.

Even with advances in care, ruptured **abdominal aortic aneurysm (AAA)** continues to be associated with high mortality. Roughly half of patients with ruptured AAAs die before reaching the hospital. For this reason, early detection and treatment of aneurysms at risk for rupture is of critical importance.

The natural history of AAAs involves three stages: development, expansion, and eventually rupture. The only known modifiable risk factor associated with progression is smoking. Other risk factors include age greater than 65, male sex, family history, and hypertension.

AAAs are variable with regard to size and growth. Some progressively enlarge over time, while others go through short periods of rapid expansion, remaining stable in between. Risk of rupture is directly correlated with increasing aneurysm size, particularly when greater than 5.5 cm, and in those patients who continue to smoke. Aneurysms below 5 cm in diameter carry a relatively low risk of rupture, except those which are rapidly expanding.

Screening and Management of Abdominal Aortic Aneurysms

The USPSTF recommends ultrasound screening for AAAs in all men aged 65 to 75 who have ever smoked. Abdominal aortic diameter greater than 3 cm is generally considered aneurysmal. Ultrasound has excellent sensitivity and specificity for the detection of AAA, but aortic measurements are not precise. Abnormal findings can be further evaluated with cross-sectional imaging (usually CTA) when needed for treatment planning. In addition to aneurysm size, it's also important to determine how much of the aorta is involved, whether the iliac arteries are involved, and to characterize the aneurysm neck.

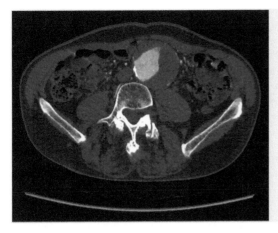

Fig. 8.7 CT of the abdomen showing an aneurysmal aorta with mural thrombus formation. (This image is provided courtesy of Matthew Czar Taon, MD, Kaiser Permanente Los Angeles.)

For asymptomatic patients diagnosed either by screening or as an incidental finding, management is driven by the risk of aneurysm rupture. Aneurysms less than 5.5 cm can be followed with surveillance ultrasound, or sometimes CT (▶ **Fig. 8.7**). Currently there is no consensus on the exact surveillance schedule, but generally speaking aneurysm size less than 4 cm can be followed with repeat ultrasound every 2 to 3 years, and those between 4 and 5.4 cm require ultrasound surveillance every 6 to 12 months. Many specialists perform CTA rather than ultrasound once an aneurysm has been identified due to the inherent operator-dependent variability with ultrasound.

Anything greater than 5.5 cm in men and 5 cm in women is an indication for elective repair of asymptomatic AAAs. Rapid expansion of the aneurysm sac (> 0.5 cm/y) is another indication for elective repair, regardless of the size. Some additional findings, including large peripheral arterial aneurysms or the presence of significant PAD (which may compromise a future aneurysm repair approach), may tip the balance in favor of elective repair.

Patients below the threshold for elective repair should be treated medically with the goal of slowing the rate of aneurysm growth and decreasing the risks associated with cardiovascular disease, particularly smoking.

Screening is an effective way to detect AAA in the high-risk population and identify those who will benefit most from repair. Unfortunately, screening is underutilized, only being pursued in about 1% of all eligible patients. Without the benefit of screening, many patients with AAA will go undiagnosed until it becomes symptomatic or ruptures.

Symptomatic, *nonruptured* AAA patients may present with symptoms related to mass effect from the aneurysm sac, compression of adjacent structures, and occasionally acute limb ischemia due to thromboemboli originating from the aneurysm.

For the patients with *ruptured* AAA who survive long enough to get to the emergency department, the typical presentation includes tachycardia, hypotension, abdominal distension, and pain radiating to the flank. They are initially triaged similar to other types of internal bleeding. If stable enough for a CT, a quick scan will help confirm the diagnosis and is helpful for preoperative purposes. Unstable patients are prepped for an ex lap without imaging. A bedside ultrasound will often suffice to confirm a ruptured AAA if there is uncertainty. In the meantime, permissive hypotension with a goal systemic BP less than 90 is usually sought.

Differentiating between aortic rupture and symptomatic nonruptured aortic aneurysm by clinical symptoms alone may be unreliable, so it's important to err on the side of caution when it is uncertain.

The options for AAA repair include a surgical or endovascular approach. Open aortic repair is a technically challenging procedure, with high morbidity and mortality. It involves exposing the aorta, obtaining proximal and distal control of the vessel, and replacing the aneurysmal portion with a prosthetic graft. **EVAR,** the minimally invasive alternative to surgical repair, is now the widely accepted first-line treatment for appropriate candidates (**Procedure Box 8.3**). The aim with EVAR is to create a seal proximally, above the aneurysm sac and distally, in each iliac artery, completely excluding flow into the aneurysm sac (▶**Fig. 8.8**).

Compared to open repair, EVAR has a shorter average procedure time, decreased blood loss, and decreased perioperative morbidity and mortality. EVAR may not be possible in patients with vascular anatomy unsuitable for endografts, depending on the manufacturer's device-specific recommendations.

General anatomical considerations when determining EVAR suitability include the following:

1. Proximal aortic neck length (segment between the most caudal renal artery and superior aspect of the aneurysm sac).
2. Angle between the top of the aneurysm sac and suprarenal aorta.
3. Distal aortic diameter/length.
4. Iliac artery diameter/length.

Each device has its own thresholds for these anatomic considerations.

After an EVAR, medical management is aimed to maintain graft patency and decrease overall risk associated with cardiovascular disease, similar to the management used for patients with peripheral vascular disease. Duration of antiplatelet therapy after EVAR is not firmly established.

Postoperative complications can include graft thrombosis, graft fracture, migration or perforation, and endoleaks (▶**Table 8.6**). **Endoleaks** allow blood to enter the excluded aneurysm sac (▶**Fig. 8.9**). This can occur in five different ways (▶**Table 8.7**). In addition,

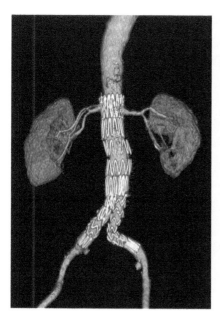

Fig. 8.8 Three-dimentional reconstruction showing an abdominal aortic aneurysm treated with an EVAR. The endoprosthetic graft with bilateral iliac limbs is shown. (This image is provided courtesy of Matthew Czar Taon, MD, Kaiser Permanente Los Angeles.)

Procedure Box 8.3: Endovascular Aneurysm Repair ⓘ

Endovascular repair of AAA is a less invasive method to decrease the risk of aneurysm growth, rupture, and death. It has replaced open surgical techniques at many centers for patients who are candidates for this technique. Preprocedural cross-sectional imaging with CTA or MRA is mandatory to ensure appropriate access vessels, to delineate landing zone characteristics, and to select the ideal grafts to have available at the time of the procedure. Additionally, patients must be willing to undergo lifelong surveillance for the development of delayed complications of endovascular repair.

While there are several devices utilized for EVAR on the market, each with its own particular procedural protocols, generally speaking, the steps are the same for most devices. The procedure begins with bilateral common femoral access; given the size of the sheaths required for these techniques, the vessels may need to be preclosed with suture-mediated closure devices or otherwise a femoral cutdown will need to be performed. An aortogram is then performed to identify the renal arteries, proximal and distal landing zones, and to confirm the previously measured graft lengths. The arteriotomy sites are then dilated, and the definitive sheaths are introduced over stiff guidewires. The ipsilateral artery is the artery that the endoprosthesis main body will be introduced through, and this side often requires a substantially larger sheath than the contralateral access.

Immediately prior to device insertion, systemic anticoagulation with intravenous heparin is initiated. The main body delivery device is then introduced over a stiff guidewire and positioned either for suprarenal or infrarenal fixation, with the fabric-covered portion just distal to the lowest renal artery, and the main body carefully deployed to expose the contralateral iliac gate (an opening in the main body into which the contralateral iliac limb is deployed). A guidewire and catheter are used to cannulate the gate from the contralateral femoral arterial sheath, which can occasionally be quite difficult due to vessel tortuosity and aneurysm size. The contralateral limb graft is then deployed over a stiff guidewire. When the contralateral iliac limb graft is deployed through the gate, there should be a short segment of overlap between the main body and the contralateral limb. The graft is then molded in place at the proximal landing zone and at the distal iliac landing zones using balloon catheters.

In some cases, the common iliac arteries are also aneurysmal, requiring extension of one or both iliac limbs into the external iliac arteries, and crossing the internal iliacs. If this is only required on one side, the internal iliac can be proximally embolized with coils or plugs (to prevent the development of an endoleak), and the stent-graft extended into to the external iliac. Operators must ensure the contralateral internal iliac artery is patent if this is performed to decrease the risk of ischemia to the pelvic organs. If both internal iliacs must be covered due to common iliac aneurysmal disease, bifurcated iliac side branch devices can be used in lieu of the conventional straight tube-graft configurations, which maintains flow to the internal iliacs while still covering the entirety of the iliac aneurysms.

At the completion of graft placement, angiography should be performed to ensure adequate positioning and seal of the graft (▶ Fig. 8.10). Finally, the arteriotomy sites are closed using either sutures, other closure devices, or using surgical techniques if a cutdown was employed.

Table 8.6 Complications after an endovascular aneurysm repair

Access-related complications	Graft-related complications
• Femoral artery pseudoaneurysm • Retroperitoneal hematoma • Arteriovenous fistula • Acute thrombosis of accessed artery	• Renal or superior mesenteric artery occlusion by the stent-graft • Renal failure, abdominal compartment syndrome

Table 8.7 Endoleaks

Endoleak	Description	Treatment
Type I	Suboptimal seals at endograft attachment sites, allowing blood to enter the aneurysm sac	Deploying another stent-graft to seal the defect
Type II	Branch vessels allow aneurysm sac filling. The most common endoleak	Transarterial embolization of the branch vessels or direct puncture of the aneurysm sac and coil or possibly liquid embolic embolization
Type III	Blood leaks into the aneurysm sac through stent-graft defects (either between the overlapping modular components or through a hole in the stent-graft itself)	Stent placed over the defect
Type IV	Blood leaks into the sac through the stent-graft material itself	None, usually self-resolves
Type V	"Endotension"; blood enters the aneurysm sac without an obvious cause. Endotension can only be diagnosed after ruling out all other causes	No good treatment

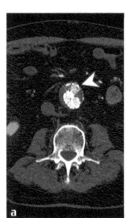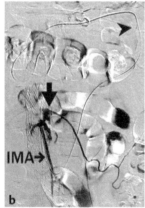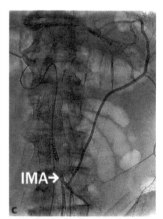

Fig. 8.9 **(a)** A surveillance CT in a 74-year-old man status post–endovascular aneurysm repair shows contrast accumulation within the aneurysm sac. **(b)** Superior mesenteric arteriogram demonstrating flow of contrast through the arc of Riolan (*arrowhead*) and into the inferior mesenteric artery (IMA), where there was retrograde filling of the aneurysm sac (*arrow*), consistent with a type II endoleak. **(c)** After coil embolization of the proximal IMA, the subsequent angiogram shows resolution of the leak.

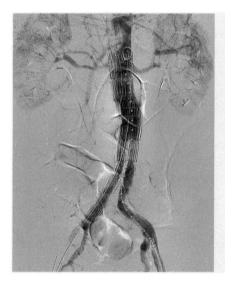

Fig. 8.10 Successful endovascular aneurysm repair with endoprosthesis positioned in the aorta and iliac stents positioned in the iliac arteries. A power injection of contrast opacifies the endograft and iliac limbs only with no opacification of the aneurysm sac. The endoprosthesis has successfully excluded the aneurysm sac from circulation. (This image is provided courtesy of Matthew Czar Taon, MD, Kaiser Permanente Los Angeles.)

if the covered stent-graft is deployed over the renal artery ostia, the patient may suffer renal ischemia and subsequent renal failure.

Post-EVAR, patients typically get surveillance CT imaging at 1, 6, and 12 months postprocedure, and annually thereafter.

Choosing EVAR versus Surgery for AAA

For asymptomatic, at-risk patients with AAAs in whom the threshold for elective repair has been reached, an elective EVAR is the procedure of choice. However, open aortic repair should be strongly considered in certain cases, such as younger, healthier patients, as they may benefit from the decreased surveillance requirements and potentially increased long-term durability.

Traditionally, all patients with ruptured AAAs would go to the OR for an open repair. As endovascular expertise has increased, more and more institutions are treating these patients' endovascularly in a hybrid OR setting with good results. There is ongoing research comparing EVAR with surgery for ruptured AAAs.

Thoracic Aortic Aneurysms

As with the abdominal counterpart, **thoracic aortic aneurysms** (TAAs) are increasing in prevalence worldwide and carry a high risk of morbidity and mortality. TAAs are increasingly being treated with endovascular techniques.

The diameter of the thoracic aorta varies by segment, normally tapering from proximal to distal. Generally, the aortic sinuses measure around 3.5 to 4 cm, while the ascending aorta and mid-descending aorta are around 2.5 to 3 cm in diameter. It is considered aneurysmal when the diameter is 50% larger than normal.

TAAs are classified by location. Ascending TAAs extend from the aortic root to the right brachiocephalic artery. Aortic arch TAAs by definition include the brachiocephalic vessels. Descending TAAs arise distal to the left subclavian artery takeoff.

TAAs by themselves usually cause no symptoms, and can remain undetected for long periods of time, only diagnosed incidentally. Large TAAs may cause symptoms related to mass effect. Nerves coursing through the mediastinum may become compressed (vagus, phrenic, recurrent laryngeal nerves, etc.) with associated neurological deficits. Aortic regurgitation can occur when there is aortic root dilation. Acute presentations of TAAs include thoracic aortic dissection and rupture.

Management of Thoracic Aortic Aneurysms

Once a patient is found to have an aneurysm, either incidentally or in the presence of symptoms, the location and size are considered. These patients tend to have other arterial aneurysms, so screening for these should be considered.

Generally speaking, the following patients should undergo evaluation for repair: (1) all symptomatic TAAs, (2) asymptomatic patients with *ascending* TAA greater than 5 cm or *descending* TAA greater than 6 cm, (3) asymptomatic patients with rapid expansion (> 0.5 cm/y), and (4) asymptomatic patients with TAAs and an associated predisposing genetic condition (e.g., Marfan's or Ehlers–Danlos). TAAs should be further worked up with CTA or MRA to map out the aortic dimensions and anatomy. Younger patients may also undergo genetic testing to check for connective tissue disorders.

Treatment options for TAAs include conservative management, surgical, and endovascular repair. The choice is based on aneurysm size, location, and presence of symptoms.

Asymptomatic TAAs that do not fall under the above "treat" categories are managed conservatively. This includes blood pressure control with a β-blocker, statin therapy, and serial cross-sectional imaging every 6 to 12 months to monitor for expansion.

If the patient is being evaluated for repair, the choice of surgery versus endovascular repair is most dependent on location of aneurysm. An unstable patient with a ruptured TAA is going to the OR. All asymptomatic, *ascending* TAAs are also going to the OR for surgical repair. The preoperative work-up for elective TAA repair is extensive and beyond the scope of this book.

Descending TAA repair is amenable to endovascular repair with a thoracic EVAR (TEVAR) (similar to an EVAR). Newer technology (branched endografts) are making TEVARs more and more viable.

Aortic Dissections

Aortic dissections occur when an intimal tear allows blood to pool within the vessel wall. The presentation can be dramatic, most commonly occurring in older, hypertensive patients who complain of tearing chest pain that radiates to the back.

When patients present to the ED with this type of chest pain, a dissection should always be on the differential. An urgent MI work-up is performed and is usually negative. At this point, most clinicians should have a high degree of suspicion for a dissection, especially in high-risk patients. Risk factors include hypertension, men in their 50s or 60s, smokers, connective tissue disease, known TAA, and those with aortic valve problems.

If the patient is stable, a CTA of the chest should be obtained. A positive study will demonstrate a dissection flap with both a true and false lumen. The dissection flap should be evaluated for the superior and inferior extent, any visible entry tears, and a determination of the origin of the aortic branch vessels from either the true or false lumen. In unstable patients, bedside transesophageal echocardiography can be performed to confirm the diagnosis.

Two commonly used classification schemes are the Stanford classification and the DeBakey classification. They're similar but the Stanford classification is more commonly used.

- Stanford A → ascending aorta and the aortic arch
- Stanford B → descending aorta
- DeBakey type 1 → ascending aorta and aortic arch; may involve descending aorta
- DeBakey type 2 → only ascending aorta
- DeBakey type 3 → only descending aorta

The first step in *all* acute dissections is lowering the blood pressure with the goal of limiting dissection extension. Intravenous β-blockers are the drug of choice. Nitroprusside can be added if additional blood pressure control is necessary, but only after β-blockers have been started. Starting a vasodilator without β-blockade can cause reflex tachycardia and potentially increased wall stress.

The next step is decided by the type of dissection and the presence or absence of complicating features. Both type A and B dissections can be complicated by malperfusion syndrome if the dissection extends into or occludes the branch arteries. Other complicating features include uncontrolled high blood pressure, unremitting refractory back pain, or rupture.

Stanford type A dissections require immediate surgical intervention. The details of the surgery will not be discussed here; just know that depending on what additional structures are involved (aortic valve, dissection extending into coronary arteries/aortic arch arterial branches, etc.), additional surgical procedures like arterial bypasses or aortic valve replacement may be required. Pure endovascular repair currently has no role in type A dissections. Some institutions are using a hybrid procedure to treat type A dissections referred to as a "frozen elephant trunk repair." For this procedure, the ascending aorta dissection is repaired surgically followed by deployment of a thoracic endograft to deal with the descending aorta dissection.

Complicated type B dissections require intervention as well, with either a surgical or endovascular repair. Thoracic endovascular stent grafts present a less morbid, minimally invasive option. TEVAR, is performed similar to the EVAR, and many of the same postprocedure complications can occur. In addition, be aware of a few more serious post-TEVAR complications. TEVARs can result in retrograde type A dissection, and stroke/paralysis can occur if the stent-graft covers too many intercostal/lumbar arteries, compromising spinal arterial supply. One way to reduce spinal cord ischemia is to insert a lumbar drain prior to a TEVAR. By reducing the CSF volume and CSF pressure, spinal cord blood flow is increased.

Uncomplicated type B dissections, on the other hand, can be managed medically. The goal is to decrease wall stress and prevent the dissection from extending or causing a catastrophic rupture. Intravenous β-blockers should be titrated to a target heart rate of 60 and systolic blood pressure of 120. Further vasodilators can be added if the β-blocker is not enough. These patients are observed closely, most often in an ICU setting.

Peripheral and Visceral Artery Aneurysms

Excluding the aorta, the most common arteries affected by arterial aneurysms are the iliac, popliteal, and splenic arteries. Many patients with aneurysms remain asymptomatic for long periods of time, and it is important to include an evaluation for popliteal/iliac artery aneurysms when performing a vascular exam in patients with peripheral vascular disease. Unfortunately, many arterial aneurysms are detected only after they rupture. Peripheral arterial aneurysms in the popliteal or iliac arteries present the additional risk of aneurysm-related thrombosis and embolization.

Iliac artery aneurysms occur commonly along with AAAs, and share the same risk factors for development. The natural history of iliac artery aneurysms is similar to AAAs; they expand progressively over time, increasing the risk of rupture. Asymptomatic iliac artery aneurysms are sometimes detected on exam as a palpable, pulsatile groin mass. When detected, further evaluation is usually performed with CTA. Ultrasound is often of limited value given how deep and tortuous the iliac arteries are in many patients.

Symptomatic patients may present after a rupture with acute groin pain and hypotension; this is a surgical emergency. Less commonly, iliac artery aneurysms may cause thromboembolic or compressive sequelae. All symptomatic patients need treatment. Treatment is also indicated for asymptomatic iliac artery aneurysms greater than 3 cm or if an aneurysm measuring less than 3 cm is rapidly expanding.

Endovascular repair with stent-graft placement across the aneurysm has become the accepted technique to treat asymptomatic or stable patients with common or external iliac aneurysms. If the aneurysm morphology is such that the stent-graft needs to be placed across the internal iliac artery, prophylactic coil embolization of the internal iliac artery is done first. This is done to prevent a type 2 endoleak. Bifurcated iliac stent-graft devices or surgical repair can also be considered if there is desire to preserve maximal pelvic arterial flow and internal iliac artery embolization is deferred.

Splenic artery aneurysms are associated with atherosclerosis, connective tissue disorders, and conditions that increase splenic arterial blood flow (liver transplantation, portal hypertension, pregnancy, etc.). Most splenic artery aneurysms are asymptomatic. When symptoms do occur, they are vague and nonspecific, including epigastric/left upper quadrant abdominal pain and malaise. Rupture presents catastrophically with initial hemodynamic instability, followed by temporary stabilization as blood collects in the lesser sac and tamponades the rupture. Eventually, the tamponade effect is lost as the expanding hematoma forces blood out of the lesser sac and the patient again becomes unstable. Unstable patients are taken to the OR for an ex lap. In these cases, the diagnosis of splenic artery aneurysm is made intraoperatively. In asymptomatic patients, the diagnosis of splenic artery aneurysm usually occurs incidentally on abdominal cross-sectional imaging.

Intervention is indicated for all symptomatic patients with splenic artery aneurysms and asymptomatic patients with splenic aneurysms greater than 2 cm. Endovascular treatment is preferred for both asymptomatic and symptomatic patients, as long as they are stable. The aneurysm sac needs to be excluded from circulation, which can be achieved with either coil embolization or placement of a stent-graft across the aneurysm. Endovascular interventions are usually successful, and surgery often is not necessary (▶ **Fig. 8.11**).

Popliteal artery aneurysms are the most commonly seen peripheral aneurysms, especially in patients with risk factors for peripheral vascular disease. Many are asymptomatic and detected during a routine vascular evaluation. A pulsatile mass may be palpated in the popliteal fossa. The diagnosis is confirmed with ultrasound.

Popliteal aneurysms can become symptomatic in several ways. While aneurysm rupture can occur (resulting in severe knee pain), it is actually *not* the most concerning sequelae, as the hemorrhage is usually confined to the popliteal fossa. Rather, intraluminal thrombosis and resulting lower extremity ischemia poses the greatest risk. Depending on the degree of luminal narrowing, some patients may present with claudication, while others develop critical limb ischemia. Acute limb ischemia can result if

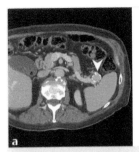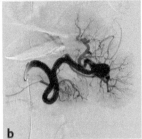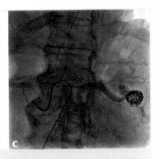

Fig. 8.11 (a) CT image shows an incidental splenic artery aneurysm. Given its size, endovascular treatment was recommended. **(b)** Digital subtraction angiography image showing the large splenic artery aneurysm. **(c)** This was successfully embolized with coils. While a covered stent can also be deployed over the neck of the aneurysm to exclude it, the tortuosity of the splenic artery precluded stent-graft placement in this case.

the aneurysm suddenly thromboses, or if thrombotic material embolizes distally. Large aneurysms can also compress surrounding structures.

Asymptomatic patients with popliteal aneurysms should be treated if the aneurysm size exceeds 2 cm. All symptomatic patients with thromboembolic manifestations should be treated. Those with claudication and critical limb ischemia should be managed the same way they are for patients with atherosclerotic disease, claudication with exercise therapy/cilostazol, and critical limb ischemia with revascularization. Acute limb ischemia should be managed with catheter-directed thrombolytics or surgical revascularization, based on the urgency of the situation.

Suggested Readings

[1] Bradbury AW. Bypass versus Angioplasty in Severe Ischaemia of the Leg (BASIL) trial: an intention-to-treat analysis of amputation-free and overall survival in patients randomized to a bypass surgery-first or a balloon angioplasty-first revascularization strategy. J Vasc Surg. 2010

[2] Guirguis-Blake JM, Beil TL, Senger CA, Whitlock EP. Ultrasonography screening for abdominal aortic aneurysms: a systematic evidence review for the U.S. Preventive Services Task Force. Ann Intern Med. 2014; 160(5):321–329

[3] Murphy TP, Hirsch AT, Ricotta JJ, et al. CLEVER Steering Committee. The Claudication: Exercise vs. Endoluminal Revascularization (CLEVER) study: rationale and methods. J Vasc Surg. 2008; 47(6):1356–1363

[4] Norgren L, Hiatt WR, Dormandy JA, Nehler MR, Harris KA, Fowkes FG; TASC II Working Group. Inter-Society Consensus for the Management of Peripheral Arterial Disease (TASC II). J Vasc Surg. 2007; 45(1) Suppl S:S5–S67

[5] Ouriel K, Veith FJ, Sasahara AA. Thrombolysis or Peripheral Arterial Surgery (TOPAS) Investigators. A comparison of recombinant urokinase with vascular surgery as initial treatment for acute arterial occlusion of the legs. N Engl J Med. 1998; 338(16):1105–1111

[6] Walker TG, Kalva SP, Yeddula K, et al. Society of Interventional Radiology Standards of Practice Committee. Interventional Radiological Society of Europe. Canadian Interventional Radiology Association. Clinical practice guidelines for endovascular abdominal aortic aneurysm repair: written by the Standards of Practice Committee for the Society of Interventional Radiology and endorsed by the Cardiovascular and Interventional Radiological Society of Europe and the Canadian Interventional Radiology Association. J Vasc Interv Radiol. 2010; 21(11):1632–1655

[7] Weaver FA, Comerota AJ, Youngblood M, Froehlich J, Hosking JD, Papanicolaou G. Surgical revascularization versus thrombolysis for nonembolic lower extremity native artery occlusions: results of a prospective randomized trial. The STILE Investigators. Surgery versus Thrombolysis for Ischemia of the Lower Extremity. J Vasc Surg. 1996; 24(4):513–521, discussion 521–523

[8] Wheatley K, Ives N, Gray R, et al; ASTRAL Investigators. Revascularization versus medical therapy for renal-artery stenosis. N Engl J Med. 2009; 361(20):1953–1962

9 Venous Disease

Andrew Klobuka, Trilochan Hiremath, and Deepak Sudheendra

The lower extremity venous circulation has two major systems: superficial and deep. The superficial veins drain the skin and direct the flow of venous blood into the deep venous system via the perforator veins. While the superficial and deep veins run longitudinally, the perforaters run horizontally (▶**Fig. 9.1,** ▶**Fig. 9.2**). Problems with flow in the perforators can sometimes propagate into the superficial veins.

The deep veins carry blood back toward the heart. In situations where the deep venous system is occluded, the superficial venous system can serve as a bypass circuit for venous return, albeit much less efficiently.

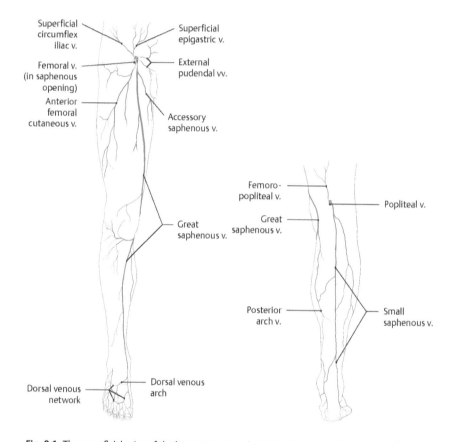

Fig. 9.1 The superficial veins of the lower extremity drain blood from the skin and superficial tissues. Venous valves prevent blood from pooling and maintain normal lower extremity hydrostatic pressure. Patients with superficial venous disease most commonly have reflux in the greater saphenous vein, but the lesser saphenous veins (including the anterior and posterior accessory saphenous in the thigh and the small saphenous in the calf) may also be involved. (Source: 1.4 Superficial Veins. In: Collares F, Faintuch S, eds. Varicose Veins: Practical Guides in Interventional Radiology. 1st Edition. Thieme; 2017. doi:10.1055/b-006-160939)

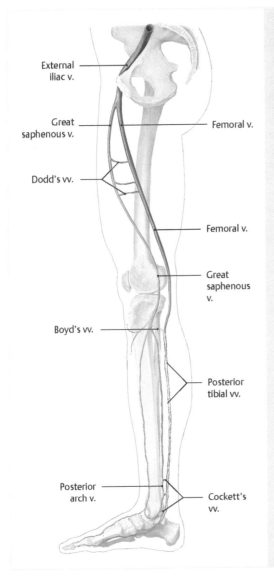

External iliac v.

Great saphenous v.

Femoral v.

Dodd's vv.

Femoral v.

Great saphenous v.

Boyd's vv.

Posterior tibial vv.

Posterior arch v.

Cockett's vv.

Fig. 9.2 Major perforators of lower extremity carry blood from the superficial veins into the deep veins. Perforators run horizontally, while the veins of the superficial and deep system run vertically. (Source: 1.5 Perforating Veins. In: Collares F, Faintuch S, eds. Varicose Veins: Practical Guides in Interventional Radiology. 1st Edition. Thieme; 2017.)

A unique feature of medium-sized veins found in the extremities is the presence of valves. Along with the normal muscular contractions of leg muscles, these one-way flaps permit blood flow only toward the heart, preventing venous blood from pooling and exerting excessive hydrostatic pressure in the extremities.

9.1 Venous Thromboembolic Disease

Venous thromboembolic disease (VTE) is a term that encompasses both deep venous thrombosis (DVT), as well as pulmonary embolism (PE). It is the third leading cause of cardiovascular death behind heart attack and stroke, and the leading cause of preventable hospital-related death.

VTE can be a complex entity, owing to a wide range of patient presentations and severities (▶Table 9.1). As you read this section, keep in mind that the key to understanding VTE management is being able to differentiate simple from complex DVT, as much of the treatment strategy hinges on this determination.

Work-up of Suspected Deep Vein Thrombosis

The symptoms most commonly associated with simple DVT are nonspecific and include extremity swelling, pain, and warmth. A swollen extremity may be caused by venous disease, lymphatic disruption, volume overload, and a number of other nonvenous conditions. Patients may have unilateral or bilateral symptoms, and in some cases may have no symptoms at all. The examination can be variable as well.

Complicating matters further, patients may be evaluated in widely different clinical settings, making it difficult to learn a single approach to diagnosis. For example, in the inpatient setting, sometimes a search for DVT will be prompted by an unexplained leukocytosis—not the type of thing you would be thinking about for a patient seen in a primary care clinic.

Given the occasionally ambiguous presentation, the patient's signs and symptoms need to be interpreted in the context of DVT risk factors to raise clinical suspicion (▶Table 9.2). Virchow's triad (venous stasis, endothelial injury, and hypercoagulable state) guides clinicians to the most common risk factors for VTE, and more exhaustive lists of risk factors generally implicate one of these three factors.

If you've spent any time in the ED, you probably have familiarity with some objective tools used to determine the probability of DVT. Measuring a D-dimer can be helpful

Table 9.1 Spectrum of VTE presentations

	DVT	PE
Acute symptoms	Lower extremity pain, swelling, edema	Hypoxemia, tachypnea
Acute complications	Phlegmasia, pulmonary embolism	RV dysfunction and obstructive shock
Chronic complications	Post-thrombotic syndrome	Pulmonary hypertension (CTEPH)

Abbreviations: CTEPH, chronic thromboembolic pulmonary hypertension; DVT, deep venous thrombosis; PE, pulmonary embolism; RV, right ventricular; VTE, venous thromboembolic.

Table 9.2 VTE risk factors

Prior DVT

Malignancy

Recent surgery

Pregnancy

Oral contraceptives

Immobilization (travel history, trauma, etc.)

Inherited coagulopathy

Smoking

Abbreviation: DVT, deep venous thrombosis.

as a screening test but needs to be used appropriately. When you order a D-dimer, you should have an understanding how the result will guide your next step. Having a D-dimer come back in the normal range ("negative") should give you confidence in ruling out DVT. Unfortunately, postsurgical and cancer patients (in whom DVT risk tends to be greatest) often have a high level of systemic inflammation and will almost always have an elevated D-dimer. In these cases, an elevated D-dimer is less useful.

The **Wells Score for DVT** is a validated metric for determining pretest probably for DVT. Essentially, those considered low or moderate risk by the Wells score should get a D-dimer, while high-risk patients should get an ultrasound and no D-dimer.

In reality, most clinicians rely on a clinical gestalt rather than a Wells score to determine when to image for suspected DVT. While not the most evidence-based approach, this is probably okay for a couple of reasons. One, an ultrasound is a relatively cheap test that can give a near definitive answer without any radiation exposure to the patient. Two, a missed diagnosis has the potential for serious complications, as will be discussed later.

Compression ultrasound is the initial imaging modality of choice. Noncompressible veins are highly suggestive for the presence of DVT. The exam will also determine the location and extent of clot burden (important for management) and can differentiate between acute and chronic DVT. Acute DVTs tend to be anechoic within larger-caliber veins, and typically do not have identifiable collaterals. Chronic DVTs are more often echogenic, within a narrow vein, and are accompanied by collaterals. Elastography is being investigated as a novel method for determining clot chronicity, but it has not yet been validated.

The sensitivity and specificity of compression ultrasound for detection of DVT is high, and nondiagnostic studies are the minority. A nondiagnostic study can be repeated a few days later to clarify the findings. Rarely, CT or MR venography is used in cases of suspected DVT involving the iliac vessels or IVC (where ultrasound compression is not possible), in some cases where the DVT is considered complicated, and occasionally for nondiagnostic ultrasounds.

Once a DVT is confirmed by ultrasound, clot burden, location, and chronicity are used to determine the treatment strategy. With simple DVTs this is relatively straightforward. Unfortunately, not all DVTs are diagnosed before complications arise. The complications that result from untreated DVT can be categorized as *local* or *embolic*.

Local Sequelae of Deep Vein Thromboses

Local complications of DVTs can develop acutely as phlegmasia, or chronically as post thrombotic syndrome (PTS).

Phlegmasia results from massive deep venous occlusion, resulting in venous congestion, cyanosis, and critical limb ischemia of the extremity. Although it represents a small minority of cases, recognition is important as phlegmasia is considered a surgical emergency. If not treated appropriately, it can quickly progress to venous gangrene and limb loss. There is a higher incidence of phlegmasia in cancer patients who develop DVT, reflecting a profoundly hypercoagulable state and higher risk of extensive thrombosis.

Phlegmasia is recognized by the presence of unique physical exam findings. **Phlegmasia alba dolens** is characterized by a pale, white-appearing limb as a result of transient arterial spasm induced by the massive venous thrombotic event. Pulses may be absent, but limb loss is unlikely at this stage. About half of the patients with phlegmasia alba dolens progress to **phlegmasia cerulea dolens**, the more serious counterpart. This results when the thrombosis involves both the deep *and* superficial venous systems. With collateral flow provided by the superficial veins compromised, venous hypertension becomes extreme. The

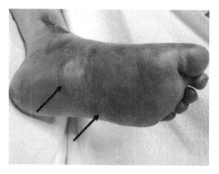

Fig. 9.3 This patient presented with a swollen, cyanotic foot, consistent with a diagnosis of phlegmasia cerulea dolens. (Source: Case 135. A 66-year-old woman with diabetes underwent a coronary bypass 11 days prior. In: Ferral H, Lorenz J, eds. RadCases: Interventional Radiology. 1st Edition. Thieme; 2010.)

appearance of the extremity progresses from pale to cyanotic (▶ **Fig. 9.3**). Venous hypertension and edema restricts arterial blood flow, leading to ischemia. Without prompt treatment, this almost invariably leads to venous gangrene, potentially requiring amputation.

Phlegmasia is a rare complication of DVT. Far more common is **PTS,** which can develop months after an acute DVT. Proximal DVTs, particularly ileofemoral, have the highest risk of causing PTS (nearly half the patients end up with PTS in 1 to 2 years). This condition is characterized by a constellation of symptoms, including pain, swelling, heaviness, fatigue, skin pigmentation, and possibly skin ulceration when severe. PTS is caused by damaged venous valves, with resulting reflux and pooling of blood in the distal veins, and ultimately venous hypertension. In mild cases, symptoms of PTS are similar to those of acute DVT, so evaluation for PTS should not be performed for at least 3 months after an acute DVT.

The diagnosis of PTS is clinical, usually apparent when classic symptoms develop several months after a documented DVT. The **Villalta scale** is a tool used to grade the severity, and can be found online for reference. Patients with a score less than 5 indicates no PTS, 5 to 14 is consistent with mild-to-moderate PTS, and 15 or more (or the presence of a venous ulcer) defines severe PTS.

The quality of life in these patients is poor, and unfortunately there is no cure for PTS. Symptom management typically involves compression stockings, leg elevation, and exercise. In experienced centers, endovascular techniques can be used to improve (but not cure) PTS symptoms. For this reason, PTS prevention is an important consideration in every patient diagnosed with a DVT.

Pulmonary Embolism

Though pulmonary embolism can result from other causes, the vast majority of PEs are a complication of DVT. Despite the association between these two conditions, PE can sometimes present in the absence of symptomatic DVT.

The pathophysiology of PE and development of symptoms involves both the circulatory and respiratory systems. When thrombus in the pulmonary artery is large enough, pulmonary artery pressure increases, resulting in increased right ventricle size and decreased cardiac output. The response to decreased cardiac output is a sympathetic nervous system mediated, compensatory increase in heart rate and systemic vasoconstriction. The thinner-walled right ventricle is not suited for pumping against high pressures in the pulmonary circulation, and right-sided heart failure can result if the pulmonary hypertension is severe enough. If the obstruction does not improve, progressive right ventricular fatigue will eventually lead to right-sided heart failure, compromised cardiac output, and systemic hypotension.

From a respiratory standpoint, the presence of thrombus results in V/Q mismatch. The parts of the lungs unaffected by the embolus receive a compensatory increase in blood flow, so much that normal ventilation can't keep up and hypoxemia develops. Platelet-derived factors released due to the presence of clot can cause edema of the healthy lung, which further worsens oxygenation. There are multiple ways in which hypoxemia develops in these patients, so it makes sense that dyspnea is the most common symptom in PE patients. Hemoptysis and chest pain are not as common, but can be seen when the PE results in pulmonary infarct.

The severity of PE can vary dramatically depending on the clot burden, as well as the chronicity and the patient's baseline cardiopulmonary health. Some may be completely asymptomatic, while others may die within minutes of an embolic event. As with DVT, pulmonary embolism produces a varied clinical picture for different patients. It's also investigated in very different settings and with different levels of suspicion. This can make it difficult to adopt one single approach to diagnosis. We'll focus on a patient presenting to the emergency room.

The differential for patients coming to the ED with dyspnea and chest pain is broad. All patients will get a basic work-up before any targeted diagnostics for PE. A chest X-ray in a patient with PE can be completely clear or may show nonspecific findings such as atelectasis. Only in a minority of cases it will show a relatively specific finding for PE, like a Hampton's hump (indicating pulmonary infarct). An ECG may demonstrate an $S_1 Q_3 T_3$ morphology, and arterial blood gas may reveal a hypocapnic, hypoxemic respiratory alkalosis. Bear in mind that even large pulmonary emboli can be present without any of these findings.

Making a clinical diagnosis of PE is difficult in all but the most obvious cases, so it usually takes a combination of risk factors and lack of better alternative diagnoses to narrow down those patients who need further work-up. Analogous to that for DVTs, there is a Wells score available for estimating the pretest probability of PE. If there is low probability, a D-dimer can be used to rule it out. If there is a high pretest probability based on the Wells criteria (score > 4), a CT pulmonary angiogram (aka PE study) is the next step. Alternatively, some clinicians use the **PERC rule**. The PERC rule is a validated set of criteria that, if met, indicate the risk of PE is sufficiently low to forgo imaging.

When used in conjunction with the Well's score for patient selection, a technically adequate CT pulmonary angiography (CTPA) is both sensitive and specific for the detection of PE, carrying a negative predictive value that approaches 100%. When the study is negative, it can often be valuable in determining an alternative cause for the patient's symptoms. When positive, it can aid in determining the severity of PE by quantifying the amount of clot and identifying any evidence of pulmonary infarct or right heart strain (▶ Fig. 9.4). Perhaps because of how useful the study has proven to be, the number of CTPAs has increased dramatically in the past two decades (including in patients who fall in the low pretest probability group).

Unlike the ultrasound for DVT diagnosis, CT exposes the patient to radiation and the risks associated with contrast administration. Additionally, liberal use of CTPA in the low-probability setting greatly increases the false-positive rate, which leads to inappropriate and avoidable treatment. This is something to keep in mind as you might find yourself in an IR practice that admits to its own service, and faced with a questionable PE in a postoperative patient.

For those patients who cannot get CTPA, due to severe contrast allergy or any other reason, a V/Q scan is another option. Pregnant patients with suspected PE get a V/Q over CTPA only when the chest X-ray is normal. A V/Q scan may be interpreted as low probability, intermediate probability, or high probability. A low-probability scan in a patient with low pretest probability needs no further work-up. A high-probability scan in a high pretest probability patient is considered positive for PE. Any other combination of discordance between the V/Q scan and the pretest probability is considered indeterminate. These patients can be further evaluated with compression ultrasound of the extremities. If DVT is identified, empiric treatment of PE is appropriate. When there is discrepancy between the ultrasound finding and the clinical suspicion for PE, these patients are evaluated on a case-by-case basis in light of the risks and benefits of treatment.

PEs are categorized as massive, submassive, or low risk. In massive PE, the patient has evidence of right heart strain and is hypotensive, often requiring inotropic support. In submassive PE, the patient has right heart strain, but is normotensive and hemodynamically stable. Low-risk patients have neither right heart strain nor hypotension, but may be symptomatic in other ways.

Right heart strain can be determined in a number of different ways. Suggestive findings on the CTPA include flattening of the interventricular septum, right ventricular (RV) enlargement, and reflux of contrast (▶ **Fig. 9.5**). Bedside ultrasound will show similar findings. Elevated biomarkers, including troponin and pro–B-type natriuretic peptide (pro-BNP), are also suggestive, especially when there are simultaneous imaging clues.

In most adequately treated PEs, pulmonary vascular physiology and right heart strain will return to normal after the pulmonary artery thrombus is resorbed by the body. In a small minority of patients, the pulmonary artery thrombus persists, organizes, and leads to a state of pulmonary hypertension. This condition is known as **chronic thromboembolic pulmonary hypertension (CTEPH)**.

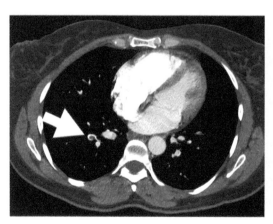

Fig. 9.4 This postoperative patient developed sudden-onset dyspnea and tachycardia overnight. CT pulmonary angiography study was obtained which showed a right-sided subsegmental pulmonary embolism (*arrow*).

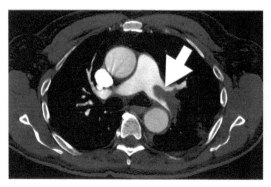

Fig. 9.5 A patient with a history of pancreatic cancer developed sudden-onset dyspnea and chest pain. After ruling out a myocardial infarct, a CT pulmonary angiography study was obtained which showed a large pulmonary embolism (PE) in the left main pulmonary artery (*arrow*). A subsequent echocardiogram identified findings of right heart strain, not unexpected for the size of this PE.

Patients with CTEPH usually have a known history of acute PE, and present with dyspnea on exertion or signs of right heart dysfunction (jugular vein distention [JVD], peripheral edema, etc.). An echocardiogram in these patients will reveal right heart strain. If suspected, CTEPH can be further evaluated with a V/Q scan. Findings of a mismatched perfusion defect is consistent with CTEPH (the same finding as for acute PE). If CTEPH is likely based on the V/Q, the patient will undergo a number of other tests to assess the degree of cardiopulmonary dysfunction.

Management of Venous Thromboembolism

The goals of DVT management include (1) symptom relief, (2) acute PE prevention, (3) recurrent DVT prevention, and (4) PTS prevention. When PE is the presenting problem, the treatment strategy includes the above, acknowledging the likelihood of concurrent DVT, but with a more pressing goal of preserving or restoring the patient's hemodynamic status.

Oral anticoagulation is the most common treatment for both DVTs and PEs. Anticoagulation does not directly break down clot, but does prevent propagation of the thrombus while the body naturally lyses it. For patients who need PE prophylaxis but cannot be anticoagulated or in whom anticoagulation has failed, an IVC filter may be an alternative. In cases of complicated VTE, certain patients benefit from venous recanalization with either endovascular therapy (catheter-directed therapy) or systemic thrombolytics.

The options available for anticoagulation include the following:

1. *Parenteral* agents such as unfractionated heparin or argatroban (for heparin allergy or history of heparin-induced thrombocytopenia).
2. *Subcutaneous* agents such as low-molecular-weight heparin (LMWH; enoxaparin) or fondaparinux.
3. *Oral* anticoagulants including warfarin (vitamin K antagonist) and direct oral anticoagulants (DOACs) such as rivaroxaban/apixaban (factor Xa inhibitors) or dabigatran (direct thrombin inhibitors).

In 2016, the American College of Chest Physicians (ACCP) released updated guidelines on antithrombotic therapy and anticoagulant selection. According to those recommendations, cancer patients requiring anticoagulation for VTE should be put on LMWH. Noncancer patients should preferentially be put on a DOAC over warfarin.

DOACs come with certain advantages over warfarin, including less drug interactions. Warfarin's drug interactions can lead to a supratherapeutic international normalized ratio (INR) and are a huge headache for clinicians. Further, DOACs do not require routine monitoring as warfarin does. This is great for patients, but it comes with the price of not being able to determine patient compliance.

A few other disadvantages of DOACs should be noted. The majority of the DOACs are renally cleared, and should be used with caution in patients with renal impairment. They are contraindicated in patients with *severe* renal impairment. Most clinicians will anticoagulate patients with end-stage renal disease (ESRD) with unfractionated heparin and warfarin (not LMWH, since it is also renally cleared). Finally, some of the DOACs do not have reversal agents, though these are expected to be available in the near future. Already, dabigatran has a reversal agent (idarucizumab). For the other DOACs (apixaban, rivaroxaban, edoxaban), prothrombin complex concentrate can be used if immediate reversal of anticoagulation is required. The half-life of the DOACs is relatively short (~ 12 hours), and generally does not require reversal in most scenarios.

While on IR, you may be asked when anticoagulation should be stopped before an elective procedure with a moderate-to-high bleeding risk. Warfarin should be stopped 5 to 6 days prior to a procedure and INR should be checked the morning of the procedure. DOACs usually can be stopped 2 to 3 days before an elective procedure. LMWH has a much shorter half-life (4–5 hours) and can be stopped the day before the procedure.

Management of Deep Vein Thromboses

Not all DVTs need to be treated (▶ Fig. 9.6). **Distal DVTs** (below the knee in the anterior/posterior tibialis, peroneal, and deep muscular veins) generally have a lower risk of embolization, and treatment is usually not necessary. There are a few key exceptions. Symptomatic distal DVTs and patients with risk factors for proximal extension *should* be treated. Risk factors for proximal extension include DVT in more than two veins, thrombus just distal to the popliteal vein, thrombus that is notably large in either diameter or length, patients with active cancer, inpatients, and those with unprovoked DVT.

Asymptomatic patients and those without risk factors for extension should get follow-up with serial ultrasound exams until resolution is ensured. **Proximal DVTs** (above the knee in the iliac, femoral, or popliteal veins) confer a higher risk of complications and should all be treated.

Simple DVTs are treated in the outpatient setting. The most common scenario when a DVT is diagnosed in the ED is for the patient to be put on LMWH until warfarin becomes therapeutic, or just simply started on a DOAC. Patients on LMWH/warfarin follow-up with their primary care physician or a specialized warfarin clinic for INR checks every couple days during this transition. DOACs have rapid onset to therapeutic activity and therefore do not need to be bridged with LMWH. For this reason, DOACs are becoming increasingly popular for treatment of simple DVTs.

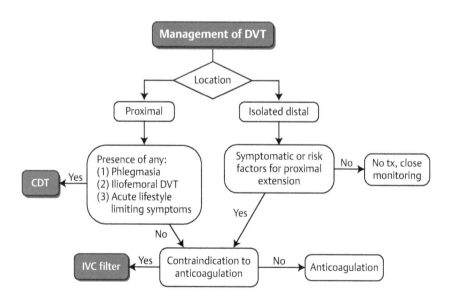

Fig. 9.6 Simplified algorithm for management of deep venous thromboses. CDT, catheter-directed thrombolysis.

The length of anticoagulation depends on a few factors. First, was the DVT provoked or unprovoked? Provoked DVTs can be attributed to an underlying cause, whether it's a prolonged hospitalization, recent surgery, or certain medications. Unprovoked DVTs occur in patients without identifiable risk factors. For a first provoked DVT, the standard anticoagulation duration is 3 months. Those with an unprovoked DVT may be extended to 6 or 12 months. Patients with recurrent DVT or provoked DVT with irreversible, persistent, or multiple risk factors, extended or indefinite anticoagulation is often the best course.

Risk of recurrence typically peaks in the first 6 to 12 months following an acute DVT, and is higher when the DVT was unprovoked. The WARFASA trial by Becattini et al in 2012 found that starting 100 mg of daily aspirin after completion of anticoagulation therapy reduces the risk of recurrence in unprovoked DVT patients, without risk of major bleeding.

After treatment is initiated, some patients are tested for genetic hypercoagulability. Thrombophilia testing should be undertaken when there is a positive family history of a genetic hypercoagulability disorder, if the patient is presenting with thromboembolism at a young age without the typical risk factors (smoking, birth control), or for thrombosis in atypical sites such as mesenteric veins.

To put things in perspective, the presence of factor V Leiden mutation, the most common genetic hypercoagulability disorder among Caucasians, carries a relative risk of VTE of less than 5, compared to the unaffected population. The relative risk of VTE from active cancer or recent surgery is on the order of 1,000. Beyond that, studies have not shown factor V Leiden to change the risk of recurrent VTE sufficiently to warrant prolongation of anticoagulation.

In most patients, anticoagulation is usually adequate for PE prophylaxis. However, anticoagulation may be contraindicated in some due to a high bleeding risk. Other patients may have worsening thrombosis despite adherence to anticoagulation. These are the patients who get referred for an **IVC filter** placement. In general, IVC filters are recommended for patients who need to be protected from a PE but anticoagulation is contraindicated or therapeutic anticoagulation has failed. Filters will be discussed in greater detail later in the chapter.

There are several other scenarios where anticoagulation for DVT treatment is insufficient, and escalation of treatment is considered. Remember, anticoagulation only prevents clot extension, it does *not* recanalize the vessel. In patients with severe, lifestyle-limiting symptoms and in patients with phlegmasia, the severity of symptoms is great enough to merit venous recanalization for expedited symptom relief and limb salvage. Options for recanalization include endovascular catheter-directed pharmacomechanical thrombolysis and surgical thrombectomy.

Catheter-directed thrombolysis (CDT) is an endovascular therapy that allows for the delivery of low doses of thrombolytic to treat DVT (**Procedure Box 9.1**). The basic idea with CDT involves use of a catheter with its tip in proximity of the clot to allow infusion of a lytic agent directly where it is needed. Once the catheter is in place, the patient is admitted to the ICU while the thrombolytic is administered. Appropriate dosing for catheter-directed tissue plasminogen activator (tPA) is 0.01 mg/kg/h (generally not exceeding a total dose of 1 mg/h). If multiple catheters are used, the dose is typically divided so that the total does not exceed 1 mg/h. The patient gets serial monitoring of hemoglobin levels, fibrinogen (varies by institution), and routine examination of the access sites during infusion. They are brought back to IR for venography after 12 to 24 hours. If repeat venography shows persistent clot burden, mechanical techniques can be used to disrupt the clot.

Mechanical thrombectomy is an important adjunct to pharmacological CDT, and is used to physically disrupt and remove clot (**Procedure Box 9.2**). Mechanical catheter-directed techniques include maceration, aspiration or suction, and rheolytic hydrolysis, amongst others.

The most common complication related to CDT is major bleeding. CDT should not be employed in patients with active bleeding, patients with a recent brain/spine surgery, or patients who have suffered a recent stroke (▶ **Table 9.3**). Another serious complication is symptomatic pulmonary embolism from thrombus manipulation. Patients with

---

Procedure Box 9.1: Catheter-Directed Thrombolysis   i

Catheter-directed thrombolysis can be performed in systemic veins, portal veins, and in the pulmonary arteries. Initial access is dependent on where the thrombus is, and should be tailored to allow the infusion catheter to cover the entire thrombus burden without portions of the catheter being covered by a sheath; multiple access sites may be required in the setting of long-segment thrombosis.

The occlusion is crossed using a catheter–guidewire combination. Once the thrombus has been crossed, angiography should be performed to verify that the catheter is intraluminal. A multi–side hole infusion catheter is then placed across the occlusion and the inner obturator wire is placed through the catheter to occlude the end hole. Thrombolytic agents are then administered slowly through the catheter, which spray outward from the side holes to lyse thrombus. The patients are brought back between 4 and 24 hours after catheter placement for thrombolysis check venography. Multiple days of lysis may be required in some patients.

Thrombolytic agents used include urokinase and tPA, with the latter far more common. The **"pulse-spray" technique** is commonly employed to deliver the lytic agents; this is where an initial bolus is delivered, followed by a continuous infusion overnight. Heparin should also be infused at slightly less than therapeutic doses through the sheath to prevent thrombus formation on the catheter or sheath. Simultaneous full-dose anticoagulation is not recommended due to the increased risk of bleeding complications.

Patients should be admitted to the ICU for close monitoring and frequent lab draws. They will be monitored for complications secondary to thrombolytic therapy, including access site or remote bleeding, distal embolization, or compartment syndrome. Platelet counts, hemoglobin, and fibrinogen levels should all be closely monitored for the duration of the lytic infusion, to help identify those patients at high risk for catastrophic bleeding.

Table 9.3 General contraindications to thrombolysis

Recent stroke, ICH, head trauma in past 3 months

CT showing ICH or large, irreversible area of infarct

Recent head/spine surgery

Presence of cerebral aneurysm, intracranial neoplasm, AVM

SBP ≥ 185 or DBP ≥ 110 mm Hg

Active internal bleeding

Bleeding diathesis (INR > 1.7, elevated PTT, platelet count < 100,000, etc.)

Abbreviations: AVM, arteriovenous malformation; DBP, diastolic blood pressure; ICH, intracranial hemorrhage; INR, international normalized ratio; PTT, partial thromboplastin time; SBP, systolic blood pressure.

Procedure Box 9.2: Mechanical Thrombectomy ℹ

Mechanical thrombectomy involves the physical disruption and removal of thrombus, and may be combined with thrombolytic agents administered during the procedure (pharmacomechanical thrombectomy). After gaining vascular access and identifying and crossing the occlusion, thrombus can be disrupted/removed in several ways.

With **suction thrombectomy**, a vacuum created by simple aspiration catheters can be used to grab onto clots and suck them through the catheter lumen, or lodge them at the catheter tip, facilitating their extraction by removing the catheter from the sheath. Dedicated vacuum-assisted thrombectomy catheters exist which utilize larger catheter lumens with reinforced material resistant to collapse under negative pressure.

Rheolytic thrombectomy utilizes a catheter which continuously instills and aspirates fluid through separate holes at the tip. This both disrupts the thrombus and creates a continuous vortex of negative pressure to remove fragmented thrombotic material. Because of the fragmentation of thrombus and rapidly flowing fluid at the catheter tip, erythrocyte lysis will occur, which carries the risk of bradycardia (due to adenosine release) and renal injury. The number of pulses is determined by the catheter diameter and whether it is used in completely thrombosed or partially flowing segments of the vasculature. Patients should be counseled that reddish- or brownish-colored urine after the procedure is a normal side effect and will decrease over time.

a history of cancer that typically results in hemorrhagic intracranial metastases (melanoma, renal cell, chorio-, hepatocellular-, thyroid, lung, and breast carcinomas) should be screened with contrast-enhanced CT or brain MRI prior to treatment.

The risk of CDT-related PE can be minimized by maintaining therapeutic unfractionated heparin levels before, during, and after the procedure with routine partial thromboplastin time (PTT) monitoring. For those patients at high risk of morbidity from PE, for example, those with poor cardiopulmonary reserve, a retrievable IVC filter can be placed prior to thrombolysis.

Large veins can also be recanalized through open **surgical thrombectomy**. This is reserved for patients with a prohibitively high bleeding risk or in whom CDT cannot be done.

In patients with DVTs, three patient populations should be considered for escalation of care to CDT:

1. Patients with phlegmasia.
2. Patients with lifestyle-limiting acute DVT symptoms not resolving on anticoagulation.
3. Patients with ileofemoral or caval thrombosis, in whom the risk for developing severe PTS is high.

In these patient populations, the benefits of venous recanalization can potentially outweigh the risks associated with the procedure.

When patients present with phlegmasia, they are immediately started on anticoagulation. However, because there is extensive thrombosis occluding blood return, anticoagulation is not enough (again, it doesn't recanalize!). The only solution is opening the deep veins with CDT or surgical thrombectomy (▶ **Fig. 9.7**).

Similarly, when a patient with a symptomatic proximal DVT continues to have symptoms despite being on anticoagulation, CDT can be considered to recanalize the vein and improve flow.

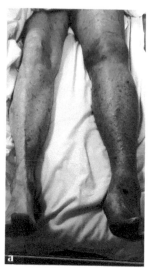 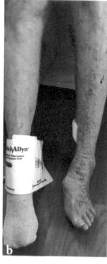

Fig. 9.7 Left-sided phlegmasia, (a) before and, (b) after catheter-directed thrombolysis. (These images are provided courtesy of Deepak Sudheendra, MD, University of Pennsylvania Medical Center.)

Recanalization with CDT is also considered when patients present with ileofemoral DVT. As mentioned, ileofemoral DVT results in the greatest risk of developing PTS, and also accounts for the most severe cases, so it makes sense to be more aggressive with treatment. However, the use of CDT for PTS prevention is somewhat controversial.

Two large clinical trials have studied whether CDT reduces risk of PTS. The CAVENT randomized controlled clinical trial by Haig et al in 2016 showed a 28% absolute risk reduction in PTS in patients treated with CDT for a first-time iliofemoral DVT. In contrast, the ATTRACT trial by Vedantham et al in 2017 failed to show evidence that pharmacomechanical CDT prevents PTS but did identify a significant decrease in PTS *severity* in those patients. The study also identified an increase in bleeding when CDT was used compared to anticoagulation alone, although none of the bleeds were fatal. Based on these results, the ATTRACT trial has dampened some of the enthusiasm for the role of CDT in treating acute DVT. Depending on who you ask, the answer will vary so we'll simply leave you with an unsatisfying "more studies are needed." Nevertheless, a strong argument can be made for employing CDT when seeing a young, otherwise-healthy patient with extensive ileofemoral DVT. These patients will reap the greatest benefits from CDT by possibly reducing the risk or severity of PTS.

Management of Acute Pulmonary Embolism

The first step in management of acute PE is determining the patient's risk (▶ **Fig. 9.8**). Low-risk patients are hemodynamically stable and have no evidence of right heart strain. The anticoagulation strategy in these patients is similar to that for simple DVT (either LMWH bridge + warfarin or DOAC). They are admitted to the floor for observation, but generally get discharged after a day or so, as long as they remain stable. Low-risk patients who are asymptomatic and have no problem with medication compliance may even be sent home from the ED on anticoagulation without admission.

Massive PEs and submassive PEs are identified as being high risk by the presence of right heart strain. They are started on a heparin drip and admitted to the ICU. Massive PEs are characterized by hemodynamic instability. Emergent pulmonary artery recanalization is

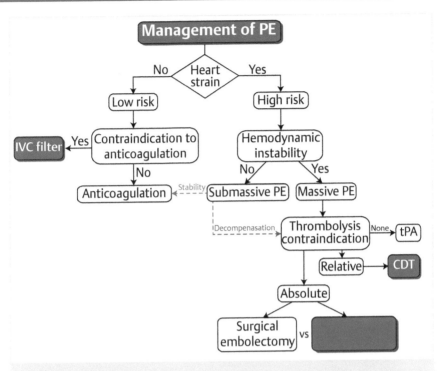

Fig. 9.8 Simplified algorithm for management of pulmonary embolisms. CDT, catheter-directed thrombolysis; tPA, tissue plasminogen activator.

important, as they can rapidly develop cardiac arrest without hemodynamic support. First-line therapy for these patients is systemic thrombolysis with 100 mg of tPA, given as a continuous infusion over 2 hours. Thrombolysis may be contraindicated in some cases (▶Table 9.3).

The use of systemic tPA therapy in cases of massive PE can rapidly reverse right heart failure, decrease mortality and the rate of recurrence. Successful lytic therapy treats the obstructing pulmonary artery thrombus, decreases pulmonary hypertension, and dissolves any residual thrombus in the deep vein from which the embolus originated.

Submassive PEs are characterized by hemodynamic stability; these patients have not yet decompensated from the right heart stress. With anticoagulation initiated, they remain in the ICU until stability is assured. After this they can be transitioned to oral anticoagulation. It's important to note that some patients may have a *high-risk* submassive PE. These patients, despite being normotensive, tend to clinically look very ill, have worrisome echo findings, and have profound hypoxia—all heralds for imminent decompensation. These high-risk patients probably benefit from pulmonary artery recanalization with lytic therapy (if there is no thrombolysis contraindication). A recent meta-analysis by Chatterjee et al in 2014 identified a lower rate of mortality, but a higher risk of major bleeding when systemic thrombolysis was used in submassive PEs. Unfortunately, identifying the high-risk submassive PE is not always easy, and the use of lytic therapy for submassive PE with moderate-to-severe RV dysfunction remains controversial. The Pulmonary Embolism Severity Index (PESI score) is a tool that is available online which can help indentify those at highest risk for short- and long-term morbidity and mortality.

Endovascular interventions for massive/submassive PEs are appropriate for patients with contraindications to systemic thrombolysis. An alternative for those with a *relative* contraindication to full-dose thrombolysis is pharmacomechanical breakdown of the thrombus with a catheter-directed, reduced dose of tPA (in the range of 20–25 mg).

If there is an absolute contraindication to thrombolytic therapy, insufficient time for tPA to take effect, or a failure of systemic thrombolysis, *mechanical* catheter-directed techniques, or surgical embolectomy is recommended.

IVC Filters

The general idea behind an IVC filter is to prevent existing or potential lower extremity thrombus from traveling to the lungs (**Procedure Box 9.3**). Even though it is typically a simple procedure, placement of an IVC filter should only be considered in cases where anticoagulation is contraindicated. A typical scenario is an elderly patient with recurrent VTE, but a high fall risk and poor candidate for anticoagulation. Sometimes the measure is temporary, as in preoperative neurosurgery or trauma patients who can't be anticoagulated for operative reasons.

There are both permanent and retrievable types of filters available. If the patient has only a short-term risk of PE (or short-term contraindication to anticoagulation), a retrievable IVC filter is recommended. A permanent filter is reserved for those with irreversible risk of PE, a lifelong contraindication to anticoagulation, or a short life expectancy where retrieval would be inappropriate.

Procedure Box 9.3: IVC Filter Placement ⓘ

Access is usually obtained via the right internal jugular vein or right common femoral vein, as these sites have a more direct path to the IVC, decreasing the incidence of filter tilt following deployment.

Prior to placing an IVC filter, caval anatomy must be assessed using caval venography. This may reveal anatomic variants including mega-cava (IVC diameter > 2.8 cm), a duplicated IVC, circumaortic renal vein, and azygous continuation of the IVC. Most of the variants don't preclude filter placement, but certain procedural adjustments may need to be made. For example, for a mega-cava, bilateral iliac filters may be necessary, while duplicated IVCs may necessitate filter placement in each cava.

Venography is also important to assess for an iliofemoral/renal/gonadal vein/IVC thrombus, as these may require a different deployment location or multiple filters. For most filters, the diameter of the cava must lie between 15 and 30 mm to ensure adequate filter expansion and wall apposition, respectively.

The site of the renal vein confluence with the IVC must be identified on each side, so that the filter can be deployed either below (infrarenal) or above (suprarenal) their ostia, decreasing the risk of renal vein thrombosis and filter tilt or migration.

Once access is secured, an introducer sheath is positioned within the IVC. The filter is advanced through the sheath to the distal end. Once appropriately positioned (most commonly with the filter tip at or slightly below the level of the lower renal vein), the filter can be deployed according to manufacturer instructions, which varies by type. You'll commonly see a pin and pull technique, where the filter is held in place and the overlying sheath is retracted, unsheathing and deploying the filter.

Prior to retrievable IVC filter placement, there should be a discussion with the patient regarding the risks of IVC filters and the importance of prompt retrieval. The longer the filter is kept in, the more likely complications may arise. This includes penetration of the caval wall and possibly the surrounding structures, migration of the strut filter, fracture, and thrombosis distal to the filter (in some cases complete caval thrombosis) (▶Fig. 9.9). The longer a filter is in place, the more challenging it can become to remove. For these reasons, IVC filters should be retrieved when they are no longer needed, for example when the patient is back on anticoagulation or when the patient is out of the VTE-risk period.

There are very few true contraindications to IVC filter placement. These include poor access to the vena cava, and anatomic constraints such as extensive caval thrombus or extrinsic compression.

Most filters that have been placed appropriately will not go on to cause any problems. Occasionally, unplanned filter removal is necessary due to a change in position of the device, loss of structural integrity, perforation, or dislodgement during other procedures (▶Fig. 9.10).

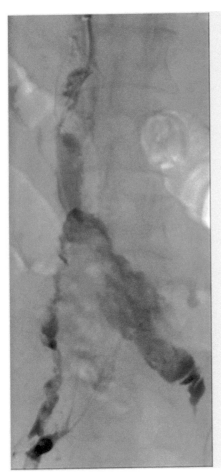

Fig. 9.9 A patient with a permanent filter in place presented with bilateral lower extremity swelling and pain. A digital subtraction venogram showed complete occlusion of the iliocaval system below the filter, consistent with extensive acute thrombosis.

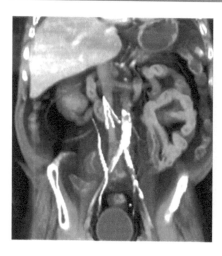

Fig. 9.10 This patient presented with vague back pain and a CT venogram was obtained. Coronal reconstruction of the CT venographic images shows a tilted filter with strut perforation through the caval wall. This filter was later removed due to ongoing pain and the risk of aortic injury.

Table 9.4 Differences between primary and secondary CVI

	Primary CVI	Secondary CVI
Pathophysiology	Idiopathic venous valve dysfunction	Insult to venous valves (acute thrombus) causes valve dysfunction
Venous system usually affected	Superficial venous system	Deep venous system
Treatment	Compression stockings, endovenous ablation/sclerotherapy	Compression stockings

Abbreviation: CVI, Chronic venous insufficiency.

9.2 Chronic Venous Insufficiency

Chronic venous insufficiency (CVI) is a consequence of venous valvular dysfunction, which leads to chronic reflux and pooling of blood in the lower extremities, and ultimately venous hypertension.

Venous hypertension results in increased hydrostatic pressure in the vein, weakening the wall, and causing abnormal dilation. This consequence of this includes some of cosmetic sequelae of venous insufficiency (telangiectasias, varicose veins, etc.). Increased hydrostatic pressure also forces fluid into the interstitium and promotes release of inflammatory mediators. The inflammatory response can lead to a more dramatic presentation of venous insufficiency including lipodermatosclerosis and venous ulcers.

Post-thrombotic syndrome, as discussed above, is an example of secondary chronic venous insufficiency. **Secondary CVI** occurs when an identifiable insult, such as thrombus or malignancy, causes damage to the venous valves and resulting in chronic venous reflux. It can occur in both the superficial and deep venous systems.

In contrast, **primary CVI** occurs due to idiopathic venous valve dysfunction, usually in the superficial venous system (▶ Table 9.4). The most commonly seen patterns are dysfunction of the saphenous veins, femoral canal perforator, external pudendal vein, and intersaphenous veins. Risk factors for primary superficial CVI include family history of CVI, obesity, occupations involving prolonged sitting or standing, superficial thrombophlebitis, and multiple pregnancies. Although CVI is seen in both men and women, women have a higher risk of developing CVI, and are more likely to seek out treatment.

Work-up of Chronic Venous Insufficiency

Patients with CVI may present to a vascular specialist with a wide range of symptoms, depending on chronicity and whether the superficial or deep systems are involved. Some patients present with only cosmetically unsavory telangiectasias (dilated intra-dermal and subdermal veins) or varicose veins (dilated, tortuous subcutaneous veins of size ≥ 3 mm). Other patients may have full-blown venous hypertension with substantial edema, burning pain, and skin tightness. Late findings of CVI include stasis dermatitis, a more severe form called lipodermatosclerosis, and sometimes ulceration. Venous ulcers tend to occur above the medial malleolus, whereas arterial ulcers typically occur directly over bony prominences, at the base of heel, over toe joints, or at the tips of digits.

When initially seeing a patient with leg swelling, systemic causes of lower extremity symptoms like heart failure, nephrotic syndrome, and cirrhosis are first ruled out.

The diagnosis of CVI is suspected by history and exam, and confirmed with ultra-sound. Compression and Valsalva maneuvers with ultrasound can accurately localize venous obstruction and reflux, as well as differentiate between superficial or deep venous insufficiency. Ultrasound should be performed in the standing position, or reverse Trendelenburg position if the patient is unable to stand, as reflux is most likely to be elicited in these positions. Reflux greater than 0.3 seconds in venous perforators, 0.5 seconds in the superficial veins, and 1 second in the deep veins is considered abnor-mal. When ultrasound is suboptimal secondary to body habitus, plethysmography is a tool that can provide an assessment of overall venous hemodynamics by measuring changes in limb volume with standing and supine positioning.

The **CEAP classification system** is the international consensus used for categorizing chronic venous disease based on Clinical signs, Etiology, Anatomy, and Pathophysiol-ogy. The "C" portion of CEAP is used most commonly as shorthand by clinicians when gauging severity (▶ **Table 9.5**).

Management of Chronic Venous Insufficiency

First-line therapy for both superficial and deep CVI is conservative management with leg elevation, graded compression stockings, and exercise. These simple measures are often enough to decrease edema and mobilize static blood in the lower extremities. Advanced disease can be treated with a variety of topical agents and appropriate wound care.

Patients with superficial CVI who remain symptomatic after a trial of conservative management (typically 3 months) are candidates for minimally invasive therapy. Tech-niques include sclerotherapy, radiofrequency ablation, and **endovenous laser ablation.**

Table 9.5 "Clinical" category of CEAP classification

C1	Small varicose veins
C2	Large varicose veins
C3	Leg edema
C4	Skin changes without ulceration
C5	Skin changes with healed ulcers
C6	Skin changes with active ulcers

The idea is to obliterate the refluxing vein and force blood into the deep veins. This requires the deep venous system veins to be competent and fully functional.

As discussed with PTS, there are unfortunately not many interventions available for CVI affecting the deep veins. Surgical options include venous bypass or vein segment transposition; both of these procedures carry significant postoperative morbidity and are rarely performed.

9.3 Catheter-Related Thrombosis

Long-term central venous access, particularly in cancer patients, is a predisposing factor for the development of **catheter-related thrombosis** (**CRT**). The initial endothelial damage from vascular access, venous stasis associated with catheter presence in the vessel lumen, and often a hypercoagulable state all contribute to thrombus formation. The risk is increased with improperly positioned catheters, when the tip is in the upper SVC, as well as left-sided catheters.

There are a few different ways in which CRT is recognized. Patients may present with symptoms of upper extremity DVT, which can include swelling, discomfort, and/or visible superficial veins as a result of collateralization. As with lower extremity DVTs, these can occasionally be associated with development of PE or post-thrombotic syndrome and should be approached with the same amount of caution.

However, the majority of patients will be asymptomatic. Thrombosis may be suspected in the event of catheter malfunction, either with infusing or with blood return. This in itself is nonspecific, possibly reflecting intraluminal clot or a malpositioned catheter, rather than true DVT. There is also a distinction between thrombus and an expected amount of fibrin coating the catheter. All catheters will eventually acquire a fibrin sheath, which is in most cases clinically insignificant. Oftentimes the presence of CRT is questioned based on an incidental finding on surveillance cross-sectional imaging for a cancer patient. This can be a challenge to deal with since it is difficult to distinguish true thrombus from fibrin sheath on CT. Fibrin sheaths are frequently overcalled as thrombus.

Management of CRT begins with prevention. When placing the central venous catheter, do your best to gain access to the vein with the first puncture to limit endothelial damage. Catheters should be sized such that the tip is positioned at the superior cavoatrial junction, preferably right-sided when possible, and using the smallest lumen size that is necessary. Prophylactic anticoagulation to prevent CRT is not supported in the literature.

When a CVC malfunctions, usually the first step is to obtain a chest radiograph to evaluate the position of the catheter. If the problem is a result of intraluminal clot or occlusive fibrin sheath, tPA may be instilled and often fixes the problem. If that doesn't work, CRT should be suspected. As with a typical DVT, duplex ultrasound is the modality of choice for evaluating potential CRT. Venography is usually reserved for scenarios when an ultrasound is equivocal and suspicion remains high.

Proven CRT, both in the case of a symptomatic patient and in cases of CVC malfunction, should be treated with anticoagulation unless there is a contraindication. If it is a cancer patient (commonly the case), LMWH is the preferred drug. Treatment length should be a minimum of 3 months, and also continued for as long as the CVC stays in place. The CVC should be removed as soon as it is no longer needed. It should also be removed regardless when there are signs of infection or symptoms persist despite anticoagulation. For those with a contraindication to anticoagulation, placement of an SVC filter can be considered, but this is controversial. Likewise, CDT may be done for select cases, though it is not firmly established as part of the treatment algorithm.

The guidelines are not as clear when there is an incidental imaging finding of possible CRT in an asymptomatic patient. If the catheter is functional, many interventional radiologists would *not* recommend anticoagulation, knowing that the finding is often just a simple fibrin sheath. Despite this, many clinicians opt to anticoagulate these patients.

9.4 Paget–Schroetter Disease

Paget-Schroetter disease (also called effort thrombosis or venous thoracic outlet syndrome [VTOS]) is a rare cause of axillosubclavian DVT. The disease occurs when the axillary or subclavian vein is constricted due to a thoracic outlet abnormality and a narrow costoclavicular junction. A common culprit is a cervical rib or hypertrophied scalene muscles.

The classic Paget–Schroetter story is a young male athlete who presents with acute arm pain and swelling after exercise or performing a repetitive activity with the arms raised overhead (e.g., swimming). Pain varies with arm position; holding the arm at chest level alleviates pain, while raising the arm above the head exacerbates symptoms. Arterial pulses are normal.

Imaging work-up usually begins with Doppler ultrasound to confirm the presence of DVT. A chest radiograph can be obtained to identify anatomic variants that predispose to thoracic outlet obstruction.

Since so many patients with Paget–Schroetter are young and otherwise healthy, the management strategy is fairly aggressive. As with lower extremity DVT, the goal of treatment for these patients is to reduce the risk of PE, PTS, and DVT recurrence. Patients are anticoagulated, unless there is a contraindication. More recent data have supported the use of CDT and venous angioplasty (▶ **Fig. 9.11**). This has been shown to reduce the risk of PTS and recurrent thrombosis. It may seem intuitive to also stent the venous segment at the point of thoracic outlet obstruction, but this is not done in practice since it can result in stent fracture and recurrent thrombosis.

After resolution of the acute DVT, patients are typically referred for surgical decompression of the thoracic outlet, sometimes even during the same hospitalization. Without surgical decompression, patients will frequently rethrombose.

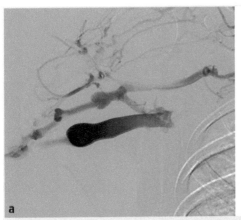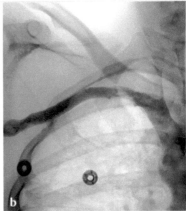

Fig. 9.11 A 26-year-old man presented with right upper extremity swelling after a weekend of painting. **(a)** Venogram performed during the procedure shows almost no flow through the right axillosubclavian vein and marked collateral formation. **(b)** After venoplasty, flow is restored to the right axillosubclavian vein and collaterals are no longer seen.

9.5 Nutcracker Syndrome

Nutcracker syndrome occurs when the left renal vein is compressed between the superior mesenteric artery (SMA) and the aorta, resulting in renal venous congestion and consequently hypertension. Most patients present with orthostatic proteinuria or asymptomatic hematuria from rupture of small congested veins in the collecting system. In severe cases of hematuria, the patient may even require blood transfusions. Other patients can present with recurrent left flank pain and/or pelvic venous congestion. This may manifest as dysmenorrhea, dyspareunia, vulvar, or scrotal varices.

The constellation of symptoms seen in nutcracker syndrome are nonspecific and overlap with several other disease processes, including malignancy. Many of these patients will get a battery of urological tests (urinalysis, ultrasound, CT urography, cystoscopy) prior to the diagnosis being made. Doppler ultrasound can be especially telling, and will show reflux in the left renal vein, along with venous collaterals. Nutcracker syndrome can be suspected on cross-sectional CT or MR studies if the left renal vein appears significantly dilated, or if there's direct evidence of renal vein compression. CT or MR venography may be used to confirm the diagnosis.

Management depends on the severity of symptoms. Patients who are asymptomatic or have mild symptoms can be observed. Patients who have clinically significant hematuria or lifestyle-limiting symptoms should be treated. The treatment of choice is endovascular stenting of the left renal vein at the site of the stenosis (▶ **Fig. 9.12**). Surgery involves transposition of the SMA or left renal vein.

9.6 May–Thurner Syndrome

May-Thurner syndrome (**MTS**) occurs when the *left* common iliac *vein* is compressed by the *right* common iliac *artery* crossing over top of it. Patients may have signs of

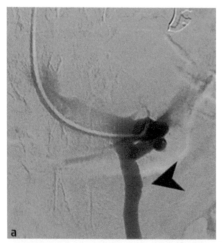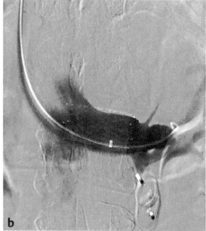

Fig. 9.12 (a) Left renal vein venogram in a young patient who presented with hematuria and left flank pain, showing absence of antegrade flow through the left renal vein, and diversion of flow into the left gonadal vein (*arrowhead*). Findings were consistent with a diagnosis of nutcracker syndrome. (b) A stent was placed across the stenosis, and subsequent venogram demonstrated normal flow through the renal vein and into the IVC. (These images are provided courtesy of Joshua Pinter, MD, University of Pittsburgh Medical Center.)

venous hypertension (swelling, pain, edema) or present with extensive left lower extremity DVT. The typical May–Thurner patient is a younger woman without any obvious risk factors who presents with left ileofemoral DVT symptoms.

Work-up for these patients usually starts the same as for any DVT, with Doppler ultrasound. Ultrasound may be able to identify a stenotic segment of the left common iliac vein and suggest the presence of MTS, although this is seldom the case due to the deeper location of the vein and the likelihood of overlying bowel gas obstructing the view. Diagnosis of MTS more often relies on high clinical suspicion, which typically leads to ordering of noninvasive venography (CTV or MRV), specifically to evaluate for the disease. In select cases, conventional venography may be indicated.

Occasionally, MTS is diagnosed (or at least suggested) based on an incidental finding on cross-sectional imaging. Asymptomatic patients do not need to be treated. For symptomatic patients, endovascular stenting is the treatment of choice (**Procedure Box 9.4**) (▶**Fig. 9.13**). There is a high rate of recurrence when these patients are treated with angioplasty only.

9.7 SVC Syndrome

External compression of the SVC results in a distinct clinical entity called **SVC syndrome**. It presents as a constellation of findings that occur secondary to obstruction of blood return from the upper extremities and head/neck (▶**Fig. 9.14**). Solid lung tumors and non-Hodgkin's lymphoma are the most common types of malignancies implicated. As the tumor enlarges, central veins becomes compressed and venous outflow obstruction results. The specific central vein affected and, consequently, the clinical

---

Procedure Box 9.4: Venous Stenting for the Treatment of May–Thurner Syndrome　　ⓘ

A common cause of isolated left lower extremity DVT, particularly in slender, young females, involves the compression of the left common iliac vein by the overlying right common iliac artery (May–Thurner compression). This may lead to acute DVT, chronic thrombotic occlusion, and pelvic varices, all of which can be treated using angioplasty and stenting when clinically appropriate.

Access is typically obtained via the left popliteal vein or below the level of the occlusion. The internal jugular vein may be used alternatively if wire access across the stenosis is not possible.

After gaining access, the stenosis is crossed with a guidewire and catheter. In the setting of acute thrombosis, thrombectomy or thrombolysis should be performed to remove the thrombus and allow assessment of the underlying venous anatomy. Intravascular ultrasound (IVUS) may be used to determine the ideal stent size by comparing the stenotic segment to areas of nonstenotic vein on the ipsilateral or contralateral side. IVUS also allows precise delineation of the site of compression, to ensure appropriate stent coverage.

Next, the vessel is predilated by balloon venoplasty. Most commonly, a self-expanding Wallstent (Boston Scientific, Natick, MA) is then placed and postdilated with a balloon of equal or slightly less diameter. Care should be taken to not cover the contralateral iliac vein outflow, and to place enough of the stent on either side of the stenosis so that it does not extrude cephalad or caudally during deployment. Poststenting venography and IVUS are then performed to ensure appropriate positioning, improvement in flow, and resolution of varices (if present).

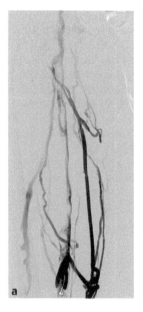
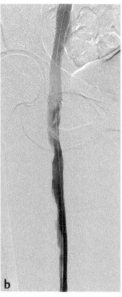

Fig. 9.13 This young female presented with acute left leg heaviness and swelling. A subsequent CT diagnosed May–Thurner syndrome. **(a)** The initial venogram shows many collateral vessels and almost no flow through the femoral vein, confirming left femoral vein thrombosis. **(b)** After thrombolysis and stenting of the stenotic segment, there is good flow through the left iliac and femoral veins. (These images are provided courtesy of Deepak Sudheendra, MD, University of Pennsylvania Medical Center.)

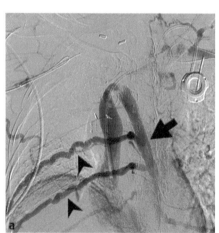
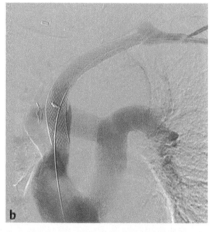

Fig. 9.14 A patient with known lung cancer presented with upper extremity and facial edema due to the compression of the SVC by tumor. **(a)** The right brachial vein has been accessed, with contrast injection revealing absence of flow through the central veins. The majority of the flow is diverted through intercostal veins (*arrowheads*), emptying into the azygos vein (*arrow*), and then finally into the lower SVC. **(b)** SVC obstruction was crossed and a stent was placed across the obstruction, resulting in restoration of SVC patency. (These images are provided courtesy of Joshua Pinter, MD, University of Pittsburgh Medical Center.)

manifestations depend on the where the tumor is. Benign etiologies such as histoplasmosis, radiation injury, and catheter associated fibrosis can also be implicated.

Typical symptoms of SVC syndrome include facial swelling, extremity edema, and visible engorgement/distension of the neck veins. Severe head/neck edema may even cause cerebral edema or lead to compression of the airway. Symptoms usually progress slowly, reflecting slow growth of the mass.

For those who present with these findings, especially in the setting of a known mediastinal malignancy, the diagnosis of SVC syndrome is almost a given. A CT with contrast can definitively provide a diagnosis and delineate the extent of stenosis.

In the past, *all* patients found to have SVC syndrome would be referred to radiation oncology for urgent radiation therapy. A change in treatment paradigm occurred when it was realized that few of these patients are actually at imminent risk, and that radiation changes to the SVC can make the endovascular treatment of recalcitrant cases more risky. Time is actually on our side as SVC syndrome is a slowly progressing process in most patients.

Nonemergent endovascular stenting is becoming widely adopted as the go-to intervention. The exception is if there is a *true* SVC syndrome emergency. True emergencies include patients who have airway or esophageal compression due to edema, or neurological symptoms from cerebral edema. In these patients, urgent endovascular stenting followed by radiation therapy is indicated. Stenting reopens the central veins, while radiation therapy reduces the underlying mass effect.

One point to note about SVC stenting is that it carries a risk of serious complications. The pericardium extends superiorly and covers a portion of the SVC, so an inferior SVC rupture can be catastrophic. Many interventional radiologists have had patients develop cardiac tamponade following SVC angioplasty. Anecdotally, the risk is reported to be greatest in patients who have had radiation to mediastinal masses. Thus, whenever stenting the SVC, it's important to be conservative with angioplasty and have covered stents and a pericardiocentesis kit ready and in the room.

Suggested Readings

[1] Chatterjee S, Chakraborty A, Weinberg I, et al. Thrombolysis for pulmonary embolism and risk of all-cause mortality, major bleeding, and intracranial hemorrhage: a meta-analysis. JAMA. 2014; 311(23):2414–2421

[2] Chiesa R, Marone EM, Limoni C, Volontè M, Petrini O. Chronic venous disorders: correlation between visible signs, symptoms, and presence of functional disease. J Vasc Surg. 2007; 46(2):322–330

[3] Comerota AJ, Grewal N, Martinez JT, et al. Postthrombotic morbidity correlates with residual thrombus following catheter-directed thrombolysis for iliofemoral deep vein thrombosis. J Vasc Surg. 2012; 55(3):768–773

[4] Haig Y, Enden T, Grøtta O, et al. CaVenT Study Group. Post-thrombotic syndrome after catheter-directed thrombolysis for deep vein thrombosis (CaVenT): 5-year follow-up results of an open-label, randomised controlled trial. Lancet Haematol. 2016; 3(2):e64–e71

[5] Kahn SR, Shrier I, Julian JA, et al. Determinants and time course of the postthrombotic syndrome after acute deep venous thrombosis. Ann Intern Med. 2008; 149(10):698–707

[6] Kearon C, Akl EA, Ornelas J, et al. Antithrombotic therapy for VTE disease: CHEST guideline and expert panel report. Chest. 2016; 149(2):315–352

[7] Khilnani NM, Grassi CJ, Kundu S, et al. Cardiovascular Interventional Radiological Society of Europe, American College of Phlebology, and Society of Interventional Radiology Standards of Practice Committees. Multi-society consensus quality improvement guidelines for the treatment of lower-extremity superficial venous insufficiency with endovenous thermal ablation from the Society of Interventional Radiology, Cardiovascular Interventional Radiological Society of Europe, American College of Phlebology and Canadian Interventional Radiology Association. J Vasc Interv Radiol. 2010; 21(1):14–31

[8] Vedantham S, Goldhaber SZ, Kahn SR, et al. Acute Venous Thrombosis: Thrombus Removal with Adjunctive Catheter-Directed Thrombolysis. Paper presented at the Society of Interventional Radiology Annual Meeting, Washington, DC; 2017

10 Dialysis Access and Interventions

Alex Lionberg, Shantanu Warhadpande, and Rakesh Navuluri

A baseline knowledge of the indications for dialysis is a good starting point for understanding how IR is involved in the care of these patients. Short-term dialysis in the acute setting and permanent dialysis for kidney failure both achieve the same goal, which is either augmentation or complete replacement of inadequate kidney function.

Acutely, the main indications for dialysis include severe acidosis, electrolyte abnormalities, fluid overload, dialyzable toxemias (such as lithium or aspirin overdose), and uremia. Determining whether the problem is severe enough to initiate dialysis is typically determined by the consultant nephrologist. If the problem is believed to be reversible, a temporary hemodialysis (HD) line for access will often suffice. In most cases these are simply placed at the bedside by the clinical service taking care of the patient. IR does not put temporary lines in unless there have been multiple failed attempts (which may indicate complex/altered venous anatomy or central venous occlusion). When there is some indication at the outset that the patient will need access for longer than a week, IR may be asked to place a tunneled hemodialysis line.

Chronic kidney disease (CKD) is common and often asymptomatic in earlier stages, with hypertension and diabetes being the two biggest risk factors for disease progression. Prudent medical management of these comorbidities can prevent or at least slow a decline in kidney function. The glomerular filtration rate (GFR) is the best overall assessment for evaluating CKD, and is estimated using serum creatinine. A GFR less than 60 for at least 3 months defines CKD. In earlier stages, CKD can be managed by the primary care physician. Patients have their GFR and urine albumin checked at regular intervals to monitor for disease progression. Referral to nephrology is indicated when GFR is less than 30 or when there is rapid progression.

Kidney failure is defined by a GFR less than 15 with symptoms or other specific criteria that would necessitate initiation of chronic renal replacement therapy. Note that patients can be labeled as having kidney failure when they reach this threshold, but this does not necessarily indicate dialysis is imminent. The designation of **end-stage renal disease** (ESRD) refers to the requirements that are met in order to qualify for Medicare coverage of renal replacement therapy.

The timing of initiating dialysis has many factors that go into it, but generally speaking the process is started only when symptoms of uremia arise, and with a GFR typically below 12. Transplant is an option for selected kidney failure candidates, but for our purposes we'll focus on the role of dialysis. Options include peritoneal dialysis (PD) and HD.

There are several types of **peritoneal dialysis**, but the concept is similar for each; dialysis solution is infused into the abdomen through a permanent catheter and allowed to dwell. Waste materials diffuse from the bloodstream across the peritoneum and equilibrate with the fluid before being removed. The exchanges are typically done multiple times a day, which can create inconvenience for the patient. Even so, outcomes for PD tend to be better than HD in the short term, and it's also cheaper. Peritoneal catheters are usually surgically placed, though placement by IR is increasing in some practice settings. Aside from this, IR does not have a significant role in the care of these patients.

With **hemodialysis**, the main challenge is establishing and maintaining vascular access. Dialysis machines require blood flow in a range somewhere between the rates seen in arteries and veins (> 300 mL/min). Another requirement is ease of access for the dialysis technicians to get the patient hooked up to the machine. Central venous access with a dialysis catheter is convenient in that it requires no needle puncture and achieves adequate flow. These lines are acceptable for short-term dialysis needs, but long-term use increases the risk of infection, making it unacceptable for chronic dialysis. The preferred route of long-term hemodialysis is an arteriovenous fistula (AVF) or graft (AVG).

AV fistulas offer a permanent and easily accessible vascular access site for dialysis patients. Most fistulas are created by vascular surgery, with directly suturing of a vein to an artery. A percutaneous IR procedure for the endovascular creation of an AVF is being studied and may become an alternative to surgical creation in the near future. Preoperative imaging of the arm with duplex ultrasound or angiography is important to size the vein and to rule out any pre-existing arterial inflow or venous outflow obstruction that might compromise fistula viability. The preferred site for fistula creation is in the distal nondominant arm (radial–cephalic). If a distal site is not possible due to vessel occlusion or inadequate vessel size, fistulas can be created more proximally (brachiocephalic, transposition brachiobasilic), but these are less desirable (▶ **Fig. 10.1**).

Prior to being used for dialysis, an AV fistula needs time to mature. The newly created fistula dilates over time to the point of becoming superficial and easily palpable. With the increased blood flow, the vein also becomes "arterialized." The walls thicken, allowing the vessel to better withstand the regular trauma that occurs with needle puncture. Bear in mind, a fistula will need to be punctured and accessed multiple times a week, for the rest of the patient's life.

An ideal fistula follows the "rule of sixes": at 6 weeks, the fistula should be 6 mm in diameter, less than 6 mm deep, 6 cm in useable length, and have flow rates that exceed 600 mL/min (▶ **Table 10.1**). In reality, time to full maturation can range between 2 and 4 months. Duplex fistula studies can be obtained to track progress.

If a suitable vein is unavailable and an AV fistula cannot be created, an **AV graft** may be necessary. AV grafts rely on a prosthetic tube to bridge the artery and vein, requiring *two* anastomoses (▶ **Fig. 10.2**). A common AV graft is the forearm loop AV graft. The arterial side of the graft is anastomosed to the brachial artery while the venous side of the graft is anastomosed to either the basilic, cephalic, or antecubital vein. AV grafts do not require time to mature and can be used immediately. In comparison to fistulas, grafts are more likely to become infected and typically have a shorter lifespan, so they should only be used if the anatomy is not suitable for an AVF.

In general, the creation of an anastomosis between artery and vein introduces a host of hemodynamic and physiologic changes within the access site and its upstream and downstream vasculature. Increased flow into the access site and anastomosed venous segment causes an increase in wall shear stress, which in turn results in dilation of the vessels at the access site. Similarly, an increase in transmural pressure stimulates proliferation of smooth muscle, leading to thickening of the vessel wall. This dilation and wall thickening are the expected changes associated with appropriate fistula maturation.

Table 10.1 Fistula rules of 6
At 6 weeks, a fistula should be…
6 mm in diameter
< 6 mm under the skin
6 cm in useable length
Flow rates > 600 mL/min

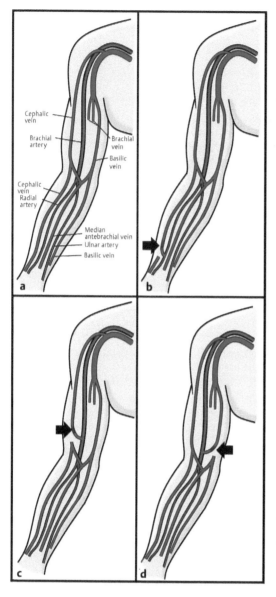

Fig. 10.1 Depiction of **(a)** normal upper extremity vascular anatomy. **(b)** A radiocephalic arteriovenous (AV) fistula. **(c)** A brachiocephalic AV fistula. **(d)** A brachiobasilic AV fistula. (These images are provided courtesy of Christopher Molloy, MD, Kaiser Permanente Los Angeles.)

10.1 Dialysis Access Dysfunction

As described, dialysis access creation leads to desirable vascular and physiologic changes necessary for fistula or graft use. However, changes in flow dynamics can also have deleterious consequences. For example, turbulence within the vessel as blood flows in and out of the dialysis access site exposes the vessel walls to an inconsistent pattern of wall shear stress. Areas of *low* wall shear stress induces a proinflammatory state and results in neointimal hyperplasia. This is one of the underlying causes of stenoses.

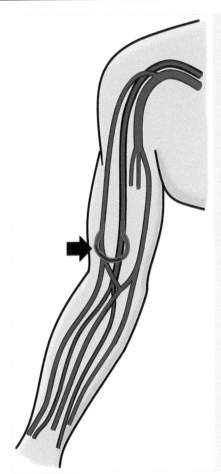

Fig. 10.2 Depiction of an arteriovenous graft between the brachial artery and the cephalic vein. (This image is provided courtesy of Christopher Molloy, MD, Kaiser Permanente Los Angeles.)

Early dialysis access dysfunction occurs anytime between fistula or graft creation and the first 3 months of use, most commonly as a result of fistula nonmaturation. A nonmatured fistula cannot be cannulated due to a combination of inadequate flow rate, suboptimal dilation of the arterialized vein, and/or a fistula depth too far below the skin.

In order for a fistula to be accessed and achieve flow rates necessary for the machine, the vessel needs to dilate. If the artery or vein chosen for the fistula are poor quality, the total dilation may be limited. Similarly, poor surgical technique may lead to incomplete dilation or a fistula that is too deep. Any additional insults on top of this, including the development of inflow or outflow stenoses, can also limit the ability of the fistula to dilate and reach a sufficient flow rate.

Grafts do not go through the process of maturation as fistulas do and can be used for dialysis relatively quickly (sometimes immediately). However, downstream neointimal hyperplasia can also occur shortly after placement due to the same physiologic changes.

Patients with matured fistulas can have varying degrees of dysfunction. Some may enjoy a relatively complication-free period, while others run into problems not long after the access is created. The dysfunction of matured fistulas and grafts can be due to stenoses anywhere along the arterial and venous limbs.

Arterial stenoses are more likely to be pre-existent rather than sequelae of access creation. The typical patient will have known peripheral arterial disease or risk factors for it (diabetes, smoking history, older age). Detection of arterial stenoses usually occurs with a nonmatured fistula and a low flow rate.

Venous stenoses are the most common reason for referral to IR. In addition to the instigating effect of turbulent flow, repetitive needle puncture of the access site causes endothelial cell damage and the release of proinflammatory cytokines, furthering the propensity for neointimal hyperplasia and stenosis in the downstream vein. Stenoses affecting the central veins can lead to venous hypertension as pooling increases hydrostatic pressure. This may result in extremity edema, prolonged bleeding time after venipuncture, and aneurysmal dilation of the access. Decreased flow rates will be noted during dialysis.

Repetitive needle punctures at the access site can weaken the vessel wall and form pseudoaneurysms (▶ **Fig. 10.3**). Increased blood flow leads to vessel dilation and aneurysm formation proximal and distal to the access site. Pseudoaneurysms are unsightly but also present a risk of rupture.

The complications above are worrisome, but do not necessarily prevent the patient from getting dialysis. In contrast, dialysis can be completely interrupted when a venous stenosis precipitates thrombosis in the fistula or graft. Hypotension, either during the dialysis session or from another process, is a known risk factor for the development of thrombosis in the setting of an underlying venous stenosis. Excessive compression of the access site after dialysis, or simply from the patient sleeping on it wrong, can also contribute. Thrombosis is detected when there is a loss of thrill or bruit over the access site. The thrombus itself is unlikely to cause any damage, but the more pressing issue is the interruption of scheduled dialysis until access can be restored.

Unfortunately, stenosis and thrombosis are a part of the natural history of fistulas and grafts for many patients. Not uncommonly, patients with matured fistulas will enter a frustrating and chronic cycle of access complication, intervention, further complication, repeat intervention, and so on.

Another unique complication associated with AV fistulas/grafts is related to hemodynamic changes within the surrounding arm vasculature. As blood flows into the fistula through the feeding artery, perfusion to distal tissues (forearm, hand, etc.) diminishes initially while collateral flow is established. This in itself usually does not result in significant issues for the patient. **Steal syndrome** occurs when too

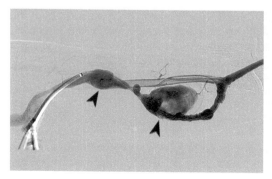

Fig. 10.3 A patient with a brachiobasilic fistula was sent to IR with low flow rates. The fistula was accessed in a retrograde fashion and an initial fistulagram revealed two pseudoaneurysms (*arrowheads*) and stenosis on the venous side. (This image is provided courtesy of Matthew Czar Taon, MD and Cuong Lam, MD, Kaiser Permanente Los Angeles.)

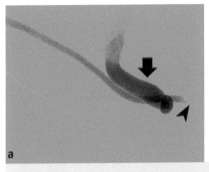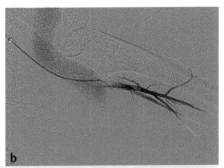

Fig. 10.4 A 37-year-old patient with a left brachiocephalic fistula presented with left hand pain during dialysis. (a) After obtaining right femoral artery access and selecting the left brachial artery, an angiogram opacified a high-flow brachiocephalic fistula (*arrow*) with little flow distal to the fistula (*arrowhead*). (b) A microcatheter was advanced slightly past the fistula with subsequent contrast injection demonstrating reflux of contrast into the fistula and persistently decreased flow in the forearm. This patient was diagnosed with steal syndrome and was referred to vascular surgery. (These images are provided courtesy of Matthew Czar Taon, MD and Cuong Lam, MD, Kaiser Permanente Los Angeles.)

much arterial flow is directed into the fistula, in effect "stealing" blood from the distal extremity (▸**Fig. 10.4**). This can result in episodic or constant ischemic pain, particularly when the arm is being used. It is more commonly seen in those with underlying atherosclerotic disease, however, it may affect those with clean arteries in the presence of a particularly high-flow fistula.

As part of a multidisciplinary team, interventional radiologists are frequently involved in addressing these problems with the goal of ensuring scheduled dialysis can go uninterrupted and the lifetime of the access is maximized. The patient's dialysis access is their lifeline. Early identification and management of these complications can have a significant impact on outcomes for dialysis patients.

10.2 Dialysis Access Monitoring and Surveillance

When patients go for dialysis, the technicians and nurses at the facility monitor for access issues. If there is a problem, it is better to identify it early so that arrangements can be made to address it before there is total dysfunction. Missing dialysis for even a couple of days due to access dysfunction can be enough to send some patients to the emergency room.

Fistulas and grafts are monitored with a focused physical exam at every dialysis session, with attention to the pulse, thrill, bruit, and overall appearance of the arm. A normal fistula or graft is only softly pulsatile and is easily compressible. Normally, elevation of the arm should cause the fistula to flatten. When a strong pulse is palpable, it indicates venous stenosis. With elevation of the arm in the presence of venous stenosis, the portion of the fistula upstream to the stenosis will not flatten.

A normal fistula should have a *continuous* thrill at the anastomosis throughout both systole and diastole (and just the arterial anastomosis for a graft). As a venous stenosis develops, the diastolic component becomes more faint and eventually the thrill will only be detected during systole. Likewise, a fistula or graft should have a continuous *low-pitched* bruit. Venous stenosis will cause the bruit to become *higher pitched*, and it will lose the diastolic component. If a bruit diminishes with elevation of the arm, it can indicate a

Table 10.2 Physical exam findings seen with fistula dysfunction

Physical exam finding	Likely pathophysiology
Prolonged bleeding after deaccess	Venous stenosis
Pulsatile quality to fistula (loss of diastolic component of thrill)	Venous stenosis
Elevation of arm diminishes bruit	Arterial stenosis
Loss of thrill/bruit	Fistula thrombosis
Erythema/warmth/fluctuance over fistula	Underlying infection
Distended, visible superficial veins over arm, neck, chest	Central venous stenosis
Extremity edema	Central venous stenosis

problem with *arterial* inflow, but arterial stenoses are much less common than venous stenoses. Complete loss of thrill and bruit is consistent with thrombosis (▶ Table 10.2).

Erythema, warmth, and fluctuance are suggestive of infection, which is much more common with grafts than fistulas. Another thing to note on exam of the arm is gross dilation of the vessels, which may represent an aneurysm or pseudoaneurysm. When there is stenosis of the central veins, the whole arm may appear swollen. It may be accompanied by distended superficial veins over the arm, neck, and chest, representing collateral formation.

In addition to monitoring the access site with physical exam, **access surveillance** is the practice of using more objective measures to monitor dialysis access health. In most practices, surveillance is done once a month. The amount of flow (Q) through the access can be measured through a number of different methods. When flow dips below 600 mL/min for grafts or 500 mL/min for fistulas, it is indicative of underlying stenosis, and per Kidney Disease Outcomes Quality Initiative (KDOQI) recommendations warrants a referral for intervention. Some advocate the use of flow measurement *downtrends* to determine appropriateness of intervention referral, rather than a discrete cutoff.

Early intervention based on dysfunction detected by surveillance is controversial. While it may sound reasonable, more recent data suggest that access interventions based on surveillance help prevent thrombosis, but do not otherwise prolong the functional lifespan of the access or reduce mortality.

One other surveillance measure you'll encounter is **venous pressure measurement**. Pressures in the venous limb often increase as there is worsening of stenosis downstream. It is not always a useful measurement, particularly with fistulas, as the presence of collaterals and accessory veins can prevent pressure from rising significantly in the presence of a stenosis. As with flow measurements, the *trend* of venous pressures is probably more informative than individual readings.

10.3 Approach to the Patient with Dialysis Access Complications

Dialysis access interventions can be challenging procedures, but there are a few steps that can make things much easier for these cases. For one, it's important to gain as much information about the problem as possible prior to starting. Patients are often referred from a dialysis center with some abnormality noted on physical exam or through access surveillance measurements. If the patient has been seen by the department previously, you'll want to review prior imaging and reports to see what's been done in the past, taking note of any stents that have been placed as well as variant anatomy. If you have no pre-existing information, it's okay to ask the patient; they often know at least what type of access has been placed.

Always perform your own physical exam of the access site and extremity. Being able to determine if the problem is in the venous or arterial limb will tell you which direction to point your needle when doing the initial access of the fistula or graft. Physical exam findings can also raise your pretest suspicion for the location of the problem.

If it looks like the access site may be infected you should cancel the procedure. Infection is the only absolute contraindication to dialysis intervention. These patients are started on antibiotics at a minimum. Antibiotics (and possibly an I&D) may be enough for superficial infections, but deeper infections usually require surgical removal and replacement of the graft. AV grafts are roughly 10 times more likely to get infected than AV fistulas. Often when an intervention is aborted due to infection, IR will place a tunneled hemodialysis line to provide alternative access while the infection is treated.

It is important to note that if there is a delay in an intervention for a nonfunctioning fistula or graft thrombosis, a dialysis central line may be necessary for urgent hemodialysis. Always know the urgency of the next dialysis session. The referring service may send the patient to you under the assumption that the procedure will restore function and dialysis will follow immediately. However, some dialysis interventions can be quite challenging and may require more than one session to solve the problem. Fluid overload and hyperkalemia should be ruled out prior to intervention. Don't assume someone else has already done this for you.

10.4 Management of Dialysis Access Complications

The main indications for dialysis access intervention include failure of a fistula to mature, signs of access dysfunction based on the monitoring or surveillance criteria described above, a completely thrombosed fistula or graft, and distal ischemia.

Dialysis access interventions are most commonly done on an outpatient basis. Some patients may be referred to IR after having a duplex ultrasound evaluation of their access, however, the majority will not. In many, the evidence of access dysfunction is convincing enough for them to be referred without a dedicated diagnostic study beforehand. It's more convenient for the patient to have diagnostic imaging done at the same time as the intervention that will be needed.

Regardless of any preceding imaging, all dialysis interventions begin with a **fistulagram** (**Procedure Box 10.1**). A fistula or graft is commonly accessed with a sheath directed in the antegrade direction (in the direction of the blood flow), and angiography is performed. If there is a pseudoaneurysm associated with the fistula, needle puncture should be at the pseudoaneurysm base, not at the apex, to reduce the risk of rupture. With antegrade access, the arterial side of the access site can be visualized by compressing the outflow vessel externally and forcing contrast to reflux into the artery (▶ **Fig. 10.5**). This is usually adequate when clinical information suggests the problem is on the venous side.

Procedure Box 10.1: Fistulagram and Dialysis Access Interventions ℹ

A fistulagram begins with accessing the dialysis site. Fistulas/grafts can be accessed in a retrograde fashion (catheter travels toward the anastomosis, against blood flow) or in an antegrade fashion (catheter travels proximally, away from the anastomosis, in the direction of blood flow). Choosing between retrograde versus antegrade access is determined by the preprocedure likely location of pathology (based on history and physical exam).

Antegrade access is indicated for interventions on the venous side of the dialysis access site (including interventions on the central veins). With antegrade access, only the venous limb is fully evaluated. A glimpse of the arterial limb can be obtained by occluding the outflow vessel with an angioplasty balloon or hemostat, and then injecting contrast; this will force contrast to reflux across the AV anastomosis (or arterial graft anastomosis) and into the artery (▶ Fig. 10.6). This provides basic information about the patency of the anastomosis/arterial limb.

Retrograde access is indicated when an intervention is needed at the AV anastomosis or within arterial limb. After obtaining retrograde access and securing a short sheath, the anastomosis can be crossed with a wire/catheter into the artery. As the catheter/wire crosses the anastomosis and courses into the artery, a characteristic loop can be seen on the fluoroscopic images. Contrast injection in the arterial limb will opacify the artery, the AV anastomosis (or graft), and the vein as the contrast follows the blood flow through the access site. The artery and arterial branch vessels *distal* to the access site can be seen. In some situations, both antegrade and retrograde access is necessary (▶ Fig. 10.7). This commonly occurs when antegrade access has been established and a reflux angiogram reveals para-anastomotic or inflow pathology, requiring subsequent retrograde access.

After the inflow and outflow have been evaluated with angiography, areas of stenosis are identified. In general, a stenosis greater than 50% of the normal vessel diameter is appropriate for intervention. Treating a stenosis is not a benign process, as the tools used have a nonnegligible risk of complications and angioplasty can be quite painful for the patient. For dialysis interventions, an important rule of thumb is to only treat stenoses that can explain the issue that prompted referral. There are also hemodynamic considerations which may sway the decision on what to treat. For example, in a patient with central venous stenosis as well as a juxta-anastomotic stenosis, opening up the juxta-anastomotic stenosis may dramatically increase outflow and could overwhelm the ability of collaterals (formed due to the central venous stenosis) to drain the arm. This could cause a previously asymptomatic central vein stenosis to become symptomatic.

Stenoses are primarily treated with angioplasty (▶ Fig. 10.8). For tight lesions, oftentimes this requires the use of a hydrophilic guidewire to cross the stenosis first, followed by exchange for a nonhydrophilic wire used to position the angioplasty balloon device. The balloon should be 1 to 2 mm larger than the normal diameter of the vessel at that location. Grafts are a fixed diameter, so balloon size should be known ahead of time (8-mm balloon for 7-mm graft). If the stenosis is recalcitrant to angioplasty, a higher pressure balloon or a cutting balloon may be used. For prolonged balloon inflation, heparin should be given as prolonged inflation causes stasis of blood and increases risk of thrombosis.

Successful angioplasty is defined by 30% or less residual stenosis. Those lesions that are successfully angioplastied but reappear shortly after may be amenable to stenting. Stents should always be self-expanding and used judiciously, as they are associated with a high rate of re-stenosis. Stent placement can also provoke new stenoses of the adjacent vessel. This may be require repeat intervention and even more stents to be placed, so it is best to use them only when necessary.

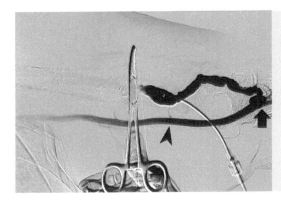

Fig. 10.5 This patient's fistula was accessed in an antegrade fashion. A hemostat was used to externally compress the outflow, and the resulting reflux of contrast opacified the AV anastomosis (*arrow*) and the brachial artery (*arrowhead*).

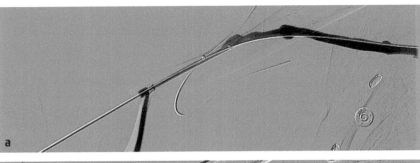

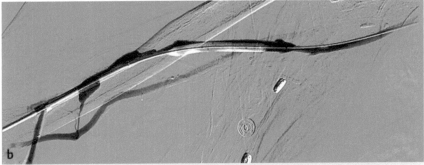

Fig. 10.6 (a) Example of antegrade access in a patient with a brachiobasilic fistula, with contrast injection occurring from the venous side and opacifying of the venous outflow. (b) Antegrade injection of contrast after occlusion of the outflow with an angioplasty balloon. Refluxed contrast opacifies the anastomosis and the distal artery. (These images are provided courtesy of Matthew Czar Taon, MD and Cuong Lam, MD, Kaiser Permanente Los Angeles.)

For dialysis access interventions, the treatment strategy differs depending on the reason for referral. Failure of fistula maturation may occur as a result of poor inflow, poor vein quality, or stenosis within the fistula—all of which can contribute to inadequate flow. Early recognition and intervention to treat the underlying cause of nonmaturation can lead to salvage of the fistula. Occasionally, despite exhaustive endovascular efforts to fix the underlying cause of nonmaturation, a surgical revision or abandonment of the fistula may be necessary. Stenoses at the fistula anastomosis and fistulas which are located too deep underneath the skin are two common causes of

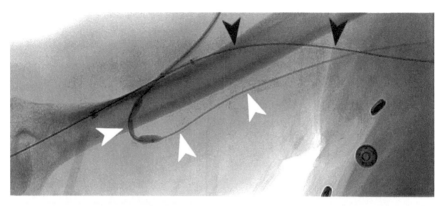

Fig. 10.7 Example of retrograde access (*white arrowheads*) *and* antegrade access (*black arrowheads*). With retrograde access, note the characteristic loop the guidewire makes as it courses through the anastomosis, into the brachial artery. (This image is provided courtesy of Matthew Czar Taon, MD and Cuong Lam, MD, Kaiser Permanente Los Angeles.)

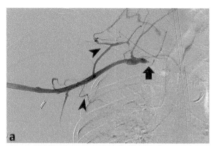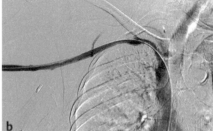

Fig. 10.8 his patient with a right brachiocephalic fistula presented with prolonged bleeding after dialysis access and low flow rates. (a) After accessing the fistula in an antegrade fashion, a venogram shows occlusion of the right subclavian vein (*arrow*) and several venous collaterals (*arrowheads*). This lesion was successfully angioplastied. (b) Post angioplasty, there is restoration of flow through the subclavian vein and disappearance of collaterals. (These images are provided courtesy of Matthew Czar Taon, MD and Cuong Lam, MD, Kaiser Permanente Los Angeles.)

nonmaturation that may be more amenable to surgery than IR treatment. Additionally, absence of a bruit soon after AVF creation suggests early thrombosis and warrants evaluation for possible surgical salvage.

Fistula/graft thrombosis can be a serious problem. In grafts, this most commonly occurs due to underlying stenosis at the *venous* anastomosis. Thrombosis can be treated with thrombolysis, often referred to as a "declot." The tools available include percutaneous, pharmacologic, and mechanical means to disrupt the thrombus. Fistula/graft thrombosis is worked up and managed urgently with the explicit goal of regaining dialysis access. There's a misconception that fistula/graft thrombosis is synonymous with impending fistula loss, but that is not the case. In some cases where there has been a delay in intervention, a thrombosis can be treated up to a month after it is detected with successful restoration of fistula function.

When a dialysis patient complains of hand pain on the same side as the access site, it should raise suspicion for steal syndrome. Referrals for hand ischemia related to a fistula may require urgent intervention when severe. These patients should first undergo angioplasty of stenoses involving the most upstream portion of the inflow (subclavian, axillary arteries, etc.). Surgical revision is sometimes required (a procedure referred to as distal revascularization and interval ligation, or DRIL).

In the case of a radiocephalic fistula, there is often retrograde flow of blood from the distal radial artery as it is stolen from the palmar arches by the access circuit. The arterial insufficiency is a function of poor flow through the ulnar artery, and so stenosis within the ulnar artery is a target for angioplasty. Another option is embolization or surgical ligation of the distal radial or ulnar artery, which will prevent the steal phenomenon in these patients.

The main complication of dialysis access intervention to be aware of is vessel rupture. Taking care to keep angioplasty balloons below burst pressure should mitigate this risk, but nonetheless rupture does happen from time to time, usually involving the venous limb. Rupture can be recognized as sudden swelling and sometimes pain that persists even with the balloon deflated. When rupture occurs, the operator should inflate the balloon at the site of rupture or just proximal to it, and always maintain guidewire access across the rupture. In many cases, simply tamponading the rupture for a short period of time will be enough to contain it. If this does not work, a stent or stent-graft can be placed over it. Unfortunately for some patients, a rupture cannot be contained, leading to thrombosis and loss of function of the access site. A rule of thumb when doing dialysis interventions is to always have the appropriate stents on hand so that a rupture can be managed if it happens.

10.5 Loss of Dialysis Access

With close attention to dialysis access function, endovascular interventions can have a significant impact on prolonging the functional lifespan of a fistula or graft. Some patients get by with relatively few interventions, while others will find their way back to IR frequently. Once a patient requires multiple stents to maintain access patency, interventions can become increasingly difficult. A thrombosis or another acute complication may occur and result in permanent loss of function of the access site, despite endovascular or surgical treatment measures.

Abandonment of a fistula or graft necessitates a temporary hemodialysis central line to allow for dialysis while a new site can be planned. A failed forearm fistula may be addressed by creation of a fistula or graft higher in the same arm or the contralateral one. Rarely, when no suitable sites are available in the arms, the lower extremity may be an option for some patients.

With repeated failures and no other options, sadly some patients will ultimately be faced with the reality of receiving dialysis through an indwelling central line for the rest of their lives. As previously mentioned, these lines are at significantly increased risk for infection. An all too common scenario is a patient dependent on a central line for dialysis who develops sepsis from a line-related infection. Infectious disease consultants often insist on removal of the infected line, to be replaced with a fresh one. This is not problematic in a typical patient, but may be a dilemma in certain dialysis patients. Since many of them at this stage have underlying venous stenosis related to prior access complications and thrombosis at the site of numerous prior central lines, there is a risk that a line could be removed and unable to be put back in. In some of these cases, the benefits of a line holiday are outweighed by the potential risk of losing access altogether. You may have to negotiate with the ID consultant to be able to do a catheter exchange over a wire as a compromise.

A relatively new option for patients who are central line-dependent is the HeRO graft (Merit Medical). The HeRO graft (Hemodialysis Reliable Outflow) has three components: an arterial component, a graft component, and a venous component. The venous component is inserted percutaneously into the internal jugular vein and, using endovascular techniques, slipped past any central venous obstruction into the right atrium (▶ Fig. 10.9). The arterial component is then surgically sutured to the brachial artery. The graft (which is the part actually cannulated during dialysis) subcutaneously connects the arterial component and the venous component.

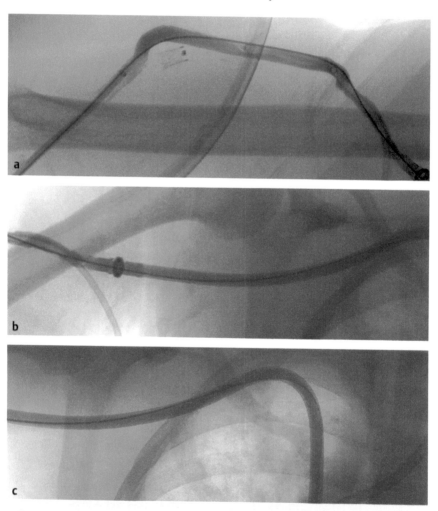

Fig. 10.9 Example of a HeRO graft with (a) the arterial component in the right arm, (b) the subcutaneous tunneled graft component, (c) the venous component entering the right internal jugular vein and coursing down into the right atrium. Note that there is no venous anastomosis.

Occasionally there will be challenging cases where dialysis access is lost *and* the patient has complete central venous occlusion, precluding the placement of a central hemodialysis catheter. Without any access, these patients cannot undergo dialysis. Options for obtaining access in patients with complete central venous occlusion include transhepatic, translumbar, or even transcollateral routes. More recently, there has been an effort to limit these options of last resort. Before using these routes, there should be an attempt to recanalize the central veins and regain the option of placing a more conventional central venous catheter.

Recanalizing central veins requires an experienced operator, as the procedure is often technically challenging and associated with a relatively high risk of complications. The initial method is using a simple hydrophilic guidewire–catheter technique to cross the lesion. The aim is to use the hydrophilic guidewire to traverse the occlusion. Once across the occlusion, the hydrophilic guidewire can then be snared from another vein (the "body floss" technique). The hydrophilic wire is exchanged for a nonhydrophilic guidewire and angioplasty/stenting can be done to open up the central veins.

Sharp recanalization involves use of a needle-tipped catheter (such as that in a TIPS kit) to pierce the occlusion and create a channel for the guidewire. **Radiofrequency recanalization** makes use of a radiofrequency device to burn through the occlusion. If the lesion can be passed from above, a snare can used from femoral access to grab and pull the guidewire/catheter to secure through-and-through access.

The use of these techniques in close proximity to vital structures within the mediastinum has the potential to be catastrophic. Preparation for any anticipated complications should be made prior to using these tools. Bailout equipment should include a large sheath, appropriately sized occlusion balloons, covered stents, a chest tube kit, and a pericardiocentesis kit.

Suggested Readings

[1] National Kidney Foundation. KDOQI Clinical Practice Guideline for Hemodialysis Adequacy: 2015 Update. Am J Kidney Dis. 2015; 66(5):884–930

[2] Khwaja K. Dialysis access procedures. In: Humar A, Sturdevant ML, eds. Atlas of Organ Transplantation. London: Springer; 2006:35-58

[3] Rodrigues L, Renaud C, Beyssen B. Diagnostic and Interventional Radiology of Arteriovenous Accesses for Hemodialysis. New York, NY: Springer; 2013

[4] Regalado S, Navuluri R, Vikingstad E. Distal revascularization and interval ligation: a primer for the vascular and interventional radiologist. Semin Intervent Radiol. 2009; 26(2):125–129

11 Genitourinary Disease

John Do, David J. Maldow, Zachary Nuffer, and Jason W. Mitchell

11.1 Uterine Fibroids

Normal menstruation is characterized by bleeding that occurs for fewer than or equal to 8 days, once every 24 to 38 days, and a volume that does not significantly interfere with quality of life. Any type of bleeding outside these parameters is considered **abnormal uterine bleeding** (AUB). Generally speaking, premenopausal abnormal uterine bleeding is less concerning than postmenopausal. AUB in a postmenopausal patient can be an indicator of an endometrial malignancy.

Some patients with uterine leiomyomas, more commonly known as **fibroids**, may come to IR as self-referrals, so it's important to have a basic understanding of the work-up for AUB, and have comfort in accurately diagnosing fibroids. A good gynecologic and obstetrical history includes the patient's pattern of menstrual cycles, vaginal bleeding outside of normal menstruation, past pregnancies, and history of infertility. Bimanual and speculum exams can be deferred if the patient has had a recent gynecological visit (< 1 month).

The differential when considering abnormal uterine bleeding in a premenopausal patient includes endometrial polyps and adenomyosis (▶ **Table 11.1**). Endometrial polyps are focal outgrowths of glandular tissue and blood vessels into the uterine cavity, typically appearing as a beefy red, friable mass. Adenomyosis is abnormal proliferation of endometrial tissue within the myometrium, characteristically resulting in a large, boggy uterus and dysmenorrhea.

Work-up for Fibroids

The diagnosis of fibroids is based on the clinical history and confirmatory imaging. Symptomatic patients most commonly present with complaints of heavy menstrual bleeding. The disruption of the endometrial surface and myometrium by these benign smooth muscle tumors contributes to menorrhagia. You may have to specifically ask about "bulk symptoms" caused by mass effect on adjacent organs, including constipation, urinary frequency, flank pain, or pelvic pain. A focused exam includes evaluation for pelvic masses, cervical lesions, and cervical tenderness.

The clinical history may be strongly suggestive for fibroids, but a pelvic ultrasound is typically necessary to confirm the diagnosis. If the uterus is quite large, there are atypical appearing fibroids on ultrasound, or if further information is needed for

Table 11.1 Causes of abnormal uterine bleeding in the premenopausal patient

Pathology	Description	Defining features
Fibroids	Benign smooth muscle tumor	Heavy menstrual bleeding, irregularly shaped uterus
Adenomyosis	Endometrial tissue in uterine muscle layer	Heavy menstrual bleeding, dysmenorrhea, large, boggy uterus on exam
Endometrial polyps	Outgrowth of endometrium into uterine cavity	Heavy menstrual bleeding

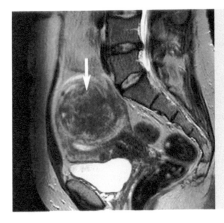

Fig. 11.1 Sagittal T2-weighted MR image of a well-circumscribed intramural fibroid in the posterior wall of the uterus. (Source: Varicoceles. In: Bakal C, Silberzweig J, Cynamon J, et al, eds. Vascular and Interventional Radiology. Principles and Practice. 1st Edition. Thieme; 2000.)

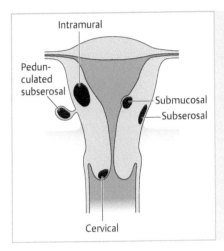

Fig. 11.2 Diagram depicting fibroids by location. (Source: Imaging Signs. In: Hamm B, Asbach P, Beyersdorff D, et al, eds. Direct Diagnosis in Radiology. Urogenital Imaging. 1st Edition. Thieme; 2008.)

treatment planning, MRI is usually the next step (▶ Fig. 11.1). MRI also has the benefit of being able to distinguish adenomyosis from fibroids. CT is sensitive for the incidental detection of fibroids but is not typically a modality used specifically for this work-up.

Fibroids are characterized by their location within the uterus: submucosal, intramural, subserosal, and pedunculated subserosal (▶ Fig. 11.2).

The majority of patients with fibroids do not need a tissue confirmation prior to treatment. A combination of clinical factors and ultrasound findings should raise suspicion for malignancy in the minority of patients that require a biopsy beforehand. This includes any postmenopausal women with uterine bleeding or a thick uterine stripe.

Management of Fibroids

Fibroids are benign, so no treatment is necessary for asymptomatic patients. For symptomatic patients, a number of medications are available as first-line therapy. Oral contraceptives or hormonal intrauterine devices can help regulate menstruation and alleviate dysmenorrhea, but they don't actually decrease the size of fibroids, and therefore have no effect on the bulk symptoms. Antiestrogenic medications can shrink fibroids but are associated with a number of side effects. For this reason, they are usually reserved for short-term preintervention purposes, as we'll discuss below. Menopause itself can reduce the size of fibroids due to a decrease in estrogenic stimuli, so perimenopausal women with bulk symptoms may prefer to wait rather than pursue intervention.

Second-line treatments include surgery (hysterectomy or myomectomy) and uterine artery embolization. **Hysterectomy** is a definitive therapy for fibroids. The surgery also benefits patients with other uterine pathology (endometriosis, adenomyosis, hyperplasia, or malignancy). **Myomectomy** is a more conservative surgical option performed hysteroscopically or laparoscopically, and involves focal resection of the fibroids. Myomectomy is limited to fibroids within the uterine cavity or on the serosal surface. Fertility is often preserved when small fibroids are treated with myomectomy. Gonadotropin-releasing hormone (GnRH) analogues (leuprolide) are given as presurgical treatment for 3 to 6 months. This causes hypoestrogenism, resulting in uterine volume reduction and amenorrhea.

Uterine fibroid embolization (UFE), also known as uterine artery embolization (UAE), is an endovascular therapy performed by IR that takes advantage of the rich blood supply of fibroids (**Procedure Box 11.1**). GnRH analogues are *not* used prior to UFE like they are for surgery; the resultant decrease in uterine artery caliber and blood flow caused by the medication make endovascular access to the uterine vessels more challenging.

Postprocedure care after a UFE is relatively straightforward. Patients are admitted for up to 24 hours following the procedure, primarily for pain control. Pelvic cramping can be moderate to severe in the first 12 to 24 hours, and typically improves after about a week with NSAIDs. **Postembolization syndrome** can be seen in up to 40% of patients, and is characterized by low-grade fever, anorexia, nausea, and malaise. Symptoms can be treated with analgesics, anti-inflammatory medications, and oral or intravenous hydration as needed. UFE patients should ideally be followed in clinic roughly 2 weeks and again 3 months after the procedure, with follow-up MRI at 6 months to assess treatment response.

Choosing between Uterine Fibroid Embolization and Surgery

Deciding between hysterectomy and UFE is difficult, but ultimately boils down to the patient's goals (▶**Table 11.2**). Do they want a definitive procedure? Do they have a desire for future pregnancy? Are they specifically interested in minimally invasive treatment?

While most studies on UFE have excluded submucosal, subserosal, and pedunculated fibroids, their treatment with UFE is not necessarily contraindicated. Some believed these types of fibroids should not be treated due to potential complications (in particular, the risk of sloughing of the necrotic fibroid into the abdomen or uterine cavity). In reality, there haven't been any significant reports to support this. Treatment of these other types of fibroids with UFE has been shown to yield similar outcomes to intramural fibroids, and many IRs no longer consider this a contraindication. On the other hand, some types of fibroids, such as pedunculated intrauterine fibroids, are more easily treated with hysteroscopic myomectomy, and there's no question the surgical approach is better.

Similarly, the total fibroid burden is not an absolute contraindication for a UFE. However, treating very large fibroids with UFE may be inappropriate. Most IRs have an anecdote or two about treatment failure, infection, or serious complication after treating very large fibroids. The upper limit of size that can be treated with UFE probably has more to do with practitioner comfortability than an arbitrary cutoff.

Procedure Box 11.1: Uterine Artery Embolization ⓘ

Uterine artery embolization is a minimally invasive treatment for uterine fibroids and may also be required in cases of abnormal placental implantation or for the treatment of refractory postpartum hemorrhage. Arterial access is obtained via the common femoral or left radial artery, and a pelvic arteriogram is performed to delineate anatomy. The anterior division of internal iliac artery is selected with a catheter and another angiogram is performed to identify the uterine artery, which is commonly hypertrophied in patients requiring this procedure. It appears long, tortuous, and anteromedial in location.

These features help to differentiate the uterine artery from other nearby vessels, including the straighter pudendal artery and the shorter/smaller-caliber cystic artery. It is critical to identify the cervicovaginal branches of the uterine artery, which supply nerve fibers to the cervix and vagina (embolization of which can precipitate cervical or vaginal necrosis, decreased sexual sensation, or inorgasmia). A microcatheter is advanced into the uterine artery distal to the cervicovaginal branches. Embolization is then performed by slowly injecting microsphere particles mixed with contrast under continuous fluoroscopic visualization. The typical particle size is 500 to 700 µm. This size decreases the risk of ovarian shunting, and has been demonstrated to cause less postembolization pain with similar efficacy when compared to smaller particles.

Embolization is repeated on the contralateral side, or alternatively both sides can be treated simultaneously in two-operator settings. The ovarian arteries may occasionally supply some or all of the patient's fibroids; this is typically suspected due to features on preprocedural imaging or in the setting of a nonhypertrophied uterine artery on iliac arteriography. The ovarian arteries can potentially be selected and distally embolized in some patients, however, the risk of ovarian failure is obviously higher for this technique. Some interventionalists always perform aortography to exclude a significant uterine supply from the ovarian arteries, while others only do this if there is suspicion for incomplete embolization from the uterine arteries.

Table 11.2 Comparing the interventions for fibroids

	Preservation of fertility	Location	Outcome
Hysterectomy	No	Any	Definitive therapy Treats other gynecological diseases
Myomectomy	Likely	*Hysteroscopic*: Submucosal *Abdominal*: Intramural Subserosal	Preserves fertility Increased risk of uterine rupture in subsequent pregnancies
UFE	Possibly	Intramural +/− Submucosal +/− Subserosal	↑ Reinterventions Shorter hospitalizations

Historically, myomectomy has been the treatment of choice for patients with severe symptomatic fibroids who want to preserve fertility. When there are multiple or very large fibroids, myomectomy may be too difficult by laparoscopic approach, and open surgery is required. Laparotomies carry greater morbidity, including longer recovery time and the risk of intra-abdominal adhesions. Regardless of the surgical technique, myomectomies do increase the risk of uterine rupture to some extent with subsequent pregnancy.

Many patients who express interest in UFE do so specifically with an interest in preserving fertility. There are patients who have successfully become pregnant after their procedure, but there's relatively little data regarding fertility after UFE beyond anecdotal reports. It's also unclear if those pregnancies are more prone to complication, though a few studies have suggested there may be worse outcomes in some pregnancies after UFE. There's quite a bit we don't know yet, and more research is needed before we can say anything definitive about the obstetric outcomes post-UFE.

One thing we do know is that the risk of premature ovarian failure and early menopause following UFE is higher in older patients, thought to be caused by shunting of embolic material into the ovarian vessels. This is important to make note of when counseling patients.

By the time a patient sees you for a UFE consult, the likelihood is he or she has already gone through a discussion of the surgical options and learned about the less invasive UFE procedure from his or her own research. Avoidance of the traditional surgical risks and longer recovery time is one of the reasons many women seek out UFE treatment. That perception does have some data to support it. According to one meta-analysis by Gupta et al in 2014, patient satisfaction and quality-of-life scores were similar in studies comparing UFE to surgery, and patients who underwent UFE had higher short-term quality-of-life scores, as well as shorter hospital stays. However, the study also found that UFE carried a significantly higher rate of symptom recurrence. Patients may not necessarily be aware of this, so it's important to explain the risk of symptom recurrence before proceeding with UFE.

From an IR perspective, the most important factor is what the patient wants. When seeing a consult, your role is to understand the patient's goals for treatment and use that to educate her on how UFE may be beneficial, as well as the associated limitations. Be prepared for situations in which the patient is a good candidate for UFE, but ultimately better off being treated surgically based on her stated preferences.

11.2 Ureteral Obstruction

Ureteral obstruction can be caused by kidney stones, stricture, or external compression from a mass or urologic malignancy. A complete obstruction often leads to hydronephrosis or hydroureteronephrosis, and may result in acute kidney injury. If left untreated, permanent loss of kidney function can result.

Acute obstruction typically presents with severe crampy lower abdominal pain radiating to the flank, most commonly due to a kidney stone. Hematuria is a common lab finding, though most emergency department physicians base the decision to pursue imaging based predominantly on clinical history. Low-dose, noncontrast CT is generally the initial imaging modality when kidney stones are suspected. The accuracy of CT is superior to ultrasound, though there is disagreement on just much of a difference exists, and if it's enough to justify the radiation exposure. Ultrasound is first line for pediatric and pregnant patients. Some advocate its use for any nonobese adult rather than CT, though this is not the norm.

Chronic obstructive uropathy is more subtle—elevated creatinine may be the only abnormal finding, a clue to deteriorating renal function. Common causes of chronic ureteral obstruction include urologic malignancies, mass effect from adjacent structures, or ureteral strictures. Renal ultrasound often demonstrates hydronephrosis, which over time can cause thinning of the renal cortex (not a feature of acute obstruction).

In general, hydronephrosis should set off warning bells for urinary tract obstruction, but it can occasionally be nonobstructive in nature. The **Whitaker test** is a urodynamic study sometimes used to differentiate between obstructive and nonobstructive dilation of the renal collecting system. This test measures the pressure difference between the renal pelvis and bladder. A needle or catheter is used to inject fluid into the collecting system under fluoroscopic guidance while pressure readings are measured in both the collecting system and bladder (with a Foley catheter). If there is an obstruction, the pressure inside the renal pelvis will progressively rise above that of the bladder. A pressure gradient greater than 15 cm H_2O is abnormal and suggests obstruction.

Management of Ureteral Obstructions

The majority of kidney stones are managed expectantly, though larger stones may necessitate intervention by a urologist, occasionally with the assistance of IR. **Percutaneous nephrostomy tube (PCN)** placement is a procedure done by IR in which a catheter is introduced through the patient's flank, into a calyx and advanced into the collecting system (▶ **Fig. 11.3**) (**Procedure Box 11.2**). Nephrolithiasis associated with evidence of infection is an indication to have an urgent PCN placed. This allows urinary tract decompression and local source control until the stone can be removed. Another indication for PCN placement is to provide access for a urologist to perform percutaneous nephrolithotomy in cases where other noninvasive measures aren't enough.

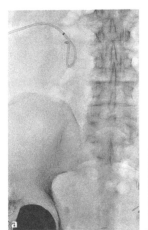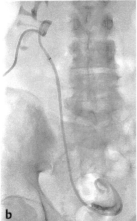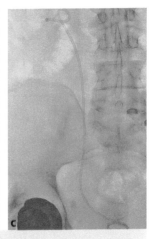

Fig. 11.3 (a) Fluoroscopic spot image of a simple percutaneous nephrostomy tube with the tip coiled in the renal pelvis. (b) The same patient after undergoing conversion to a percutaneous nephroureterostomy with the proximal drain coiled in the renal pelvis and the distal drain coiled in the bladder. Note that percutaneous access is maintained. (c) The drain was later fully internalized to a nephroureteral stent. The proximal pigtail is coiled in the renal pelvis and distal pigtail is in the bladder. There is no longer percutaneous access to the drainage system. Access for removal or replacement is done by urology via cystoscopy.

Percutaneous nephrostomy, nephroureteral stenting, and double-J ureteral stenting are procedures performed by interventional radiologists for the treatment of urinary obstruction or infection, or to facilitate urinary diversion in the setting of distal leak or malignancy. The patient is typically positioned prone, although lateral oblique positioning can be employed for patients unable to assume the prone position due to body habitus, recent abdominal surgery, or breathing difficulty. The procedure can be accomplished using ultrasound or fluoroscopic guidance, which involves placement of an 18- to 22-gauge needle into a posterolateral calyx in the middle or inferior pole of the kidney. Upon visualization of urine drainage from the needle, additional confirmation of intracalyceal positioning can be performed by the injection of contrast, which will opacify the collecting system. When there is concern for urinary infection, care should be taken not to overdistend the collecting system, which can cause translocation of bacteria into the bloodstream and precipitate sepsis. A wire is coiled in the renal pelvis and the tract dilated, to facilitate upsizing to a larger-caliber nephrostomy tube.

In cases where a ureteral obstruction can easily be crossed by a wire, a PCNU tube is placed instead of a PCN tube. This extends from the patient's skin, through the ureter, and terminates in the bladder. This type of catheter can potentially be capped on the outside, allowing internalized drainage across the obstruction from the renal pelvis to the bladder. The advantage of this is maintaining the ability to exchange the tube over a wire, which is usually done every 8 to 12 weeks to maintain patency. In contrast, a completely internalized double-J ureteral stent requires cystoscopic exchange by urology.

Mild hematuria is common after these procedures and should clear within 48 to 72 hours. Gross or persistent hematuria should not occur, and may indicate a vascular injury during tube placement, potentially requiring additional imaging and/or embolization.

If the obstruction is secondary to a narrowing or stricture in the ureter, ureteroplasty and/or stent placement can bypass the obstruction and allow urine to pass from the kidney into the bladder. Urologists can place a stent across the obstruction in a retrograde fashion by introducing it through the urethra. In certain cases when the retrograde approach has failed or is infeasible, IR may be asked to place the stent in an antegrade approach, similar to how the PCN is introduced. Stents can be placed as an internal–external drain, referred to as a **percutaneous nephroureterostomy** (PCNU), or can be completely internalized (▶ **Fig. 11.3**). PCNU preserves access such that IR can bring the patient back to do exchanges percutaneously, whereas internalized stents necessitate any future stent exchanges to be performed in a retrograde fashion by urology.

11.3 Lower Urinary Tract Obstruction

Benign prostatic hyperplasia (BPH) is a common cause of lower urinary tract symptoms in adult males. History alone will often be suggestive of the diagnosis. Patients complain of urinary frequency, hesitancy, weak stream, retention, and nocturia. On a digital rectal exam, the prostate is smooth, symmetric, and enlarged. The American Urologic Association symptom score or the **International Prostate Symptom Score (IPSS)** can be used to track symptoms over time and determine the best course of management. Both can be found online.

Some advocate measuring a prostate-specific antigen (PSA) to screen for prostate cancer when working up BPH, though this is a controversial topic. The PSA can be elevated for a number of different reasons, so this should be taken into account when faced with an abnormal result.

Patients with the combination of BPH symptoms and an elevated creatinine should get an ultrasound or CT urogram to evaluate for more proximal obstruction involving the bladder, ureters, or kidneys. Transrectal ultrasound and postvoid residual volume (PVR) are studies used to classify the severity of obstruction and guide treatment.

Management of Benign Prostatic Hyperplasia

Behavioral modification is recommended for all patients with BPH. This includes voiding in a seated position, avoiding fluids prior to bedtime, reducing consumption of mild diuretics (alcohol, coffee, etc.), and double voiding to empty the bladder as much as possible.

Medical therapy is initiated according to a patient's symptom score. Mild-to-moderate symptoms (IPSS 0–19) are treated with an α_1 antagonist (terazosin, doxazosin). Severe symptoms (IPSS ≥ 20) or failure of monotherapy warrant addition of a 5α-reductase inhibitor (finasteride), which blocks conversion of testosterone to dihydrotestosterone. For irritative urinary symptoms (i.e., urgency, frequency, and incontinence), an anticholinergic agent can also be initiated.

More aggressive therapy should be considered when patients on maximum medical therapy fail to achieve an adequate response over 1 to 2 years, or for those who cannot tolerate medical therapy, or have progression of disease despite therapy.

Surgical options include prostatectomy or **transurethral resection of the prostate (TURP)**. Prostatectomy is the most aggressive option, carrying significant morbidity, However, it is a definitive treatment. TURP involves insertion of a scope into the urethra and removing the problematic prostate tissue through cautery and dissection. Urinary incontinence and retrograde ejaculation are relatively common after TURP.

Prostatic artery embolization (PAE) is an emerging IR procedure that provides an alternative to surgery (**Procedure Box 11.3**). Embolizing the prostatic artery has been shown to decrease prostatic volume and improve BPH symptoms. Prostate cancer should be ruled out with a PSA screen and transrectal biopsy (if necessary) before proceeding with PAE.

Systematic reviews of PAE have shown significant improvements in quality of life and symptom scores with the procedure. The typical complications associated with TURP are avoided with PAE. While the data for PAE are promising, the procedure is relatively new and not yet firmly established in major treatment guidelines. For now, PAE may be presented as an option for patients who are poor surgical candidates or who are not willing to undergo the more invasive surgical procedures.

11.4 Gonadal Vein Insufficiency

Gonadal vein insufficiency presents as a varicocele in men and pelvic congestion syndrome (PCS) in women.

A **varicocele** is dilation of the pampiniform plexus due to valvular incompetence or compression of the testicular vein (▶ **Fig. 11.4**). Symptomatic varicoceles may present with achy scrotal pain (worse when standing), heaviness, testicular atrophy, and reduced fertility. Because of the longer drainage pathway for the left testicular vein and its relationship to the left renal vein, the majority of varicoceles are left sided. A new right-sided varicocele can be a clue that there is a pelvic or abdominal mass that is compressing the vein and should prompt further evaluation with cross-sectional imaging.

Procedure Box 11.3: Prostatic Artery Embolization

PAE is performed to decrease prostatic volume and improve urinary retention in the setting of BPH. PAE is a novel procedure which shows excellent promise as a minimally invasive alternative therapy to transurethral resection of the prostate, and is associated with fewer complications. The procedure is performed similarly to uterine artery embolization, starting with pelvic and internal iliac arteriography.

Prostatic arteries are more variable in origin, course, and number per side. Because of this variability, most operators utilize cone beam CT (CBCT) to identify the prostatic arteries and confirm catheter location. Frequent use of CBCT is important for ensuring that the candidate vessel only supplies the prostate, as many other vessels will supply adjacent structures such as bladder or rectum. Prostatic arteries can arise from the internal iliac artery directly, from the internal pudendal artery, obturator artery, or other visceral arteries in the pelvis.

Each prostatic artery is selected with a microcatheter, and angiography is performed to assess vessel size, flow characteristics, and distal vascularity. Embolization with particles is carried out to the point of sluggish forward flow/near stasis, and a completion angiogram is done to confirm devascularization. Embolization is then repeated on the contralateral side.

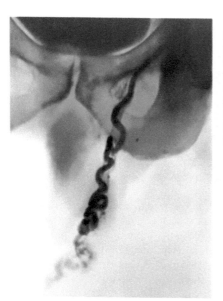

Fig. 11.4 After left renal vein catheterization, a venogram was performed while the patient beared down. Valsalva maneuver induced reflux of contrast into a dilated testicular vein, confirming the diagnosis of varicocele. (Source: Varicoceles. In: Bakal C, Silberzweig J, Cynamon J, et al, eds. Vascular and Interventional Radiology. Principles and Practice. 1st Edition. Thieme; 2000.)

Ovarian vein (and sometimes iliac vein) incompetence can result in the formation of varices around the uterus and ovaries (▶ **Fig. 11.5**). This can manifest as a constellation of symptoms known as **pelvic congestion syndrome**. Women will typically present with chronic, achy pelvic pain, worse when standing. In addition, a dilated ovarian vein can occasionally compress the ureter.

For both varicocele and PCS, Doppler ultrasound is used to evaluate for other causes of scrotal or pelvic pain and to confirm the diagnosis. With a varicocele, the veins of the pampiniform plexus are enlarged, measuring at least 2 mm during Valsalva maneuver. With PCS, the size of varices is believed to be less important than the evidence of reflux on duplex ultrasound, since the size will vary by patient position, phase of respiration, and amount of abdominal pressure.

Despite the utility of ultrasound, imaging diagnosis remains controversial. Some practitioners only rely on MR or CT venogram to demonstrate the presence of varices and dilation of the gonadal veins. Others will proceed directly to angiographic venogram without preceding imaging if the history and physical exam are strongly suggestive.

Management of Gonadal Vein Insufficiency

Varicoceles are treated symptomatically with scrotal support and NSAIDs. Reasons to pursue more definitive treatment include infertility, testicular atrophy in young patients (catch-up growth of the atrophic testis after treatment is possible), and pain that does not respond to conservative therapy. Treatment options include surgical ligation and **testicular vein embolization**. Both surgical and endovascular treatment are highly efficacious. Unilateral treatment of the left testicular vein is often sufficient, particularly for infertility. The main advantages of endovascular treatment are shorter recovery and less morbidity.

PCS can also be treated conservatively with NSAIDs and/or pharmacologic suppression of ovarian function. When conservative treatments are inadequate, endovascular treatment may be a good option for the patient. Gonadal vein embolization offers a high clinical success rate with few complications (▶ **Fig. 11.5**) (**Procedure Box 11.4**).

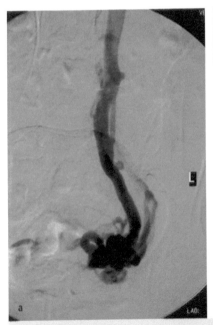 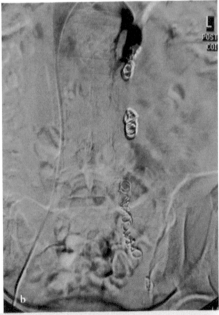

Fig. 11.5 (a) Fluoroscopic image obtained after contrast injection in the left renal vein while patient performed a Valsalva maneuver. Pooling of contrast in the ovarian vein can be seen. This patient had long-standing chronic pelvic pain. (b) Pain improved after coil embolization of the dilated gonadal vein. Sources: (a) Imaging. In: Siskin G, ed. Interventional Radiology in Women's Health. 1st Edition. Thieme; 2009. (b) Treatment. In: Siskin G, ed. Interventional Radiology in Women's Health. 1st Edition. Thieme; 2009.

To minimize gonadal radiation exposure, continuous fluoroscopic imaging and digital subtraction angiography of the testis or ovaries are avoided wherever possible, and pulsed (low-dose) fluoroscopy is used in combination with careful collimation.

Access is commonly obtained via the right common femoral vein or the right internal jugular vein; a variety of catheters have been utilized for this procedure, including several renal and gonadal vein-specific catheters. Contrast is injected into the renal vein or vena cava while the patient bears down, allowing for identification of valvular incompetence and venous collaterals, especially those that originate from the renal hilum or paralumbar region. These can bypass the gonadal vein and increase the chance of recurrence.

Embolization is usually performed with a combination of metallic coils and the sclerosant sodium tetradecyl sulfate (STS). After selecting the gonadal vein, a coil pack is formed in the caudal gonadal vein at the level of the inguinal ligament. STS mixed with contrast and air or Gelfoam is then injected, and an additional nest of coils is placed to trap the sclerosant within the vein. Repeat venography is performed at multiple levels, working backward from the inguinal ligament to the left renal vein or IVC. The idea is to identify any collaterals that parallel the primary gonadal vein that could hypertrophy and cause persistent or recurrent symptoms. If more collaterals are identified, these are selected and treated with additional sclerosant and coils. The treatment is carried back to the level of the left renal vein or IVC until all veins/collaterals have been treated.

The gonadal veins are prone to spasm from guidewire manipulation, which may necessitate pausing the procedure temporarily, administration of nitroglycerin, or occasionally rescheduling the procedure for a different day.

Care should be taken to avoid sclerosant reflux into the scrotum or periuterine collaterals, which can cause considerable discomfort.

Suggested Readings

[1] Bulman JC, Ascher SM, Spies JB. Current concepts in uterine fibroid embolization. Radiographics. 2012; 32(6):1735–1750

[2] Ignacio EA, Dua R, Sarin S, et al. Pelvic congestion syndrome: diagnosis and treatment. Semin Intervent Radiol. 2008; 25(4):361–368

[3] Kandarpa K, Machan L, Durham JD. Handbook of Interventional Radiologic Procedures. Philadelphia, PA: Wolters Kluwer; 2016

[4] Kuang M, Vu A, Athreya S. A systematic review of prostatic artery embolization in the treatment of symptomatic benign prostatic hyperplasia. Cardiovasc Intervent Radiol.

12 Neuro IR

Juan Domingo Ly Liu, Mangaladevi Patil, and Joseph J. Gemmete

12.1 Ischemic Stroke

It is an exciting time for neurointerventionalists. Back in 1995, the NINDS trial demonstrated a clear benefit to the use of intravenous tissue plasminogen activator (tPA) for acute stroke. This remained the standard of care for acute stroke intervention for two decades, until several trials published in 2015 showed improved outcomes with the use of endovascular thrombectomy compared to medical management alone. This has ushered in a new era, with updated treatment algorithms for stroke. Neurointerventional radiologists, interventional neurologists, and neurosurgeons may each have a role in providing these interventions, but this will vary between institutions. With the growth of interventional stroke therapy, IR trainees should aim to develop a good understanding of the diagnosis and triage of patients with acute neurological emergencies.

Approach to a Patient with Suspected Stroke

The work-up of a suspected stroke begins before the patient arrives at the hospital. The patient's history is assessed by first responders using the Cincinnati Prehospital Stroke Scale or the Los Angeles Prehospital Stroke Screen. Higher scores on either scale will prompt first responders to activate the stroke protocol at the receiving hospital.

The first decision when the patient arrives in the emergency department is determining if it is truly a stroke. There are many stroke mimics, including encephalitis, seizures, or metabolic disturbances. Typically, the emergency department physician and stroke neurologist work together to make that determination.

Patients with sufficient concern for stroke get a noncontrast head CT as soon as they roll into the ED to exclude intracranial hemorrhage. If suspicion is high enough, some institutions also perform a CTA of the head and neck while the patient is still in the CT scanner.

Management of Ischemic Stroke

Tissue plasminogen activator (tPA) is the first-line standard of care for ischemic stroke patients that meet the inclusion criteria. The NINDS trial (1995) demonstrated the efficacy of tPA in reducing neurologic disability if given within a 3-hour window of symptom onset. The ECASS III trial (2008) expanded upon this by showing the efficacy of tPA given up to 4.5 hours after symptom onset. The current guidelines state that if the patient is an intravenous tPA candidate and symptom onset is less than 4.5 hours, the patient should receive tPA—anything beyond that, tPA is not an option.

A number of questions need to be answered as soon as possible to figure out if the patient should get tPA. Initial candidacy is determined by time from last-known-well, symptom severity, and noncontrast head CT findings (▶Table 12.1). Timing of stroke onset can be difficult to determine, as many patients awake from sleep with symptoms. Symptom severity is determined using the National Institutes of Health (NIH) Stroke Scale. CT images are evaluated for presence of hemorrhage at a minimum, and signs of early ischemia if present. After intracranial hemorrhage has been ruled out, other criteria are then reviewed to exclude patients with a prohibitively high risk of complication from tPA.

Table 12.1 Inclusion/exclusion criteria for tPA for stroke

Inclusion criteria
Ischemic stroke
Symptom onset < 4.5 hours from last-known-well
Exclusion criteria
Recent stroke, ICH, head trauma in past 3 months
CT showing ICH or large, irreversible area of infarct
Recent head/spine surgery
Presence of cerebral aneurysm, intracranial neoplasm, AVM
SBP ≥ 185 or DBP ≥ 110 mm Hg
Active internal bleeding
Bleeding diathesis (INR > 1.7, elevated PTT, platelet count < 100,000, etc.)

Despite being the first-line therapy for acute ischemic stroke, systemic thrombolytic therapy has not been shown to be equally effective in every intracranial vessel. A study from 2010 by Bhatia et al showed that stroke patients with large vessel occlusions had the lowest rates of vessel recanalization following systemic tPA administration, and also the poorest neurological outcomes among all groups studied. This prompted a search for additional techniques to improve outcomes in patients with large vessel occlusions. Advances in mechanical thrombectomy proved to be the solution.

While mechanical thrombectomy has been performed for acute ischemic stroke since the early 2000s, several negative trials precluded its widespread acceptance. MR CLEAN (2015) was the first trial to show the superiority of early mechanical thrombectomy compared to tPA alone in the treatment of proximal anterior large vessel occlusion. It was the largest and most inclusive of five simultaneous trials focusing on thrombectomy. After MR CLEAN was published, all other ongoing trials were stopped early due to overwhelming evidence (ESCAPE in North America, EXTEND-IA in Australia, SWIFT PRIME, and REVASCAT in Spain); however, the data collected from those trials were also strongly supportive. This new evidence has revolutionized the way ischemic stroke is treated.

In situations where tPA is less efficacious, mechanical thrombectomy excels; it benefits patients who have large vessel occlusions, and it is the *only* intervention potentially available to those who are not tPA candidates. As an added advantage, thrombectomy has a longer window for use in stroke patients.

Once the decision has been made to give tPA or not, the next step is to determine if the patient is a candidate for thrombectomy. Three factors are taken into consideration: location of the clot, time from symptom onset, and imaging findings. CTA is usually the go-to for identifying large vessel occlusions, as well as providing a road map for endovascular treatment. Clot in the proximal anterior circulation is most amenable to mechanical thrombectomy. This includes the internal carotid artery (ICA), M1/M2 branches of the middle cerebral artery, and A1/A2 branches of the anterior carotid artery.

Initial guidelines recommended mechanical thrombectomy for an anterior circulation stroke up to 8 hours from the time of symptom onset. In 2018, the DEFUSE 3 trial by Albers et al showed that this window can be extended to as much as 16 hours in select patients. The trial made use of perfusion imaging, which essentially looks for evidence of salvageable ischemic damage (also called penumbra), and differentiates it from irreversible damage. The larger the penumbra, the greater theoretical benefit from intervention. While the earlier trials demonstrated the efficacy of new endovascular techniques and devices, the most recent studies are further guiding decisions by selecting patients who have the highest benefit-to-risk ratio. With the prospect of a longer intervention window, mechanical thrombectomy is only going to take on a more prominent role in stroke therapy, with the potential to create a significant impact on the care of these patients.

The Food and Drug Administration (FDA) has approved three main types of mechanical thrombectomy devices: coil retrievers, aspiration devices, and stent retrievers ("stentrievers")—the latter two being more common. All three have the same basic function, which is removal of an occlusive thrombus within the artery (**Procedure Box 12.1**). Complications of these devices include intracerebral hemorrhage, subarachnoid hemorrhage (SAH), distal embolization, dissection, perforation, and non-revascularization.

Patients treated with mechanical thrombectomy are admitted to the ICU for 24 hours following the procedure. Blood pressure is tightly controlled to maintain normotension, and serial neuro examinations done to monitor for signs of deterioration. If there is a decline in neurologic function, a head CT is obtained to look for hemorrhagic conversion or cerebral edema.

For all patients, regardless of intervention, risk factors for stroke recurrence or propagation are addressed during the hospitalization. Aspirin is usually started within 24 hours. Medical management for hyperlipidemia and diabetes is optimized. Active smokers are counseled on smoking cessation. An exercise regimen is prescribed to

---

Procedure Box 12.1: Mechanical Thrombectomy for Ischemic Stroke   i

Mechanical thrombectomy is a technique used for treating ischemic stroke. The procedure requires two special pieces of equipment: a balloon guide catheter (BGC) and a stent retriever. In order to arrest forward flow through the affected artery, the BGC employs a balloon at its tip; when inflated, the balloon occludes the vessel at a point proximal to the thrombus and prevents distal embolization of thrombus fragments during the procedure by stopping flow.

After obtaining femoral arterial access, the ICA is selected and a diagnostic angiogram performed to identify the site of intracranial vessel occlusion. The BGC is parked proximal to the clot with the balloon deflated. Through the lumen of the BGC, a microwire is deployed and navigated to the site of the thrombus. The occlusion is then crossed by the microwire and microcatheter. The microwire is removed and the microcatheter exchanged for the stent retriever device, deployed at the site of thrombus. The stent is left in place for 5 minutes, which allows the thrombus to incorporate into the interstices of the metallic stent.

The balloon on the BGC is inflated to arrest forward flow. The stent retriever and incorporated thrombus is then retracted into the BGC. While retracting the BGC with stent retriever enclosed, a syringe on the back end is gently aspirated to assist in thrombus removal (▶ **Fig. 12.1**). After removing the stent retriever and trapped thrombus, the BGC is vigorously aspirated to remove any residual components of thrombus in the catheter or treated vessel, as these could embolize and create untreatable distal occlusions.

The balloon on the BGC is then deflated and a diagnostic angiogram is repeated. Because of the manipulation of the vessel, intracranial vasospasm can develop; this is treated with intra-arterial verapamil or nicardipine, and the angiogram is repeated to confirm resolution. Once revascularization has been obtained, strict blood pressure control is essential to decrease the risk of reperfusion hemorrhage.

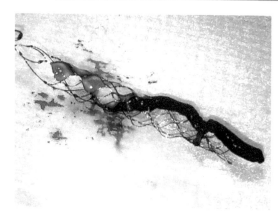

Fig. 12.1 Photograph of stent retriever shows thrombus which was removed from a patient's middle cerebral artery. (This image is provided courtesy of Dr Joseph J. Gemmete, MD, University of Michigan Health System.)

improve overall cardiovascular health. A bedside or fluoroscopic swallow evaluation is done before a diet is prescribed. Physical/occupational therapy and possibly the physical medicine and rehabilitation service should be consulted to begin the rehabilitation process. Finally, screening for atrial fibrillation and carotid disease can be done to assess the risk of embolic events.

For secondary prevention of stroke in patients with noncardioembolic stroke, guidelines recommend the patient take aspirin, clopidogrel, ticagrelor, or a combination drug comprised of aspirin and extended-release dipyridamole. In cases of cardioembolic stroke secondary to atrial fibrillation, an anticoagulation strategy can be determined based on that patient's CHADS-VASC score.

12.2 Carotid Artery Stenosis

Carotid stenosis secondary to atherosclerotic disease is considered a preventable cause of ischemic stroke, so it's important to take notice of it, especially in high-risk patients. There's two different ways carotid stenosis can be discovered: either an asymptomatic patient is diagnosed by screening ultrasound, or neurologic symptoms (transient ischemic attack, syncope, amaurosis fugax, stroke) prompt a search for underlying disease.

Understanding the severity of a patient's stenosis has become an increasingly complicated task as we gain new knowledge about how to treat these patients. If you've learned anything about any of the landmark carotid stenosis trials, you probably remember that the percentage of stenosis is important for stratifying patients. The gold standard for measuring that percentage is angiography, but it is an invasive test and is not routinely used for that measurement alone. Ultrasound, CTA and MRA are noninvasive methods that can be used to approximate the stenosis with relative accuracy. We classify stenosis as mild (< 50%), moderate (50–69%), or severe (≥ 70%).

A number of factors contribute to the strategy for treatment of carotid stenosis including degree of stenosis, presence or absence of symptoms, patient age and comorbidities, as well as an institution's surgical complication rate. The algorithm for sorting all this out is not as clear-cut as it is for treating stroke, so you should focus instead on understanding the most general guidelines.

Regardless of the severity of carotid stenosis, medical management is the first step. Maximum medical therapy includes both medication (blood glucose control, hypertension, cholesterol, and antiplatelet drugs) as well as lifestyle changes (exercise, smoking cessation, and diet modifications). In select cases, revascularization may be considered in addition to optimal medical therapy. The two options for revascularization are carotid endarterectomy (CEA) and carotid artery stenting (CAS).

Carotid endarterectomy is the gold standard invasive intervention for carotid artery stenosis. For endarterectomy to be an option, the lesion must be accessible (i.e., not too high in the neck). Patients who have undergone previous neck surgery or who have been exposed to previous head and neck radiation are considered higher-risk candidates, and surgery is generally avoided. The patient must also be healthy enough to undergo surgery.

Carotid artery stenting is a minimally invasive endovascular procedure that can be performed by vascular surgeons, interventional cardiologists, interventional neuroradiologists, and interventional radiologists, depending on the practice setting (**Procedure Box 12.2**, ▶ **Fig. 12.2**). CAS can be considered as an alternative to CEA in most cases. Some specific indications that favor CAS over CEA include lesions too high for CEA, recurrent stenosis after CEA, treatment of patients with prior head and neck radiation, and those with prohibitively high surgical risk.

Outcomes of major trials also help determine when CAS is appropriate. One of the associated risks inherent to stenting is iatrogenic stroke due to embolizing plaque debris. The development of distal embolic protection devices have helped to minimize this risk. These devices use either a balloon or filter deployed distal to the lesion to be treated, which blocks debris from traveling into the major intracranial vessels.

Choosing between CEA, CAS, or Optimal Medical Therapy Alone

The treatment of *asymptomatic* carotid stenosis with revascularization over the past 20 years has been guided by the results of a few major trials that took place in the 1990s. The studies showed there was a significant reduction in risk of stroke when CEA was performed for 60% or greater carotid stenosis. However, this finding has been met

---

Procedure Box 12.2: Carotid Artery Stenting   i

The goal with CAS is to increase blood flow to the downstream vessels supplied by the stenotic vessel, decrease the risk of plaque fragmentation and thrombosis or embolization, and thereby reduce the risk of stroke.

After obtaining arterial access through the common femoral artery (CFA), an aortogram of the aortic arch is performed. The affected common carotid artery is selected and angiography performed to evaluate vessel diameter, stenosis severity, and downstream perfusion. The stenosis is then crossed with a guidewire, and an appropriately sized **embolic protection device (EPD)** is deployed distal to the stenosis in a straight segment of the vessel. This will capture embolic debris that may mobilize at the time of stenting.

Predilation of the lesion is performed with a balloon, taking care to monitor for baroreceptor-mediated bradycardia (which may require Valsalva maneuvers or pharmacologic intervention with atropine or glycopyrrolate to reverse). A self-expanding metallic stent is then positioned across the stenosis, deployed, and postdilated. A follow-up angiogram is done to assess residual stenosis and embolic debris burden within the protection device; significant debris within the EPD may require insertion of an aspiration catheter prior to EPD retrieval to prevent the emboli from escaping. The EPD is then retrieved and completion carotid and cerebral angiography performed to confirm revascularization.

with skepticism in more recent years. The medical therapy arm of these trials does not reflect the nearly two decades worth of advances in drug efficacy and evidence-based treatment goals.

With current optimal medical therapy, some believe that the risk of stroke from carotid stenosis is as low as the periprocedural operative risk associated with revascularization. Others still advocate intervention for asymptomatic patients, but reserve it for those with more severe stenosis, in the 80% or greater range (▶ **Fig. 12.3**).

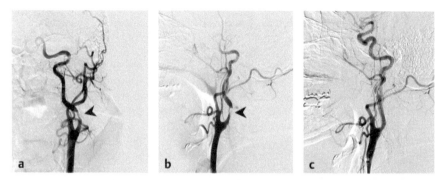

Fig. 12.2 Patient presented with a transient ischemic attack and was found to have a left internal carotid artery (ICA) stenosis. Digital subtraction angiography images show an 80% stenosis of the left ICA in the **(a)** Anteroposterior view and **(b)** lateral view. **(c)** After left carotid artery stenting, there is restoration of flow through the left ICA.

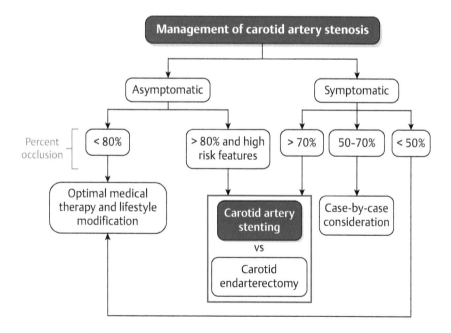

Fig. 12.3 Simplified algorithm for management of carotid artery stenosis.

Stenosis severity itself is a rather weak predictor of future events, but along with other findings can help identify patients who likely benefit from revascularization. Certain plaque characteristics identified with ultrasound or MRI, including predominantly lipid rich, ulcerated or hemorrhagic types, are higher risk and may tip the balance in favor of intervention. This is probably the best approach until there are new data comparing revascularization to current medical therapy. The CREST-2 trial, started in 2014, will hopefully provide better guidance by comparing optimal medical therapy alone to both CEA and CAS. The trial is expected to be completed within a few years of the publication of this text.

Symptomatic patients are typically identified by carotid ultrasound in the setting of a recent stroke, amaurosis fugax, or transient ischemic attack (TIA). As with asymptomatic carotid stenosis, landmark trials in the 90s demonstrated the overwhelming efficacy of CEA in reducing stroke or death in symptomatic patients with greater than 70% carotid stenosis (most notably the NASCET trial).

Since then, carotid artery stenting has emerged as a less invasive alternative to CEA. In the early 2000s, the SAPPHIRE trial compared CEA to CAS with use of a distal embolic protection device. The study found no significant difference in the incidence of death, stroke, or myocardial infarction (MI) in symptomatic patients at 1-year post-treatment. However, CAS did show a lower rate of revascularization compared to CEA during this same time period. The caveat to this trial is that it enrolled only patients considered high risk for surgery. The efficacy of CEA versus CAS for *average* surgical risk patients was compared by the original CREST study published in 2010. This study found that both CEA and CAS were similar in the primary end point (periprocedural stroke, death, MI), though the periprocedural stroke rate was somewhat higher after CAS, and periprocedural MI was higher following CEA. It also showed that the risk of stroke or death was higher for CAS in the subset of patients over 70 years old.

Based on the currently available data, *symptomatic* patients with greater than 70% stenosis will benefit from revascularization. Symptomatic patients between 50 and 69% stenosis are approached on case-by-case basis. Good surgical candidates with a greater than 5-year life expectancy, treated by a surgeon with less than 6% periprocedural stroke or death rate, and men in particular may benefit from revascularization. Studies have failed to show the same benefit for treatment of women in this group. Symptomatic patients below 50% stenosis are treated with medical management only.

After determining whom to treat, the next question is with what intervention? Revascularization with surgery versus stenting is not a clear-cut decision. CEA is preferred but CAS is the procedure of choice when there are contraindications to CEA due to lesion location, a patient's surgical risk, or history of radiation to the neck. Based on the available data, CEA is more beneficial for patients over the age of 70, and when there is a life expectancy of at least 5 years. When patients don't fall neatly into one category or another, the decision will likely be determined by the local expertise. While CEA has been around longer, increasing operator experience, coupled with continuous technological advances in the field, such as embolic protection devices and flow-reversal technology, have made CAS an increasingly attractive alternative for symptomatic carotid artery stenosis.

For the *asymptomatic* patients, it's unclear if any intervention beyond optimal medical therapy is necessary. For now, those asymptomatic patients with severe stenosis and other high-risk indicators may be considered for either CEA or CAS. These treatment algorithms will be updated as more research becomes available.

12.3 Cerebral Aneurysms

A **cerebral aneurysm** may be encountered incidentally on brain imaging or angiography, or occasionally by screening in patients with a family history of aneurysms. A history of autosomal dominant polycystic kidney disease or connective tissue disorders is also an indication for screening. In most cases, however, a cerebral aneurysm goes undiagnosed until the time of rupture. These patients typically display signs and symptoms of SAH ("worst headache of my life"). They can also present with neurologic deficits due to mass effect or thromboembolism. A cerebral aneurysm should be included in the differential for any patient who presents with suspicious new or chronic neurologic complaints.

Regardless of how the aneurysm is found, it should be further evaluated with CTA. This is the best modality to delineate the aneurysm size, shape, and location—all of which will help guide further management. Treatment considerations are different for ruptured and unruptured aneurysms.

Management of Ruptured Cerebral Aneurysms

Patients with ruptured aneurysms are admitted to the ICU. Medical management goals include blood pressure control (goal BP < 160/90), maintenance of euvolemia, reversal of anticoagulation, seizure prophylaxis, and treatment of elevated intracranial pressure (ICP). Oral nimodipine and a statin are started shortly after admission, which can decrease the risk of symptomatic vasospasm.

In patients with concern for elevated ICP, external ventricular drains (EVDs) can be placed at the bedside. Also known as a ventriculostomy, an EVD is a catheter placed through a burr hole on the side of the skull, which terminates in the lateral ventricle or foramen of Monro. It measures ICP and drains cerebrospinal fluid (CSF) (along with any blood in the ventricular system). If there are signs of impending herniation, a craniotomy is performed to evacuate intracranial hematoma and relieve ICP.

Once the patient is stabilized, there is a question of whether to do an intervention or not. This is highly dependent on the patient's clinical status. The **Hunter and Hess grading system** is used to score the patient's clinical status after a ruptured SAH. Favorable grades (1–3) are most likely to get a significant benefit from intervention. For those with clinical grades (4–5), the neurologic deficit is severe enough that the benefit of intervening is limited. A discussion with the family and physician team is usually necessary in order to determine if more aggressive treatment is within the patient's best interest. Families will often opt for more of a palliative approach in these cases.

When intervention is pursued, the choice is endovascular coiling versus surgical clipping. Endovascular coiling induces thrombosis and excludes the aneurysm from circulation (**Procedure Box 12.3**). Major risks during endovascular coiling include thromboembolic events and rebleeding. Surgical clipping involves directly visualizing the aneurysm sac and placing a clip across the neck of the aneurysm, thereby excluding the sac from circulation. Clipping can be associated with complications including rebleeding, intracranial hemorrhage, and new neurologic deficits related to parenchymal retraction.

The International Subarachnoid Aneurysm Trial (ISAT) was a multicenter, randomized trial published in 2005 that compared surgical clipping and endovascular coiling for the treatment of ruptured cerebral aneurysms. The study showed that endovascular coiling resulted in decreased mortality, greater independent survival, and better functional independence compared with surgical clipping. As a result of this study, the guidelines now recommend an endovascular approach over clipping in those patients who are candidates. The exceptions are wide-neck or giant aneurysms, which may be too difficult to treat with endovascular coiling.

Procedure Box 12.3: Endovascular Coiling for Cerebral Aneurysm ⓘ

The goal of endovascular treatment is to prevent flow within the aneurysm by either filling it with embolic material or by excluding it through the use of the stent, thereby depressurizing the abnormal segment of vessel and decreasing the risk of rupture (▶ **Fig. 12.4**). Simple coiling is a method for treating narrow-necked aneurysms, and involves catheterizing the aneurysm with a microcatheter and deploying metallic coils directly into the aneurysm to fill its lumen. This decreases inflow and promotes clot formation.

If the aneurysm neck is too wide to allow for coil packing, other techniques can be employed. One method includes the placement of a microcatheter within the aneurysm and then inflation of a balloon across the neck prior to coil deployment, preventing prolapse into the parent vessel until they are tightly packed and unlikely to migrate. Stent-assisted coiling involves the deployment of a metallic stent across the neck and then catheterization of the aneurysm through the interstices of the stent prior to coil deployment, effectively trapping the coils within the aneurysm.

Flow-diverting stents may also be used without coiling; these devices have a greater surface area and decreased porosity, which directs blood through the stent and away from the aneurysm sac. In some situations, a fully covered stent may be deployed across the aneurysm neck. However, appropriately sized covered stents required for the treatment of cerebral aneurysms are not always readily available. Regardless of the technique, treated aneurysms should be surveilled with follow-up imaging to confirm occlusion and exclude recanalization due to coil compaction or incomplete treatment.

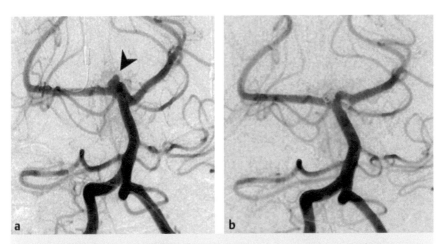

Fig. 12.4 DSA image in the anterior–posterior projection showing a right vertebral artery angiogram. A basilar apex aneurysm is visible **(a)** before and **(b)** after coil occlusion. (These images are provided courtesy of Dr Joseph J. Gemmete, MD, University of Michigan Health System.)

Management of Unruptured Cerebral Aneurysms

For unruptured cerebral aneurysms detected incidentally or on screening studies, the treatment strategy is less well established. Management options include conservative management, endovascular treatment (coiling +/– stenting), and surgical clipping.

The decision of when and how to intervene depends on (1) the size and location of the aneurysm, (2) age of the patient, and (3) risk factors for rupture. These factors include personal and family history of rupture, presence of daughter sacs, poorly controlled hypertension, and smoking status.

Several major studies have helped in the creation of the current guidelines for an unruptured cerebral aneurysm. The first International Study of Unruptured Intracranial Aneurysms (ISUIA) trial in 1998 concluded that patients without prior history of SAH presenting with an unruptured, anterior circulation cerebral aneurysm less than 7 mm do not require treatment. A second ISUIA study published in 2003 basically confirmed findings from the first ISUIA trial, concluding that larger aneurysm size (> 7 mm) was a clear risk factor for rupture. The authors also found that patients with aneurysms of the middle cerebral artery (MCA) or anterior cerebral artery (ACA) had better outcomes following surgical clipping than endovascular coiling. Take this with a grain of salt, however, as endovascular technology has improved significantly since then.

The following general guidelines can be used for determining the treatment strategy for unruptured aneurysms, though actual practice patterns will likely differ based on clinician preference (▶ **Fig. 12.5**). For aneurysms *less than 7 mm*, conservative management is preferred. This includes blood pressure control, smoking cessation, and serial CTA/MRA every few years to track growth. Intervention can be considered on a case-by-case basis for those smaller than 7 mm in the presence of multiple risk factors.

For aneurysms *larger than 7 mm*, intervention should be considered. Older patients and those with significant comorbidities may be better off managed conservatively, though any aneurysm greater than 10 mm is usually better off treated.

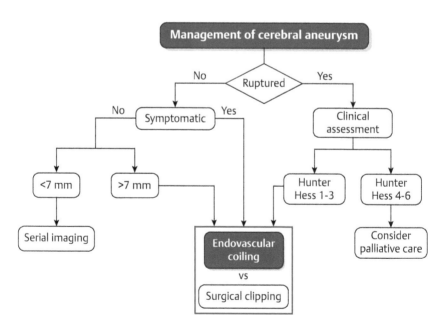

Fig. 12.5 Simplified algorithm for management of cerebral aneurysms.

12.4 Cerebral Arteriovenous Malformations

An **arteriovenous malformation (AVM)** is an abnormal tangle of blood vessels which connect arteries and veins without a normal intervening capillary bed (▶ **Fig. 12.6**). This tangle is called the nidus. As blood flows from the arteries to the draining veins, higher pressures cause the vessels to dilate and become tortuous. The abnormal hemodynamics result in weakening of vessel walls, leading to aneurysm formation and rupture. As with cerebral aneurysms, the risk of rupture is the key concern with AVMs. For this reason, the approach and management is quite similar, though there are a few important differences.

Cerebral AVMs are congenital, reflecting a failure of capillary formation during early embryogenesis, and are also usually sporadic. They can also develop in rare hereditary syndromes, such as hereditary hemorrhagic telangiectasia (aka Osler–Weber–Rendu syndrome) and Sturge–Weber syndrome. AVMs may be diagnosed in childhood or well into adulthood.

AVM ruptures can be catastrophic, and not uncommonly fatal. These patients present with symptoms typical of a SAH (though the bleed may in fact be intraparenchymal). Sometimes the presentation is less dramatic when the AVM leaks blood rather than ruptures. The presence of an AVM can serve as an epileptogenic focus and result in seizures. Any of these presentations can lead to further evaluation with brain MRI and confirmation of the diagnosis. More often than not, however, cerebral AVMs do not directly cause any symptoms. In some cases, asymptomatic patients may be detected incidentally on neuroimaging for an unrelated reason (trauma, headache, etc.).

While CTA and MRA can often suggest the presence of an AVM, the gold standard for evaluation is angiography, which allows the clinician to characterize the feeding arteries, draining veins, and the nidus itself. Angiography is usually reserved for treatment planning.

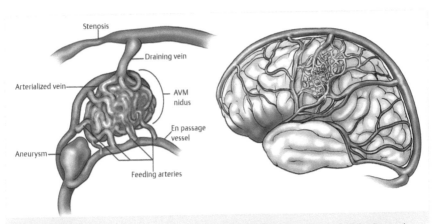

Fig. 12.6 Arteriovenous malformation demonstrating a nidus along with arterial feeders and draining veins; note the proximal cerebral aneurysm. (Source: Patient and Lesion Selection. In: Bendok B, Naidech A, Walker M, et al, eds. Hemorrhagic and Ischemic Stroke. Medical, Imaging, Surgical and Interventional Approaches. 1st Edition. Thieme; 2011.)

Management of a Patient with an Arteriovenous Malformation

The treatment strategy for cerebral AVMs differs between those who have already experienced a bleed and those who have been diagnosed incidentally. Ruptured AVMs carry a high risk of a rebleeding, and should almost always be treated.

The risk of bleeding for an AVM that has never bleed before is lower, in the range of 1% per year. In general, deciding which asymptomatic patients to treat is a matter of weighing the risk of a future bleed to the risk of performing the intervention. In older patients, the risk of conservative management may be considered low enough that treatment is unnecessary. In contrast, young patients have a much longer period of time for a bleed to occur, and so they more often undergo prophylactic treatment.

Smaller AVMs have been shown to bleed at a *higher* rate than larger ones (opposite of that for a typical cerebral aneurysm). Deeper location within the brain portends a higher risk of bleeding, but the associated surgical risk is also higher for these. Risk of treatment also takes into account the location of the AVM in relation to brain centers with critical function, referred to as "eloquent" areas. The **Spetzler Martin Scale** is a grading tool that is used to help weigh the risk of future bleed against the risk of treatment.

Treatment for cerebral AVMs is all-or-nothing. Surgical resection allows for an immediate cure. Partial treatment by reducing the size of the AVM does not decrease the risk of bleeding, and may actually increase it. Endovascular embolization is not used primarily, but as an adjunct to induce shrinkage of the AVM preoperatively, which makes for a safer surgery at a later point (**Procedure Box 12.4**). Oftentimes, multiple embolizations are repeated to achieve this goal prior to resection.

For AVMs that are unresectable due to location or are high risk otherwise, stereotactic-guided radiosurgery is the next best treatment option. Radiation therapy induces fibrosis of the AVM, which in turn reduces risk of rupture. The process of fibrosis is slow, sometimes taking years, so there remains a risk of bleeding during this lag time. Radiosurgery tends to be more effective for smaller AVMs than for large ones.

Procedure Box 12.4: Endovascular Treatment of Cerebral AVMs   i

Cerebral AVMs are often complex, with multiple feeding arteries and draining veins. Unfortunately, coil embolization of the feeding arteries is unlikely to lead to successful AVM eradication, as smaller arteries which were previously not seen or were too small to treat will hypertrophy and continue to feed the malformation. Therefore, treatment of the nidus itself is essential for success.

After gaining arterial access and performing a cerebral angiogram, a microcatheter is navigated under image guidance into an artery supplying the AVM, in close proximity to the nidus. A magnified digital subtraction angiogram is then performed to assess the feeding and draining vessels, flow rates, and areas of major venous shunting. Upon confirming the downstream vessel leads directly to the AVM, embolization of the AVM is then performed with ethylene vinyl alcohol (EVOH) Onyx (ev3, Irvine, CA) or n-butyl cyanoacrylate (nBCA) glue (Codman Neurovascular, Raynham, MA). The goal is to occlude the AVM nidus. Careful consideration of the embolic agent characteristics is tailored to the vessel size and flow rates, such that the embolic agent will become trapped before washing out into the draining veins.

Major risks of this procedure include nontarget embolization into a nearby artery (which may supply the brain or other head and neck structures) or into the venous circulation, eventually ending up in the pulmonary arteries. In addition to obstructing flow within the vessels and nidus, these agents incite an intravascular inflammatory reaction which precipitates vascular fibrosis and durable occlusion of the AVM.

12.5 Head and Neck Bleeds

Head and neck bleeds most commonly occur due to trauma or malignancy. The ICA and vertebral arteries supply the brain, while the external carotid artery (ECA) supplies tissues of the face, neck, scalp, and orbits. Endovascular techniques can be used to treat various carotid artery–associated bleeds, the most important of which to know are epistaxis and carotid artery blowout.

Epistaxis can occur anteriorly from the Kiesselbach plexus (an ICA/ECA anastomosis) or posteriorly from the branches of the facial or maxillary arteries (both ECA branches). Trauma (e.g., nose-picking) is the most common cause of epistaxis. Mucosal erosion due to infection or dry weather, coagulopathy, and local tumors can all increase the risk of epistaxis.

Epistaxis can usually be managed conservatively. Management begins with nose-pinching and tamponading the small vessels. This is especially efficacious for anterior, easily accessible bleeds. If bleeding persists despite manual pressure, cauterization with silver nitrate or electrocautery is indicated. If hemostasis is still not achieved, nasal packing can be performed. Only after nasal packing fails are invasive interventions considered. Though not always the case, bleeds originating from the posterior nasal cavity more often require escalation of care to invasive interventions.

One option is surgical ligation of the culprit branch of the ECA. This was the definitive treatment for many years. IR can achieve the same effect through endovascular embolization, with the sphenopalatine artery (branch of the maxillary artery) being a common target. Embolization is successful in stopping the bleed in the majority of cases.

Care should be taken when embolizing to ensure only the target ECA branch vessel is embolized. The ECA has numerous anastomotic connections with the internal carotid and vertebral arteries, many of which are not clearly seen during angiography. The cranial nerves are also at risk. Even a small amount of nontarget embolization can have dire consequences.

Carotid blowout syndrome (CBS) is a potentially emergent problem that affects head and neck cancer patients treated with surgery and radiation therapy. Radiation to the neck can lead to adventitial fibrosis of the common carotid artery and its branches, weakening the vessel wall. On top of this, postsurgical changes can result in flap necrosis or mucocutaneous fistulas overlying the vessels. In some cases, direct invasion of a tumor into the vessel can also be the inciting factor. The end result is a predisposition to carotid artery rupture, which can happen years or even decades after treatment. A commonly cited study by Maran et al found an overall CBS incidence of approximately 4% of all patients who have undergone radical neck dissection.

CBS is categorized into three types according to severity. Type I, "threatened," is prior to hemorrhage, when there are signs on exam or imaging that indicate a rupture is likely. Type II, "impending," is when hemorrhage occurs but ceases on its own or with packing. This is considered a warning sign that a more severe bleed is imminent. Type III, "acute carotid blowout," is defined by massive hemorrhage that does not stop after packing.

The diagnosis of acute CBS is suspected when a head and neck cancer patient presents to the ED with profound bleeding from the oropharynx or sometimes a wound over the neck. When there is rapid bleeding from the mouth, it can be difficult to differentiate between CBS and an upper GI bleed, especially when the patient has a history of GI bleed or risk factors. In either case, the first step is securing the airway and resuscitation.

If it is determined that acute carotid blowout is more likely based on history and exam, the mouth should be packed and neuro-IR consulted. Angiography is the gold standard for confirming the diagnosis of type II and III CBS, and allows for treatment when appropriate. Patients who present with threatened CBS and some type II patients who are stable will get CTA rather than angiography. CTA can identify a pseudoaneurysm and occasionally active extravasation of contrast.

Surgical treatment of CBS has fallen out of favor due to high mortality and a significant rate of postprocedural neurological damage. Furthermore, post-treatment changes to the neck predispose to poor healing after surgery. Surgery is reserved for cases where endovascular therapy is unavailable or has failed.

The gold standard treatment for acute or impending CBS is endovascular therapy with either coil or detachable balloon occlusion, or stent-graft deployment. Occlusion of the carotid artery can be done without neurological sequelae as long as the circle of Willis is patent and the contralateral carotid is also not affected. In nonemergent cases, balloon occlusion can be tested by leaving the balloon inflated and doing a neuro examination to ensure no deficits arise. If the patient has no problems after 30 minutes of balloon occlusion, it is safe to permanently occlude the vessel. In theory, the use of stent-grafts carries a lower risk of neurological insult, but there are some reports of recurrent hemorrhage due to inadequate coverage of the entire length of at-risk artery.

Currently, there is not much data comparing occlusion to grafting for CBS. Some advocate the use of occlusion for nonemergent cases, where there is time to perform a balloon occlusion test beforehand. Stenting may be more appropriate for those who fail the balloon occlusion test, or in emergent cases where it cannot be performed.

One other point to keep in mind is that many of these patients are terminally ill. Whenever possible, the goals of care conversation with the family should be initiated prior to attempting any intervention.

One other indication for head/neck embolization is preoperative devascularization of head and neck tumors, which can limit blood loss during resection. Studies have shown that preoperative embolization decreases the number of transfusions, operative time, surgical exposure, and perioperative complications.

12.6 Vertebral Body Compression Fractures

Vertebral body compression fractures are a relatively common cause of acute debilitating back pain in the elderly. These are often a consequence of underlying osteoporosis or metastatic disease. Osteoporotic fractures are not always preceded by trauma. Focal back pain is the usual presenting symptom, but it's not uncommon for these to be discovered incidentally. Painful fractures range from mild to incapacitating, and symptoms may develop weeks, months, or even years after the initial fracture. On exam, there is usually midline focal tenderness to palpation over the spinous process of the affected vertebra.

Vertebral body compression fractures are defined by vertebral body height loss of greater than or equal to 15%. Adjacent vertebral bodies can be used for a rough comparison. The most common location is from levels T9 to L2. Radiographically, the appearance may take the form of a wedge fracture, biconcave deformity, endplate irregularity, or complete collapse. Complex fractures with retropulsion of bone fragments or epidural hematoma formation may result in neurological deficit.

Plain films of the spine are often sufficient to make the diagnosis, particularly in the lower thoracic and lumbar levels. Both CT and MRI can provide a more comprehensive evaluation of the anatomy and degree of compression, as well as to evaluate for spinal canal compromise. MRI is also the most sensitive for distinguishing between acute and chronic compression fractures.

In the absence of neurologic symptoms, a trial of pain medications, activity modification, and bracing should be the initial strategy. Medical therapy starts with NSAIDs or acetaminophen, and escalated to opioids only if needed. Patients may be referred for intervention at the time of diagnosis, or more commonly after having failed conservative management.

Surgery is indicated if there is vertebral column instability or nerve/cord compression with neurologic deficits. Surgical correction tends not to be a great option given the often poor bone density in patients with osteoporosis or tumor infiltration.

Percutaneous vertebral augmentation is the insertion of cement or coils into the fractured vertebral body. Vertebral body augmentation is indicated when pain is poorly controlled after a trial of conservative management for at least a couple weeks. The goal of the procedure is symptomatic relief, but it can also help to stabilize the spine and reduce the risk of progression of the fracture.

The two main techniques are **vertebroplasty** and **kyphoplasty** (**Procedure Box 12.5**). Both involve injection of cement, but kyphoplasty adds an additional step of deploying a high-pressure balloon within the vertebral body, creating a void, and injecting cement in a controlled manner (▶ **Fig. 12.7**). Theoretically, the additional step with kyphoplasty reduces kyphosis caused by the fracture, and injecting cement at a lower pressure reduces the risk of cement extravasation.

It's not always clear-cut which of the two is the better approach, so for your purposes just understand the difference between the two. A third, relatively recent addition that you might hear about is something called a **Kiva device**, which research has shown to have some advantages over kyphoplasty. When the Kiva device is used, less cement is required and the treated vertebral body has biomechanical properties closer to that of natural bone. Previous trials have demonstrated that this technique is less likely to lead to the development of new adjacent compression fractures.

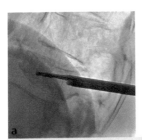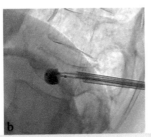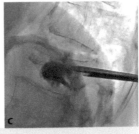

Fig. 12.7 (a) Kyphoplasty procedure with needle access into the anterior third of the vertebral body. **(b)** The bone tamp has been inflated to create a void within the vertebral body, allowing for **(c)** cement injection into the cavity at a lower pressure.

Percutaneous vertebroplasty starts with positioning the patient prone (ideal) or in the lateral decubitus position. The vertebral body is localized using *biplanar fluoroscopy* (providing simultaneous anterior–posterior as well as lateral fluoroscopic images). An appropriate needle is then selected; options range from 11-gauge in the lumbar segment to 13- or 15-gauge in the thoracic segment. The most common approach is transpedicular; the needle is advanced through the pedicle and into the vertebral body, which avoids paravertebral structures and the spinal canal. It is critical to avoid entry of the needle into the spinal canal, which risks neurologic injury. One of the detectors is positioned to look down the barrel of the pedicle to confirm the needle is not violating the pedicular cortex, while the other is positioned laterally to monitor the needle's anterior progress. The needle is advanced to the anterior third of the vertebral body, and cement is injected under continuous fluoroscopic monitoring, stopping when the cement reaches posterior third of the body. The goal is to evenly distribute the cement and provide vertebral body stabilization, while avoiding extrusion of cement into the paravertebral space or spinal canal.

Kyphoplasty is performed in a similar manner as vertebroplasty with an additional step of creating a void within the anterior vertebral body by deploying an inflatable bone tamp (IBT) through the introducer needle. A specialized kyphoplasty balloon insufflator (which requires very high pressures) is used to inflate the balloon. Once balloon inflation has been performed, the balloon is removed and cement injected to fill the void. Kyphoplasty is often performed via a bilateral transpedicular approach.

Kiva device uses a 6-gauge needle, which is advanced into the anterior third of the vertebral body. Loops of nitinol coil are deployed in the vertebral body (serving the same function as a guidewire). A plastic coil ring is advanced over the nitinol coil. Cement can then be injected through the plastic coil rings (▶ **Fig. 12.8**) with filling occurring only *within* the plastic coil rings.

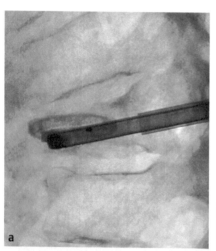 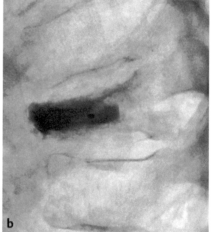

a   b

Fig. 12.8 **(a)** Lateral spot fluoroscopic images show two coils of the KIVA device within the T7 vertebral body. **(b)** Cement has been injected and can be seen inside the coil rings. The KIVA device allows for more controlled injection of the cement. (These images are provided courtesy of Dr Joseph J. Gemmete, MD, University of Michigan Health System.)

Suggested Readings

[1] Barnett HJM, Taylor DW, Haynes RB, et al. North American Symptomatic Carotid Endarterectomy Trial Collaborators. Beneficial effect of carotid endarterectomy in symptomatic patients with high-grade carotid stenosis. N Engl J Med. 1991; 325(7):445–453

[2] Berkhemer OA, Fransen PS, Beumer D, et al. MR CLEAN Investigators. A randomized trial of intraarterial treatment for acute ischemic stroke. N Engl J Med. 2015; 372(1):11–20

[3] Brott TG, Hobson RW II, Howard G, et al. CREST Investigators. Stenting versus endarterectomy for treatment of carotid-artery stenosis. N Engl J Med. 2010; 363(1):11–23

[4] Clark W, Bird P, Gonski P, et al. Safety and efficacy of vertebroplasty for acute painful osteoporotic fractures (VAPOUR): a multicentre, randomised, double-blind, placebo-controlled trial. Lancet. 2016; 388(10052):1408–1416

[5] Connors JM, Jurczak W, Straus DJ, et al. ECHELON-1 Study Group. Brentuximab vedotin with chemotherapy for Stage III or IV Hodgkin's lymphoma. N Engl J Med. 2018; 378(4):331–344

[6] International Study of Unruptured Intracranial Aneurysms Investigators. Unruptured intracranial aneurysms—risk of rupture and risks of surgical intervention. N Engl J Med. 1998; 339(24):1725–1733

[7] Mohr JP, Parides MK, Stapf C, et al. international ARUBA investigators. Medical management with or without interventional therapy for unruptured brain arteriovenous malformations (ARUBA): a multicentre, non-blinded, randomised trial. Lancet. 2014; 383(9917):614–621

[8] Molyneux AJ, Kerr RS, Yu LM, et al. International Subarachnoid Aneurysm Trial (ISAT) Collaborative Group. International subarachnoid aneurysm trial (ISAT) of neurosurgical clipping versus endovascular coiling in 2143 patients with ruptured intracranial aneurysms: a randomised comparison of effects on survival, dependency, seizures, rebleeding, subgroups, and aneurysm occlusion. Lancet. 2005; 366(9488):809–817

[9] National Institute of Neurological Disorders and Stroke rt-PA Stroke Study Group. Tissue plasminogen activator for acute ischemic stroke. N Engl J Med. 1995; 333(24):1581–1587

[10] Nogueira RG, Jadhav AP, Haussen DC, et al. DAWN Trial Investigators. Thrombectomy 6 to 24 hours after stroke with a mismatch between deficit and infarct. N Engl J Med. 2018; 378(1):11–21

[11] Valavanis A. Preoperative embolization of the head and neck: indications, patient selection, goals, and precautions. AJNR Am J Neuroradiol. 1986; 7(5):943–952

[12] Van Meirhaeghe J, Bastian L, Boonen S, Ranstam J, Tillman JB, Wardlaw D. FREE investigators. A randomized trial of balloon kyphoplasty and nonsurgical management for treating acute vertebral compression fractures: vertebral body kyphosis correction and surgical parameters. Spine. 2013; 38(12):971–983

13 Pediatric IR

Rajat Chand, Victor Nicholas Becerra, Nicholas Zerona, Ashley Altman, and James K. Park

Generally speaking, treatment used in adult IR can be applied to most pathology seen in the pediatric population. There are some differences, however, in the more extensive involvement of the anesthesia team, the increased attention to minimizing radiation exposure, and the importance of a multidisciplinary approach to treating pediatric patients.

Procedures that would generally require minimal sedation or local anesthesia for adults often require deep sedation or general anesthesia for pediatric patients. Neonates and infants can often have minor procedures such as lumbar puncture or peripherally inserted central catheter (PICC) insertion with the use of oral sucrose for mild analgesia. Distraction techniques (toys, music, etc.) can be provided by child life experts during the procedure. Older children, on the other hand, may require sedation or general anesthesia even for minor procedures. The developmental stage of the child also should be considered in planning the procedure. As such, anesthesiologists are far more involved in pediatric IR than in adult IR.

13.1 Vascular Anomalies

There are two types of vascular anomalies: vascular *tumors* and vascular *malformations* (▶ Table 13.1). The most common type of vascular tumor in the pediatric world is the benign **infantile hemangioma.** Infantile hemangiomas show up in the first year of life, commonly on the skin, in the liver, or within the GI tract. Most infantile hemangiomas proliferate in the initial few months of life then regress.

Infantile hemangiomas generally do not cause issues, and are managed medically with β-blockers. IR rarely plays a role in the management of vascular tumors, and is usually only involved when the hemangioma results in a large vascular shunt. If large enough (typically a liver hemangioma), shunting can potentially lead to high-output cardiac failure. Another indication for intervention is if the hemangioma is in a sensitive location, near the airway, eye, etc.

In contrast, vascular malformations are a relatively much more common source of referrals for pediatric IR. Vascular malformations are due to errors in vascular morphogenesis rather than proliferation of the endothelial cells. Vascular malformations are classified as either *low-flow* or *high-flow* lesions, referring to the movement of blood through the malformation. From an IR standpoint, it's helpful to maintain this organization in your head since it reflects the significant difference in how these types of malformations are treated.

Table 13.1 Vascular anomalies seen in children

Vascular tumors	Vascular malformations
Infantile hemangiomas	High-flow malformations: 1. Arteriovenous malformations 2. Arteriovenous fistulas
Capillary hemangiomas	Low-flow malformations: 1. Venous malformations 2. Lymphatic malformations

Low-Flow Vascular Malformations

Low-flow malformations include capillary, venous, and lymphatic malformations. While capillary malformations are generally treated by dermatologists and plastic surgeons, venous and lymphatic malformations are seen by pediatric IR.

Venous malformations (VMs) are the most common vascular malformation. They can occur anywhere in the body, but most commonly in the head/neck or extremities. VMs arise due to a deficiency of smooth muscle cells lining the vessel wall, which consequently causes the vein to dilate and form vascular lakes. The malformations are present at birth, but are typically not detected until they grow (often during puberty).

A VM can present in a number of different ways. Once big enough, the patient or a parent might see the lesion underneath the skin. Superficial VMs look like soft blueish masses, and can sometimes bleed. They tend not to be as well-circumscribed as vascular tumors. Deeper VMs within intramuscular, intraosseous, or even intracranial compartments may not be directly visible. As these deeper malformations grow, they can lead to pain and swelling. There is also a predisposition for thrombus formation since blood can be stagnant within VMs.

Lymphatic malformations (LMs), in contrast, are usually detected at birth as soft, compressible masses in the head/neck area or sometimes in the limbs. The most common type of LM is a cystic collection of lymph that is caused by obstruction of the lymphatic channels. The natural course of lymphatic malformations is one of expansion and contraction. Expansion is often the result of a certain stimuli (bleeding or infection of the lesion), while contraction can occur spontaneously as lymph drains out of the lesion.

Diagnosis of the low-flow malformations is predominantly clinical. Physical exam of a patient presenting with the symptoms described above is often enough to make the diagnosis in the hands of an experienced clinician. Key exam findings can differentiate a VM from an LM. When VMs are compressed and released, they refill with blood quickly. They also tend to get bigger if the involved body part is placed in a dependent position. Differentiating between them is not always clear-cut, as certain malformations have components of both.

Imaging is performed when the diagnosis needs confirmation or for treatment planning. Imaging characteristics can sometimes help differentiate between VMs and LMs. The tendency for thrombus formation with VMs sometimes leads to formation of intralesional phleboliths, which may be a clue on plain films or cross-sectional studies. Ultrasound of a venous malformation most commonly shows a heterogeneous, but mostly hypoechoic compressible mass, with little or no Doppler flow. Lymphatic malformations are similar, but can be unilocular and may have internal septations. MRI is required to fully delineate the extent of tissue involvement for both VMs and LMs, and is done after an initial ultrasound (▶ **Fig. 13.1**). A venous malformation will appear on MRI as cyst-like vascular channels that are hyperintense on T2-weighted images. LMs that have had prior hemorrhage may show a fluid–fluid level. MRA or conventional angiography of low-flow malformations in most cases will look relatively normal, so these are not very useful for diagnosis. Direct puncture and contrast administration will define the lesion during IR treatment.

Both lymphatic and venous malformations may become problematic due to their location. They can be cosmetically displeasing if superficial, or compress nearby vital structures. Each also has its own unique complications. Lymphatic malformations carry a risk of infection, while venous malformations are prone to thrombose and become painful. Any of these issues are considered indication for treatment.

Since vascular malformations are relatively rare, most cases will be sent to a regional referral center and approached by a multidisciplinary team to determine a treatment plan. This often includes pediatrics, plastic surgery, orthopedics, and IR. Referrals for vascular malformation treatment not uncommonly are sent to us with an incorrect diagnosis, so the first step is reviewing the outside studies to confirm the identity of the lesion and determine if there is an indication for treatment. Conservative measures and reassurance are reasonable for many of these patients.

Low-flow malformations that require intervention can be treated with surgery, IR sclerotherapy, or a combination of both. The basic concept behind sclerotherapy for low-flow malformations is to inject an irritant substance into the malformation (▶ **Fig. 13.2**). This causes injury to the endothelial cells, inducing fibrosis and involution. The procedure is ultrasound-guided, fluoroscopy-guided, or occasionally CT-guided.

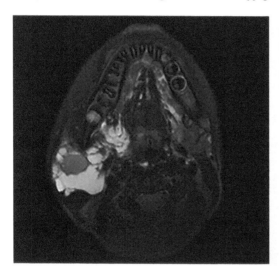

Fig. 13.1 T2-weighted MRI image of the head showing a lymphatic malformation (lymphatic collection is T2 bright) in the right mandibular area.

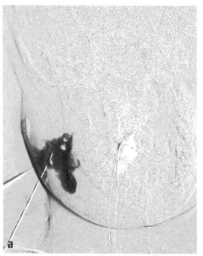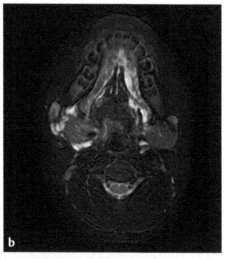

Fig. 13.2 **(a)** Fluoroscopy image shows needle access and contrast injection into the right mandibular lymphatic malformation (same patient from ▶ **Fig. 13.1**). Subsequent injection of a sclerosant, bleomycin, resulted in fibrosis and, eventually, **(b)** malformation regression.

For VMs, the sclerosing agent used is either ethanol or sodium tetradecyl sulfate (STS). Ethanol is the more effective of the two, but is associated with worse side effects and is rather painful for conscious sedation patients. The same can be used for LMs, as well as a doxycycline-based sclerosant. Usually patients are brought back for multiple sclerotherapy sessions to achieve symptomatic relief.

In the past it was thought that surgical resection of the malformation was always preferred, since sclerotherapy is not considered curative. More and more, institutions now favor sclerotherapy as first-line therapy for many patients due to the benefits of a minimally invasive approach. Some infiltrative malformations are simply not amenable to surgery due to the functional or cosmetic defects associated with resection.

High-Flow Vascular Malformations

High-flow malformations are much less common than low-flow malformations, and consist of the **arteriovenous malformation** (AVM) and **arteriovenous fistula** (AVF). The defining feature for both is an abnormal connection between arteries and veins without an intervening capillary bed. In AVMs, this connection is characterized by a tangled mesh of dilated arteries and veins, referred to as a nidus. In AVFs, the connection is a single shunt between artery and vein. While AVFs can be congenital, the majority are acquired after trauma or iatrogenic injury, and are therefore rare in the pediatric population.

AVMs are congenital malformations that can occur practically anywhere in the body, with the head and neck being most common. In infants, they typically start out small and escape detection unless found incidentally. As with all vascular malformations, they can grow as the patient grows. Inciting factors such as trauma, puberty, or pregnancy can induce rapid expansion. They do not regress as some of the low-flow malformations do.

The initial presentation of a patient with an AVM varies widely depending on the size of the lesion and the location, but symptoms generally do not develop until it has grown significantly. Dilation of the involved vessels can lead to spontaneous bleeding or rupture, which is especially worrisome with cerebral AVMs (discussed separately in Chapter 12). Though rare, AVMs in the stomach or bowel can be a cause of bleeding that often goes undetected by conventional diagnostic tools.

Another problem with enlarging AVMs is the hemodynamic consequences of vascular shunting. In the absence of a capillary bed, lower resistance can lead to preferential blood flow through the AVM, known as "vascular steal phenomenon." Tissues distal to the AVM can become ischemic in this way. In the most extreme cases, shunting can lead to high-output heart failure as cardiac output rises to meet the demand.

Symptomatic *extremity* AVMs can present as a soft mass with skin discoloration. Some patients may only have vague pain. If large enough to result in vascular steal, the distal extremity may experience skin ulceration or necrosis as a result of ischemia. Symptomatic *pulmonary* high-flow lesions behave differently. In contrast to the peripheral AVM left-to-right shunt, large pulmonary AVMs can result in a *right-to-left* shunt as blood from the pulmonary artery is shunted to the pulmonary veins (▶ **Fig. 13.3**). Once symptoms arise, patients may present with hemoptysis, dyspnea, or hypoxia. Patients are also at risk for paradoxical emboli due to the right-to-left shunt. The risk is greatest in pulmonary AVMs greater than 3 mm.

The diagnostic approach to high-flow malformations is similar to that of low-flow malformations. In the pediatric population, ultrasound is the initial imaging modality of choice. Ultrasound can readily detect peripheral AVMs, with color flow and arterialized venous waveforms. MRI of the lesion will be dark on both T1 and T2 sequences, with enlarged feeding and draining vessels, and serpentine flow voids reflecting the higher rate of blood flow. AVMs do not appear as a mass (differentiating them from low-flow malformations and vascular tumors), but may have surrounding edema due to mass effect. Conventional angiography is typically only done at the time of intervention, but will easily identify an AVM by its rapid shunting through multiple channels.

Because of a strong association between pulmonary AVM and **hereditary hemorrhagic telangiectasia** (HHT), these patients are usually screened for pulmonary AVMs with an echo and bubble study to detect a right-to-left shunt.

As with other vascular malformations, intervention for AVMs is only indicated for symptomatic patients, and only when conservative management is insufficient. Surgery does have a role in resection of some localized AVMs, but for the most part the treatment is embolotherapy. The treatment strategy for AVMs is elimination of the nidus. If the feeding and draining vessels are treated but the nidus remains intact, collateralization will reconstitute the AVM. What makes this problematic is that no two AVMs are the same, beseeching the interventionalist to come up with an individualized approach to every case (and highlighting the importance of the multidisciplinary team). The exact strategy will vary depending on the anatomy of the AVM, including the configuration of feeding arteries and draining veins.

In general, the approach is to use balloon occlusion or a blood pressure cuff to slow down blood flow through the AVM, such that the nidal vessels can be embolized. Often a variety of different embolic agents are used, and percutaneous direct access to the nidus may be necessary. In all but the simplest cases, the treatment is staged with the patient brought back for multiple sessions until there is adequate symptomatic relief.

Pulmonary AVMs greater than 3 mm should be prophylactically embolized, as the risk of paradoxical emboli increases over time. Symptomatic pulmonary AVMs should also be treated. The treatment of choice for pulmonary AVMs is coil embolization (▶ **Fig. 13.3**). The pulmonary artery is catheterized and the feeding arteries embolized as close to the nidus as possible. Particles should *not* be used as they can enter the

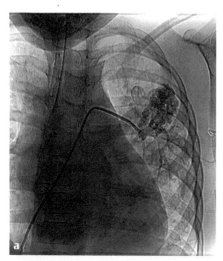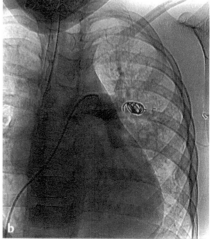

Fig. 13.3 (a) Fluoroscopic image shows a contrast injection through a left pulmonary artery catheter with subsequent opacification of a pulmonary arteriovenous malformation. (b) Post-treatment with coil embolization.

systemic circulation and cause nontarget embolization. In the vast majority of cases, coil embolization is successful. Recurrence can happen, however, as the lesion recruits additional vessels through angiogenesis. Patients are usually followed with CT angiography of the chest at 6 and 12 months postprocedure.

13.2 Osteoid Osteomas

An **osteoid osteoma** (OO) is a benign bone tumor characterized by a central bone-forming lesion, also referred to as a nidus, with surrounding reactive sclerosis. The classic presentation is a teenage male with an aching pain that worsens at night and is relieved by NSAIDs. The tumors usually develop in the long bones or spine. Pain is caused by irritation of the intraosseous nerve endings by high levels of prostacyclin and prostaglandin.

Physical exam is often unhelpful in the diagnosis of osteoid osteoma. On plain films, the osteoid osteoma appears as a partially calcified central lucency, with surrounding cortical thickening and medullary sclerosis. Given the initially indolent course, symptoms may be present for months before an osteoid osteoma reveals itself radiographically. Making the diagnosis based on a plain film can be challenging, especially when the lesion is in an atypical location. Second-line imaging is usually done with bone scan or CT. Bone scan will show increased activity in the nidus and less intense activity in the surrounding reactive bone. CT will show the nidus and boundaries of the sclerotic bone. It is the most precise modality for preprocedure planning (▶ **Fig. 13.4**). MRI often has a variable appearance, and is not ideal for evaluation of osteoid osteomas.

First-line treatment of an osteoid osteoma begins with conservative management. Some tumors spontaneously resolve over time, so pain control with NSAIDS and observation is a reasonable approach. Unfortunately, many patients fail conservative management due to the intolerable pain. Treatment for these patients is with either surgical resection or thermal ablation.

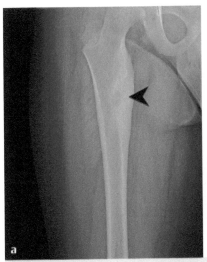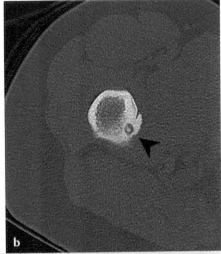

Fig. 13.4 **(a)** Plain frontal radiograph and **(b)** axial CT of the right femur showing a right femoral osteoid osteoma with classic imaging features. Note the central, radiolucent nidus with surrounding sclerosis.

Surgery involves open excision of the nidus and curettage of the lesion. More recently, a minimally invasive CT-guided radiofrequency ablation (RFA) procedure performed by IR has become the preferred option. It involves inserting an ablation probe into the nidus and heating the area to the point of osteonecrosis. This is generally a same-day procedure which is usually very well tolerated and offers near immediate pain relief. Recurrences are infrequent, but they can be retreated with RFA if need be.

Surgery may be necessary for some lesions in close proximity to vital structures, where thermal ablation cannot be done safely. For example, some vertebral lesions are too close to the spinal canal for RFA. In general, the ablation zone should be maintained at least 1 cm away from at-risk structures.

Suggested Readings

[1]   Ghanem I. The management of osteoid osteoma: updates and controversies. Curr Opin Pediatr. 2006; 18(1):36–41

[2]   Shovlin CL, Letarte M. Hereditary haemorrhagic telangiectasia and pulmonary arteriovenous malformations: issues in clinical management and review of pathogenic mechanisms. Thorax. 1999; 54(8):714–729

[3]   Van Aalst JA, Bhuller A, Sadove AM. Pediatric vascular lesions. J Craniofac Surg. 2003; 14(4):566–583

Index

Note: Page numbers set in **bold** or *italic* indicate headings or figures, respectively.

Index